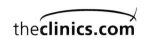

PSYCHIATRIC CLINICS

OF NORTH AMERICA

Dissociative Disorders:
An Expanding Window into
the Psychobiology of the Mind

GUEST EDITOR
Richard A. Chefetz, MD

March 2006 • Volume 29 • Number 1

SAUNDERS

An Imprint of Elsevier, Inc.
PHILADELPHIA   LONDON   TORONTO   MONTREAL   SYDNEY   TOKYO

W.B. SAUNDERS COMPANY
A Division of Elsevier Inc.

1600 John F. Kennedy Boulevard • Suite 1800 • Philadelphia, PA 19103-2899

http://www.theclinics.com

PSYCHIATRIC CLINICS OF NORTH AMERICA
March 2006
Editor: Sarah E. Barth

Volume 29, Number 1
ISSN 0193-953X
ISBN 1-4160-3514-1

Reprints. For copies of 100 or more, of articles in this publication, please contact the Commercial Reprints Department, Elsevier Inc., 360 Park Avenue South, New York, New York 10010-1710. Tel.: (212) 633-3813 Fax: (212) 462-1935 e-mail: reprints@elsevier.com

The ideas and opinions expressed in *Psychiatric Clinics of North America* do not necessarily reflect those of the Publisher. The Publisher does not assume any responsibility for any injury and/or damage to persons or property arising out of or related to any use of the material contained in this periodical. The reader is advised to check the appropriate medical literature and the product information currently provided by the manufacturer of each drug to be administered, to verify the dosage, the method and duration of administration, or contraindications. It is the responsibility of the treating physician or other health care professional, relying on independent experience and knowledge of the patient, to determine drug dosages and the best treatment for the patient. Mention of any product in this issue should not be construed as endorsement by the contributors, editors, or the Publisher of the product or manufacturers' claims.

Psychiatric Clinics of North America (ISSN 0193-953X) is published quarterly by W.B. Saunders, 360 Park Avenue South, New York, NY 10010-1710. Months of publication are March, June, September, and December. Business and Editorial Offices: 1600 John F. Kennedy Blvd., Suite 1800, Philadelphia, PA 19103-2899. Accounting and Circulation Offices: 6277 Sea Harbor Drive, Orlando, FL 32887-4800 Periodicals postage paid at New York, NY and additional mailing offices. Subscription prices are $180.00 per year (US individuals), $305.00 per year (US institutions), $90.00 per year (US students/residents), $215.00 per year (Canadian individuals), $370.00 per year (Canadian Institutions), $250.00 per year (foreign individuals), $370.00 per year (foreign institutions), and $125.00 per year (international & Canadian students/residents). Foreign air speed delivery is included in all *Clinics'* subscription prices. All prices are subject to change without notice. **POSTMASTER:** Send address changes to *Psychiatric Clinics of North America*, Elsevier Periodicals Customer Service, 6277 Sea Harbor Drive, Orlando, FL 32887-4800. Customer Service: 1-800-654-2452 (US). From outside of the US, call 1-407-345-4000.

Psychiatric Clinics of North America is covered in *Index Medicus, Current Contents/Social and Behavioral Sciences, Social Science Citation Index, Embase/Excerpta Medica,* and PsycINFO.

Printed in the United States of America.

GUEST EDITOR

RICHARD A. CHEFETZ, MD, Private Practice of Psychiatry; Advanced Psychotherapy Training Program, Washington School of Psychiatry; Institute of Contemporary Psychotherapy & Psychoanalysis; Washington Psychoanalytic Center; Distinguished Visiting Lecturer, William Alanson White Institute of Psychiatry, Psychoanalysis, and Psychology; Co-Director, Dissociative Disorders Psychotherapy Training Program, International Society for the Study of Dissociation; Past President, International Society for the Study of Dissociation; Washington, District of Columbia

CONTRIBUTORS

JUDITH G. ARMSTRONG, PhD, Clinical Associate Professor of Psychology, University of Southern California, Los Angeles, California

ILARIA BIANCHI, MA, Doctoral Student, Catholic University of the Sacred Heart, Department of Psychology, Milan, Italy

ELIZABETH S. BOWMAN, MD, Consulting Psychiatrist, Indiana University Epilepsy Clinic; Adjunct Professor of Neurology, Indiana University School of Medicine, Department of Neurology, Indianapolis, Indiana

BETHANY L. BRAND, PhD, Associate Professor of Psychology, Towson University, Towson, Maryland

LISA D. BUTLER, PhD, Senior Research Scholar, Department of Psychiatry & Behavioral Sciences, Stanford University School of Medicine, Stanford, California

CATHERINE C. CLASSEN, PhD, Associate Professor, Department of Psychiatry, University of Toronto; Academic Leader, Trauma Therapy Program, Department of Psychiatry, Sunnybrook & Women's College Health Sciences Centre; Director, Women's Mental Health Research Program, Centre for Research in Women's Health, Toronto, Ontario, Canada

CONSTANCE DALENBERG, PhD, Professor of Psychology, Alliant International University, San Diego, California

PAUL F. DELL, PhD, Director, Trauma Recovery Center, Psychotherapy Resources of Norfolk, Norfolk, Virginia

LISSA DUTRA, EdM, MA, Doctoral Student, Department of Psychology, Boston University, Boston, Massachusetts

NIGEL P. FIELD, PhD, Associate Professor, Pacific Graduate School of Psychology, Palo Alto, California

JANINA FISHER, PhD, Instructor and Senior Supervisor, The Trauma Center, Boston, Massachusetts

A. STEVEN FRANKEL, PhD, JD, Adjunct Professor of Law, Golden Gate University School of Law, Lafayette, California; Clinical Professor of Psychology, University of Southern California, Los Angeles, California

PAUL A. FREWEN, MA, Doctoral Candidate, Department of Psychology, The University of Western Ontario, London, Ontario, Canada

JENNIFER ALOE KAHLER, PsyD, Licensed Clinical Psychologist, The CENTER: Posttraumatic Disorders Program, The Psychiatric Institute of Washington, DC, Washington, District of Columbia

RICHARD P. KLUFT, MD, Clinical Professor of Psychiatry, Temple University School of Medicine, Philadelphia, Pennsylvania; Private Practice in Psychiatry and Psychoanalysis, Bala Cynwyd, Pennsylvania

RUTH A. LANIUS, MD, PhD, Associate Professor, Departments of Psychiatry and Neuroscience, The University of Western Ontario; Director, Traumatic Stress Service and WSIB Traumatic Stress Service Workplace Program, London Health Sciences Centre, London, Ontario, Canada

RICHARD J. LOEWENSTEIN, MD, Medical Director, The Trauma Disorders Program, Sheppard Pratt Health Systems; Clinical Associate Professor, Department of Psychiatry, University of Maryland School of Medicine, Baltimore, Maryland

KARLEN LYONS-RUTH, PhD, Associate Professor, Harvard Medical School, Cambridge Hospital, Department of Psychiatry, Cambridge, Massachusetts

PAT OGDEN, PhD, Founder and Director, Sensorimotor Psychotherapy Institute, Boulder, Colorado

CLARE PAIN, MD, FRCPC, Assistant Professor, Department of Psychiatry, University of Western Ontario, Canada; Assistant Professor, Department of Psychiatry, University of Toronto, Toronto, Canada

COLIN ROSS, MD, Founder and Director, Colin A. Ross Institute for Psychological Trauma, Richardson, Texas

VEDAT SAR, MD, Professor of Psychiatry and Director, Clinical Psychotherapy Unit and Dissociative Disorders Program, Medical Faculty of Istanbul, Istanbul University, Istanbul, Turkey

MICHELLE R. SCHUDER, PhD, Instructor in Psychology, Harvard Medical School, Cambridge Hospital, Department of Psychiatry, Cambridge, Massachusetts

ELI SOMER, PhD, Associate Professor, School of Social Work, University of Haifa; Director of Training, Maytal—Israel Institute for Treatment and Study of Stress, Haifa, Israel

JOAN A. TURKUS, MD, Psychiatric Consultant and Co-Founder, The CENTER: Posttraumatic Disorders Program, The Psychiatric Institute of Washington, DC, Washington, District of Columbia; Private Practice, Falls Church, Virginia

KAREN G. WAY, PhD, Clinical Psychologist, Private Practice, Highland Park, New Jersey; Clinical Psychologist, Raritan Bay Mental Health Center, Perth Amboy, New Jersey

PATRICIA WOODS, RN, CPMHN(C), Trauma Therapy Program, Department of Psychiatry, Sunnybrook & Women's College Health Sciences Centre, Toronto, Ontario, Canada

CONTENTS

Three models of DID were evaluated: (1) DSM-IV's classic model of DID (i.e., multiple personalities + switching + amnesia), (2) Dell's subjective/phenomenological model of DID, and (3) the sociocognitive model of DID. DSM-IV narrowly portrays DID as an alter disorder, whereas the subjective/phenomenological model portrays DID as a far more complex dissociative disorder. The sociocognitive model portrays DID as a socially-constructed, iatrogenic condition. The subjective/phenomenological model of DID successfully predicted 23 specific dissociative symptoms of DID, whereas the DSM-IV model and the sociocognitive model could not predict these symptoms. The data revealed the DSM-IV model to be a deficient portrayal of DID that is overly focused on alters. The sociocognitive model of DID was shown to be frankly incorrect.

Metaphors that are used to describe a problem often have the effect of setting the problem—that is, framing the difficulty to be solved in such a way that some solutions are more thinkable than others. The common metaphors used to describe pathologic dissociation have this effect, subtly directing both clinicians and patients in understanding and treating the disorder. Two primary metaphor categories accommodate many of the problem-setting metaphors for dissociation: (1) the self is a thing that is divided, multiplied, or perforated by trauma; and (2) the self is an agent who dissociates, turning attention away from trauma and external relationships. Although both metaphor categories testify to the human experience of interpersonal malevolence, the verb-based metaphors of personal agency are more congruent with goals of treatment.

This article presents evidence supporting the primacy and ubiquity of dissociation in normal human experience and argues that normative (nonpathological) dissociative experiences represent manifestations of absorption and its attendant features in the facilitation of different mental activities. Forms of normative dissociation (absorption in activities, daydreams, fantasies, and dreams) and their possible functions in daily life (processing, escape, and reinforcement) are discussed as are pathological parallels and implications for the putative dissociative continuum. Greater appreciation of the pervasiveness, mechanisms, and utility of normative dissociation and its place in the normal stream of consciousness can inform understanding of pathological dissociative states.

Data from longitudinal attachment studies of families at social risk indicate that disorganized attachment behaviors in infancy are important precursors to later dissociative symptomatology. This early vulnerability is related to patterns of parent-infant affective communication observable by the end of the child's second year. These longitudinal relations do not occur because of the occurrence of later trauma or abuse, which suggests that the quality of primary attachment relationships may partially account for why some people exposed to later trauma develop dissociative symptoms and others do not. It remains unclear whether the early relationship is predictive due to the onset of an internal process of mental segregation in infancy or to enduring patterns of parent-child dialog that continually reinforce the child's segregated and contradictory mental contents.

Clinicians who treat individuals who are chronically traumatized recognize that the Diagnostic and Statistical Manual of Mental

Disorders, Fourth Edition does not provide an adequate diagnostic category to capture the range of symptomatology with which these individuals frequently present. Borderline personality disorder and posttraumatic stress disorder often are considered the best diagnostic options. Alone or together, however, these categories neither describe the full range of symptomatology for individuals suffering as a result of chronic traumatization nor provide an adequate framework for understanding etiology or treatment. New diagnostic categories are needed to account for the range of symptom constellations that result from chronic traumatization.

SECTION 2: RESEARCH AND EVALUATION

This article reviews studies of the neural correlates of dissociative experiences, as assessed by positron emission tomography and functional magnetic resonance imaging, with reference to van der Kolk and colleagues' definitions of primary, secondary, and tertiary dissociation. Key cortical structures involved in these processes include the medial prefrontal, anterior cingulate, somatosensory, and insular cortex, and the thalamus. Distinctive neural correlates of primary and secondary dissociative experiences in individuals who have posttraumatic stress disorder are regarded as supporting state-phase models of animal defensive reaction to external threat. Disconnection of neural pathways normally linking self-awareness with body-state perception, occurring as a result of childhood trauma, may occasion the development of tertiary dissociative identities. Suggestions for future research are discussed.

Dissociative disorders almost always co-occur with other psychiatric disorders. The lack of dissociative disorder sections in widely used general psychiatric assessment instruments, however, has contributed to their being overlooked for many decades. Recent studies have demonstrated the presence of significant dissociative comorbidity for several psychiatric disorders, and provided clues about the etiology, clinical phenomenology, treatment, and natural course of these disorders. Its link to childhood trauma makes dissociation important for evaluation of stress-diathesis in general psychiatry. Dissociation has the potential of contributing to the development of new models of mental functioning and novel treatment modalities in psychiatry based on the principles of a new science: psychotraumatology.

offered in this article aims to explore commonalities across cultural variations in phenomena involving altered states of consciousness. This article discusses native dissociation along two major classifications: nonpossession trance and possession trance.

International research has documented the universality of dissociative disorders. Not only are dissociative disorders common in various countries but they are also clinically similar in different cultures. Differences may exist, however, between starting points of interest among dissociation researchers in various countries. Beside dissociative identity disorder, somatoform dissociation has been a major study area in The Netherlands, Turkey, and Germany. Dissociative psychosis was the starting point for dissociation studies in Turkey, whereas depersonalization disorder currently is the most studied dissociative disorder in the United Kingdom. The backlash movement remains limited to North America.

SECTION 3: TECHNIQUE

Ego strengthening and skill building are valuable therapeutic interventions in clinical work with patients who have dissociative disorders. These interventions include psychoeducation; pacing and containment; grounding skills; an understanding of traumatic reenactment; safety planning; installation of an internal healing place; journaling and artwork; and "talking through" and "internal meeting" (specifically for dissociative identity disorder). These interventions are to be used judiciously within the psychodynamic framework of psychotherapy.

Traumatized individuals demonstrate a number of complicated and debilitating signs, symptoms, and difficulties consisting primarily of bodily responses to dysregulated affects. To address these bodily based symptoms of trauma and the psychologic components, the authors propose that it is possible to weave sensorimotor understandings and techniques into existing psychodynamic or cognitive-behavioral models of therapy. In sensorimotor psychotherapy, it becomes possible to address the more primitive, automatic, and involuntary functions of the brain that underlie traumatic and post-traumatic responses. After clients observe and report the interplay of their physical sensations, movements, and impulses and notice their internal reactions, meaning making emerges, with subsequent transformation of habitual response tendencies.

The treatment of dissociative identity disorder (DID) is facilitated by therapists' being prepared to work directly with alters. Interventions that access and involve the alters in the treatment are vital components of the successful treatment of DID and should be a part of the therapeutic armamentarium of those who treat this patient population. This article defines alters, describes alter system development, and provides a rationale for accessing and working directly with the alters.

This article discusses two in-depth clinical vignettes from the stabilization phase (stage one) of the treatment of dissociative identity disorder. Presented are representative problems and interventions to manage dangerousness to self or others, to begin the establishment of the therapeutic alliance, to work with persecutory or violent alters, to interpret the traumatic transference, to help the patient separate past from present, and to teach the patient basic symptom containment skills. In addition, practical strategies to help reframe the patient's posttraumatic cognitive distortions to further the goals of stabilization are discussed.

FORTHCOMING ISSUES

RECENT ISSUES

PSYCHIATRIC
CLINICS
OF NORTH AMERICA

Psychiatr Clin N Am 29 (2006) xv–xxiii

Preface

Why Should You Read These Articles on Dissociative Processes?

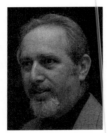

Richard A. Chefetz, MD
Guest Editor

Most mental health clinicians have not had formal training in dissociation or dissociative disorders, a sad fact of current professional life—sad because it means that if you are a mental health clinician, your treatment of people with the following histories (among others) may lack full efficacy:

- all self-harming behaviors;
- all addictions;
- eating disorders;
- conversion disorders;
- pseudoseizures;
- childhood sexual abuse;
- childhood physical abuse;
- childhood neglect and emotional abuse;
- growing up in a household as a witness to repeated violent behaviors;
- hearing voices with goal-directed, nonbizarre messages or conversation;
- "rapid-cycling" mood change occurring multiple times in a day or hour;
- attention-deficit problems that are inconsistent or situational;
- chronic posttraumatic stress disorder;
- chronic depersonalization or derealization;
- prolonged or multiple life-threatening hospitalizations in childhood;
- profound body dysmorphic symptoms; and
- borderline personality adaptations.

doi:10.1016/j.psc.2005.12.001   *psych.theclinics.com*

I am not saying that everyone with these kinds of histories will have a dissociative disorder. What I am saying is that dissociative processes are often the engine that drives these histories into childhood and adult psychopathologies. To borrow from a favorite childhood story, the dissociative process is the "little engine that could." If you don't know how dissociative processes work, then you don't know how to ask your patients about some of the central symptoms of their lives—and because most of these symptoms have been lifetime experiences, these people are not likely to volunteer that they are troubled by what they consider normal for them. If they do become conscious of their dissociative symptoms, they often believe their symptoms are a sign of "craziness" that would cause them to be "locked up in the loony bin" rather than be taken seriously, respected, and helped. People will most often hide their dissociative processes if they are aware of them. If they are not aware, then you will have to be smart enough to ask about these processes before you will have a chance of gently opening—just a little—the lid of their very own private Pandora's box, in which their mind is hidden.

What are dissociative processes?

- Depersonalization (defined below)
- Derealization (feeling that the world is unreal)
- Microamnesia (repeatedly forgetting what was just said, or somehow knowing what was just said by recalling it as if it had been read in a newspaper rather than just experienced as a "lived" event) and macroamnesia (includes forgetting "outside the range of normal experience" [1])
- Identity confusion (not knowing one's name)
- Identity alteration ("I'm Mary, not Jane.")

Dissociation is that process in which normally related psychologic experiences and events are detached from each other and result in a distortion of experience with both subtle and profound alterations in interpretation of the meaning of personal and interpersonal events. For example, depersonalization (an out-of-body experience or feeling "unreal") [2] is generated by a psychologic detachment for sensing being embodied, being located in "my body." When a person cannot feel their bodily senses, then they can't feel their feelings either; they become emotionally numb, a hallmark of posttraumatic disorders. Depersonalization can be thought of as a desperate unconscious control mechanism for squelching overwhelming effects like terror, horror, utter helplessness, and so forth. A standard—and sad—report of depersonalization is having a recollection of floating on the ceiling watching "as I was raped. The person below was me, sort of, but I wasn't there. But I was. It was all very confusing. I just feel numb about it now."

When knowledge is isolated (corollary to isolated affect, emotional numbness), a person may experience a storm of painful effect, complete with sobbing, hyperventilation, and so forth, but not have any sense of a context for why they are feeling so distressed. ("It makes me feel crazy to be taken over by all this weeping and not have a clue why I'm even crying!") Similarly, veterans from military conflicts return home to people they have loved, know they should feel more "moved" emotionally, but simply "feel nothing"—the affect is isolated, and they have posttraumatic numbness, a dissociative symptom. Likewise, a powerfully successful businessman is rarely able to sleep when traveling. Unconsciously he experiences his hotel room, one of many on a long hallway, as too close a match for one of many hospital rooms he occupied as a child with recurrent near-fatal medical events. He spends his nights depersonalized, feeling unreal, in a panic, sleepless. A drug-addicted housewife can't remember why she snorted another round of cocaine. "I told myself I wasn't going to do it, and then I watched myself reach for that line and lift it to my face, the whole time yelling inside my mind to stop, but my arms weren't under my control!" The teenage girl in the emergency room, after cutting her upper arm, reported that "It's nothing. It stopped bleeding, so who cares? I didn't feel anything. I just got calm and felt better after I saw the blood. I don't remember cutting my arm, but I do know I didn't feel it." The bulimic says, "My stomach was so painfully full that my whole body hurt. That's when I went to throw up, and this weird and wonderful fog filled my head like everything was just a dream. I must have fallen asleep. When I woke up I knew what I had done, but in a weird way it didn't feel like I had done it, I just knew I felt better, calm. Finally. It's what always happens. I hate throwing up, but the calm afterward is just fine with me."

A new model of mind for the twenty-first century: states of mind

Over 100 years ago, Sigmund Freud collaborated with Joseph Breuer to write a treatise on hysteria [3] at about the same time that Pierre Janet picked up his own pen [4]. Hysteria baffled contemporary neurologists. No wonder! With a name that meant "wandering womb," hysteria seemed to be a disease of women that men could not understand. Janet wrote about the disaggregation of the personality, while Freud and Breuer took him on in the preface of their *Studies on Hysteria*, declaring that what was a so-called "double consciousness" was essentially a mistaken description of the process of repression and a weakness of the ego. Freud's disciples, including James Strachey and Joan Riviere, brought psychoanalysis to the English-speaking world at the same time that Eugene Bleuler coined the term *schizophrenia* ("split mind") [5], and the work of Janet was eclipsed as the divisions in the dissociative mind became conflated with schizophrenia. It was not until the 1980s that this error began to be corrected with a new literature on what was then called *multiple personality disorder* [6,7]. Now, over 100 years later, there are no good experimental models of repression, while evidence for disaggregation of mental processes—or *dissociation*—is a rapidly enlarging scientific and clinical literature. Contemporary psychoanalysis and psychiatry are moving far away from Freud's structural theory, id, ego, and super-ego, and embracing studies on the self and relational psychology, and an exploding literature on attachment. The study of the dissociative disorders is opening a large door into the study of mind. A confluence of work in a number of disciplines has arrived at the conclusion that a parsimonious "model of mind" is that of "states of mind" as the basic building blocks of mind [8–21]. The advantages of a "states of mind" or "states of being" model, are spelled out in the articles presented in this issue. Of particular importance is that with attention to the language of the therapy (see the article by Way in this issue), patients with dissociative and other psychiatric disorders immediately understand what their therapists are saying about their minds.

Some important questions

How do dissociative processes work? What is the neurobiology that underlies dissociative experience? What happens to an individual's subjectivity in dissociative experience? What does "I" feel like when you can't remember what your name is? Is there some kind of normal dissociative process? Wouldn't these processes, when unrecognized, skew psychiatric research through misdiagnosis? If borderline adaptations are filled with dissociative process, wouldn't it be more useful to reformulate borderline and posttraumatic processes with a knowledge of dissociative processes? How do I learn to think intuitively about these processes so that I can "get into the mindset" of my patients and use these processes to their advantage, or at least halt their destructiveness? What about intervening with the out-of-control, self-destructive patient with a full-blown dissociative disorder and altered personalities? You don't expect me to believe there are other people inside my patients, do you? (Not only is that not expected of you, it would simply be wrong to reify a subjective experience rather than call that shift in subjectivity to the patient's attention and study their experience with them.) How do I intervene to work with a potentially violent dissociative patient? How do I understand and work with alter phenomena? Is it really appropriate to agree with the patient when they tell me their name is different than their given name? Doesn't that just make things worse? Aren't I feeding a delusion? Is there something about the particular use of language, descriptive metaphor, in the treatment of the dissociative disorders that predicts or limits what we understand about a mind, or how to help someone with these problems?

What can you learn about in the pages that follow?

The 16 articles in this issue are organized into three main sections: theory, research and evaluation, and technique. The theory section is led by Paul Dell's revisionist model of the dissociative disorders as the picture of a mind suffering from relentless intrusions of dissociated affects, knowledge, and so forth. Over a decade of work on his multidimensional inventory of dissociation has informed this view that emphasizes how individuals suffer from intrusive experience into every aspect of executive functioning. Whether you agree with him or not, he sifts dissociative experience through a very fine mesh and provides a marvelous tour of the dissociative mind. Karen Way then provides a unique vantage point from which to consider dissociative phenomena and experience by understanding how the metaphors that describe persons with dissociative disorders influence our views of mind as subject and object. She explores the notions of the self as a thing that is divided versus the self as an agent in the world that turns inwardly, away from traumatic experience and relatedness, but nevertheless cannot escape the past. She discusses her conclusion in detail: verb-based metaphors are more consistent with the goals of treatment. Lisa Butler explores the realm of normative dissociation. She combines her knowledge of dissociation and hypnosis to develop a line of inquiry that exposes the extent to which dissociative processes are part of our everyday lives. Being absorbed in reading this paragraph and having lost track of your surrounding environment is an example of everyday dissociation. Check out what she has to say. You'll learn that a dissociative process is not just something that occurs as a result of a traumatic experience—it is part of the basic operating systems in our mind. Dissociation helps us to focus and concentrate. The challenge is to not lose our bearings. Of course, paradoxically, in the face of trauma, losing one's bearings may be preferable to staying focused on unbearable trauma from which there is no escape. Lyons-Ruth and colleagues discuss how it is the specific qualities of the parent–infant dialog that are most predictive of adult dissociative disorders. The notion that traumatic experience is always at the root of dissociative adaptation seems not so sure in the face of this work. Trauma may be associated with adult and childhood dissociation, but it is the particular quality of the patterns of parent–child communication that are most predictive of dissociative coping styles. It is the "hidden trauma" of profound interpersonal emotional dysfunction that may fuel basic dissociative processes. It is within this context that Catherine Classen and colleagues responded to my invitation and wrote a reformulation of borderline and posttraumatic disorders by describing a posttraumatic personality disorder. Based on an exploration of insecure attachment that is disorganized versus organized, this article is a marvelous font toward understanding a confluence of conditions that are related to both trauma and profound relational failures. Whereas type D attachments (disorganized/disoriented pattern) are clearly consistent with the phenotype of adult dissociative disorders, the emotionally dismissive parent of the type A attachment (avoidant pattern) and the preoccupied parent of the type C attachment (anxious/ambivalent pattern) clearly show up in the behavior of borderline and posttraumatic patients. With trauma histories so prevalent in our borderline patients, isn't it time to think about reformulating the borderline construct as well as chronic posttraumatic adaptations into something that is more parsimoniously structured? You will learn a lot from their careful reformulation.

The research and evaluation section leads off with an article by clinician-scientists Frewen and Lanius. They review studies of the neural correlates of dissociative experiences, as assessed by positron emission tomography and functional MRI through the organizing principles of what some writers have called primary, secondary, and tertiary dissociation. They show how the key cortical structures involved in these processes include the medial prefrontal, anterior cingulate, somatosensory, and insular cortex, as well as the thalamus. Distinctive neural correlates of primary and secondary dissociative experiences in individuals who have posttraumatic stress disorder support state-phase models of animal defensive reaction to external threat. They speculate that disconnection of neural pathways normally linking self-awareness with body-state perception, occurring as a result of childhood trauma, may occasion the development of tertiary dissociative identities. In another article, Vedat Sar and Colin Ross discuss how the lack of attention to and knowledge about the dissociative disorders can lead to misadventure and misleading results in psychiatric research. It has always astonished me that even though the diagnosis of schizophrenia relies heavily upon hearing voices, most researchers do not screen for dissociative disorders. With psychotherapeutic interventions for schizophrenia de-emphasized, the tragedy of misdiagnosis of a dissociative disorder as a schizophrenic disorder is accentuated. Sar and Ross provide some interesting ideas to consider with regard to diagnosis and research.

Brand, Armstrong, and Loewenstein discuss how psychologic assessment can assist in the diagnosis of dissociative identity disorder (DID) as well as treatment planning for dissociative patients. They outline a battery that can assess the extent of dissociation, review the research on dissociation on various psychologic tests, and present new Rorschach data on severely dissociative patients that can be useful in planning treatment. Their work is on the frontier of the best in clinical research. As a group, their clinical skill is extraordinary. I hope you will take some time to digest their wisdom. Likewise, Frankel and Dalenberg offer a sterling review of the forensic psychology literature that is designed to be a reference guide for study by the practicing clinician. They address the role of the forensic mental health professional in the context of court-related evaluations of claims of dissociative disorders, the possible relationships between such claims and the issues to be decided by the trier of fact, research developments that may bear on the forensic evaluation of DID from biological, psychologic, and social data sources, and provide a checklist of issues about which forensic evaluators should be prepared to respond on direct and cross-examination.

For the consultation liaison clinician in you, spend some time looking at Elizabeth Bowman's comprehensive review of the relationship between pseudoseizures and dissociative processes. Bowman is one of the world's leading authorities on this topic. If you have ever treated a patient with pseudoseizures, then you know that moving the patient's understanding of what ails them from a medical model of their problem to a psychologic model requires the utmost skill. Cross-reference this with the Turkish experience in the ubiquitous presentations of conversion disorder, and you begin to see the potential for understanding a whole range of neuropsychiatric presentations based on dissociative process.

You will enjoy Eli Somer's discussion of culture-bound syndromes related to dissociative process. The expression of dissociative process is guided somewhat by culture, and Dr. Somer discusses this in detail. There is a wide range of dissociative process visible in behavioral syndromes in both sophisticated and more primitive societies. To round out this section on research and evaluation, Vedat Sar starts with the Turkish experience and adds an international roster of literature and research on the dissociative disorders. While some critics have said that dissociative disorders were a North American phenomenon, all one might need do to end the controversy is to combine the insights of Somer and Sar.

The last section will be a special treat for clinicians who are eager to learn more about the application of theory. Turkus and colleagues have put to paper many years' experience as they spell out the basics of a coherent treatment from psychoeducational approaches, through grounding techniques, to fostering inter alter communication. Their contribution is filled with clinical wisdom. Pain, Ogden, Fisher, and Ryder spell out an important element of treatment, how to integrate a knowledge of the sensorimotor neurobiologic processes into the treatment of trauma. Many clinicians focus on dissociation of affect and knowledge as the main topic of a treatment. These clinicians show how sensorimotor and even cerebellar dissociations are a powerful mode of inquiry into healing a mind filled with experience that outstripped the capacity to speak and describe overwhelming adversity with words. Somatic approaches to treatment are invaluable. While their approach may not seem immediately applicable to routine psychotherapy, read closely and you will see that even without special training, you can adapt their technique and still maintain appropriate clinical boundaries in the treatment of the traumatized person.

The last two articles in this issue are both a *tour de force*. Rick Kluft has written a kind of "everything you ever wanted to know about alter personalities but were afraid to ask" article. In many ways, Kluft is the father of this field. His knowledge is extraordinary. I hope you enjoy reading his work as much as I did. Rich Loewenstein's clinical wisdom comes alive in "DID 101." Having trained under his supervision, all I can say is that he continues to delight me with his creativity and his uncommon good sense. No matter what your level of skill, you will learn something from this blow-by-blow illustrative dialog of working with two particularly challenging patients, one initially in restraints, and the other skillfully self-destructive and previously impervious to intervention.

No editor works in a vacuum. Everybody has a life. I particularly wish to thank my wife, Kathryn Chefetz, LCSW, a psychoanalyst who "gets" dissociative disorders and who has tolerated (mostly) the time that has been taken from our relationship and family for me to complete this project. I only hope to live up to the high standard she sets for intellectual honesty and compassionate involvment in doing the work of complex treatments. She is a valued colleague. Thank you for your support, Kathryn. I also want to thank my editor, Sarah Barth, for allowing me to put together 16 rather than the usual 14 papers for an issue of this type. I want to thank my authors for their hard work, and for their respectful challenges to my editorial input that made producing this publication both a pleasure and a learning experience. They are an extraordinary group of clinicians and researchers. Lastly, I wish to thank my colleagues at the International Society for the Study of Dissociation. You have provided me with many worthy challenges, but most of all with your warmth and friendship. When Rich Loewenstein edited the last issue of the *Psychiatric Clinics of North America* on this subject in 1991, many of the authors, and this editor, were still early on in the learning curve for understanding complex dissociative disorders and dissociative processes. The growth of this field in the last 15 years has been extraordinary. I look forward to the next 15 years, and to the advances that will lead to better treatments, faster healing, and resolution of pain for our patients. We need to assure, as best we can, that our patients can complete treatment and then go on to lead productive lives in a growth-promoting community. Fantasy? No, not at all. I believe the vast majority of our patients can do this work when their clinicians are well educated. Time to get back to work and make this belief a reality. Please join me.

Richard A. Chefetz, MD
4612 49th Street NW
Washington, DC 20016, USA

E-mail address: r.a.chefetz@psychsense.net

References

[1] American Psychiatric Association. Diagnostic and statistical manual of mental disorders. 4th edition [text revision, DSM-IV-TR]. Washington DC: American Psychiatric Association; 2000.

[2] Simeon D. Depersonalizaiton disorder: a contemporary overview. CNS Drugs 2004;18: 343–54.

[3] Breuer J, Freud S. Studies on hysteria. Volume 2. London: The Hogarth Press; 1895.

[4] Janet P. The major symptoms of hysteria. New York: Macmillan; 1907.

[5] Bleuler E. Dementia praecox or the group of schizophrenics. New York: International Universities Press; 1911.

[6] Kluft RP, editor. Childhood antecedants of multiple personality. Washington, DC: American Psychiatric Press, Inc.; 1985.

[7] Putnam FW. Diagnosis and treatment of multiple personality disorder. New York: Guilford
     Press; 1989.
[8] Siegel DJ. The developing mind: toward a neurobiology of interpersonal experience. New
     York: Guilford Press; 1999.
[9] Emde RN. Positive emotions for psychoanalytic theory: surprises from infancy research
     and new directions. J Am Psychoanal Assoc 1991;39(Suppl):5–44.
[10] Main M, Morgan H. Disorganization and disorientation in infant strange situation behav-
     ior: phenotypic resemblance to dissociative states. In: Michelson LK, Ray WJ, editors.
     Handbook of dissociation: theoretical, empirical, and clinical perspectives. New York:
     Plenum Press; 1996. p. 107–38.
[11] Nijenhuis ERS. Somatoform dissociation: major symptoms of dissociative disorders.
     J Trauma Dissociation 2000;1:7–32.
[12] Stern DN. The interpersonal world of the infant. New York: Basic Books; 1985.
[13] Bromberg PM. Standing in the Spaces. Hillsdale (NJ): The Analytic Press; 1998.
[14] Chefetz R, Bromberg P. Talking with "Me" and "Not-Me": a dialogue. Contemp Psycho-
     anal 2004;40:409–64.
[15] Damasio A. The feeling of what happens: body and emotion in the making of consciousness.
     New York: Harcourt Brace; 1999.
[16] Gleaves D, May M, Cardena E. An examination of the diagnostic validity of dissociative
     identity disorder. Clin Psychol Rev 2001;21:577–608.
[17] Hilgard ER. Divided consciousness: multiple controls in human thought and action. New
     York: John Wiley & Sons; 1986.
[18] Horowitz MJ, Fridhandler B, Stinson C. Person schemas and emotion. J Am Psychoanal
     Assoc 1991;39(Suppl):173–208.
[19] Krystal H. Integration and self healing: affect, alexithymia, and trauma. Hillsdale (NJ): An-
     alytic Press; 1988.
[20] Ledoux J. The emotional brain. New York: Simon & Schuster; 1996.
[21] Liotti G. Disorganization of attachment as a model for understanding dissociative psy-
     chopathology. In: Solomon J, George C, editors. Attachment disorganization. New York:
     Guilford Press; 1999. p. 291–317.

ELSEVIER
SAUNDERS

Psychiatr Clin N Am 29 (2006) 1–26

PSYCHIATRIC
CLINICS
OF NORTH AMERICA

A New Model of Dissociative Identity Disorder

Paul F. Dell, PhD*

*Director, Trauma Recovery Center, Psychotherapy Resources of Norfolk,
330 West Brambleton Avenue, Suite 206, Norfolk, VA 23510, USA*

The *Diagnostic and Statistical Manual of Mental Disorders, Fourth Edition-Text Revision* [1] (DSM-IV-TR) describes the classic features of dissociative identify disorder (DID) that are widely known in the general culture. According to the DSM-IV-TR description, a person who has DID switches from one personality to another; each personality has its own identity; and the host personality has amnesia for the activities of the other personalities. I have argued that this description of DID is deficient because it omits most of the dissociative phenomena of DID [2–4] and focuses solely on alter personalities.

This article presents data from 220 persons who have DID and explores how those data fit with three contrasting models of DID: (1) the DSM-IV's classic picture of DID (ie, multiple personalities + switching + amnesia), (2) Dell's subjective/phenomenological model of DID [4], and (3) the sociocognitive model of DID. The DSM-IV narrowly portrays DID as an alter disorder, whereas the subjective/phenomenological model portrays DID as a far more complex dissociative disorder that is characterized by recurrent dissociative intrusions into every aspect of executive functioning and sense of self.[1] The subjective/phenomenological model of DID subsumes the DSM-IV model of DID, but not vice versa. The sociocognitive model argues that DID is a socially-constructed, iatrogenic condition.

The dissociative phenomena of dissociative identity disorder

Thirteen dissociative symptoms of DID have been well-replicated. These 13 dissociative symptoms have been reported by 8 to 32 empirical studies of

---

[1] This article does not address the psychological mechanism of these dissociative intrusions (ie, self-states or alter personalities); that topic requires a separate paper [4].

* 101 Brattle Street, Apt. 3, Cambridge, MA 02138.
E-mail address: PFDell@aol.com

Table 1
Thirteen well-documented dissociative symptoms of dissociative identity disorder

Symptom	Empirical studies
Straightforward dissociative symptoms	
Amnesia	32
Conversion	28
Voices	22
Depersonalization	20
Trances	17
Self-alteration	16
Derealization	14
Awareness of the presence of alters	10
Identity confusion	10
Flashbacks	8
Psychotic-like dissociative symptoms	
Auditory hallucination	13
Visual hallucinations	11
Schneiderian first-rank symptoms	14
'Made' actions	6
Voices arguing	5
Voices commenting	4
'Made' feelings	3
Thought withdrawal	2
Thought insertion	2
'Made' impulses	1

Empirical studies are the number of empirical studies that have reported the occurrence of that dissociative symptom in persons who have dissociative identity disorder.

DID (Table 1). The subjective/phenomenological model accounts for these symptoms, but the DSM-IV model does not.[2]

Three items in Table 1 are psychotic symptoms (auditory hallucinations, visual hallucinations, and Schneider's first-rank symptoms), but I contend that there are many patients whose auditory hallucinations, visual hallucinations, or first-rank symptoms are dissociative in nature rather than psychotic (see later discussion).

Straightforward dissociative symptoms

Amnesia

Amnesia is the most frequently reported dissociative symptom of DID [3–35]. At least 10 different manifestations of amnesia have been reported in persons who have DID: (1) time loss [3,6,10,11,14–18,20,24,25,27,32, 33,35]; (2) fugues [3,5,7,10–14,20–22,24,27,29,31,32,36]; (3) being told of disremembered actions [3,10,11,13,14,16,17,19,27,32,35]; (4) temporary loss of well-practiced knowledge or skills [3,10,13–16,18,25,35]; (5) finding objects

---

[2] DSM-IV accounts for 2 of the 13 well-replicated dissociative symptoms of DID.

among one's possessions [3,10,13,14,27,32]; (6) amnesia for childhood [24,27,32]; (7) amnesia for personal identity [6,35]; (8) strangers know the person [27,32]; (9) objects are missing [27,32]; and (10) finding evidence of one's recent actions [3,6,14].

Amnesia is one of the five diagnostic symptoms of dissociation that the Structured Clinical Interview for DSM-IV Dissociative Disorders–Revised (SCID-D-R) [33] measures. Amnesia is also one of the two factors of pathological dissociation on the Dissociative Experiences Scale (DES) [54]. Despite its robust replication in the empirical literature on DID, amnesia did not become a diagnostic criterion for DID until the DSM-IV [37]. DSM-IV provides a vague definition of amnesia. Detection of amnesia would be greatly facilitated if the DSM included well-validated examples of amnesia in DID (such as those in the previous paragraph).

Conversion symptoms

The second most commonly documented dissociative symptom of DID is somatoform conversion (and other somatoform symptoms) [3,6,7,10–16,20–22,24,27,30–32,35,36,38–45]. Conversion symptoms have been considered to be somatoform dissociative symptoms since at least the time of Janet [46]. Nevertheless, despite cogent criticism and convincing empirical evidence [47–51], the DSM-IV classifies conversion disorder as a somatoform disorder, rather than a dissociative disorder. The *International Classification of Diseases, Tenth Edition* (ICD-10) [52], on the other hand, classifies conversion symptoms as *dissociative [conversion] disorders* (F44). The somatoform disorders section of DSM-IV states that dissociative and conversion symptoms commonly occur in the same individual. The dissociative disorders section of DSM-IV lists conversion symptoms among the associated descriptive features of DID.

Voices

The third most commonly documented dissociative symptom of DID is hearing voices [3,5–7,10,11,13–16,18–20,22,24,25,27,31,32,35,36,53]. These voices are usually, but by no means always, located "in the head." A small minority of persons who have DID deny hearing voices; some of the latter actually do hear voices, but they have reframed or rationalized them (eg, "it's me," "it's just my conscience"). Nevertheless, some persons who have DID genuinely do not hear voices. The descriptive text in DSM-IV mentions voices, but seems to (inaccurately) limit the presence of voices in DID to command hallucinations (ie, "a voice giving instructions") [1].

Depersonalization

Depersonalization is the fourth most frequently documented dissociative symptom of DID [3,5–12,14,21–24,27,31,33–36]. Depersonalization is one of the five diagnostic symptoms of dissociation that the SCID-D-R assesses.

Depersonalization/derealization is also one of the DES's two factors of pathological dissociation [54,55]. The DSM-IV account of DID makes no mention of depersonalization.

Trance states

The empirical literature on DID has repeatedly documented the presence of trance states (ie, periods of nonresponsiveness during which the person manifests a blank stare) [3,5,6,11,14–20,24,25,27,31,35,36]. Although the occurrence of trance states is thoroughly documented in the adult and child literature on DID, the DSM-IV makes no mention of trance states in DID.

Self-alteration

Self-alteration is the sixth most frequently documented dissociative symptom of DID. [3,5,6,8,11,14–20,25,33–35]. Self-alteration is not synonymous with switching from one personality to another. Self-alteration is the subjective experience of undergoing sudden, inexplicable, and often ego-alien changes in one's sense of self. These experiences are obviously similar to depersonalization, but they do not have depersonalization's quality of generalized detachment and alienation. In self-alteration, for example, one does not feel so much detached from one's body, thoughts, or urges as one feels that one's body, thoughts, or urges belong to someone else. Identity alteration is one of the five diagnostic symptoms of dissociation that the SCID-D-R assesses. DSM-IV focuses on visible switching from one personality to another; it makes no mention of the experience of self-alteration.

Derealization

Derealization has repeatedly been reported by persons who have DID [3,6,8–11,14,23,24,27,32–34]. Derealization is one of the five diagnostic symptoms of dissociation that the SCID-D-R measures. Depersonalization/derealization is also one of the DES's two factors of pathological dissociation [55]. The DSM-IV account of DID makes no mention of derealization.

Awareness of the presence of other personalities

Awareness of the presence of other personalities has been widely reported in the empirical literature on DID [16–20,24,25,27,32,35]. Such awareness is a common occurrence in DID. Moreover, many patients who have DID hear or see what some personalities say or do when they are "out." Many clinicians have incorrectly assumed that a person who has DID can never be aware of the activities of another personality. This assumption, which is supported by the classic view of DID, is often cited as a reason for ruling out the diagnosis of DID (ie, if the patient remembers what an alter personality did or said, then the patient, supposedly, does not have DID) [56]. The Dissociative Disorders Interview Schedule (DDIS) [64] and the SCID-D-R inquire about the person's subjective awareness of other personalities. The

DSM-IV does not mention that patients who have DID typically have subjective awareness of other personalities.

Identity confusion

Identity confusion is often reported in persons who have DID [3,8–10,14,17,32–35]. Identity confusion is one of the five diagnostic symptoms of dissociation that the SCID-D-R measures. The DSM-IV account of DID makes no mention of identity confusion.

Flashbacks

Flashbacks are common for persons who have DID [3,10,14, 18,24,27,32,35]. Similarly, posttraumatic stress disorder (PTSD) has been reported to be extensively comorbid with DID [10–12,15,24]. The DDIS and the SCID-D-R inquire about flashbacks. DSM-IV lists flashbacks as an associated descriptive feature of DID.

Psychotic-like dissociative symptoms

In the 1980s, researchers of DID were acutely aware that many cases of multiple personality had received a prior diagnosis of schizophrenia [6,7,9,22,27,31,36,53,57]. Accordingly, research in the 1980s often focused on psychotic-like symptoms of DID (which could lead to an erroneous diagnosis of schizophrenia).

Auditory hallucinations

At least 13 studies have documented the presence of auditory hallucinations in patients who have DID [5–7,11–13,18,20,21,24,25,35,36]. Authors of studies reporting auditory hallucinations have typically provided little description or explication of the clinical phenomena that they included under this rubric, which is unfortunate because at least three different referents for auditory hallucinations are present in a population of patients who have DID. These are: (1) hearing the voices of alter personalities, (2) the auditory component of dissociative flashbacks, and (3) genuinely psychotic auditory hallucinations. I suspect that most of the 21 studies that have reported auditory hallucinations in persons who have DID are referring to hearing the voices of alter personalities. This interpretation of voices in DID would seem to underlie the DSM-IV-TR's view of auditory hallucinations in DID: "an identity that is not in control may nonetheless gain access to consciousness by producing auditory ... hallucinations (e.g., a voice giving instructions)" [1].

Visual hallucinations

Eleven studies have reported that patients who have DID experience visual hallucinations [6,7,11–13,18,20,21,24,35,36]. The same problem exists in these reports as in reports of auditory hallucinations; the authors of the studies have provided very little description or explication of the clinical phenomena they included under this rubric. In a population of patients who have DID, at least three possible referents for visual hallucinations exist: (1) seeing or visualizing alter personalities (either in the mind or externally), (2) the visual component of dissociative flashbacks, and (3) genuinely psychotic visual hallucinations. In my experience with patients who have DID, genuinely psychotic visual hallucinations are uncommon, but they may occur if a person who has DID develops reactive dissociative psychosis [58] or another (comorbid) psychotic disorder. On the other hand, visual flashbacks and seeing alters are common experiences. Seeing or visualizing an alter seems to underlie DSM-IV-TR's view of visual hallucinations in DID: "an identity that is not in control may nonetheless gain access to consciousness by producing ... visual hallucinations" [1].

Schneiderian first-rank symptoms

Fourteen studies have reported the occurrence of Schneiderian first-rank symptoms [59] in persons who have DID [5,18,24,26–32,38,53,60,61]. Another eight studies have reported the occurrence of specific first-rank symptoms in patients who have DID, including voices arguing [10,13,14,20], voices commenting [6,10,14,20], "made" feelings [3,10,35], "made" impulses [10], "made" actions [3,6,10,20,35,36], thought withdrawal [3,6], thought insertion [3,6], thought broadcasting [6,10], and delusional perception [6,36].

Kluft [53] was the first to document the frequency of the 11 Schneiderian first-rank symptoms in a well-diagnosed series of DID cases. He reported that eight of the first-rank symptoms (voices arguing, voices commenting, "made" feelings, "made" impulses, "made" actions, influences on the body, thought withdrawal, and thought insertion) were common in DID, but that three of the first-rank symptoms (thought broadcasting, audible thoughts, and delusional perception) did not occur in DID. Although other researchers have occasionally reported thought broadcasting, audible thoughts, and delusional perceptions in patients who have DID [6,10,18,26,36], I concur with Kluft that such symptoms are not phenomena of DID. Instead, these symptoms may occur if a patient who has DID undergoes a true psychotic episode (eg, major depressive episode with psychotic features, reactive dissociative psychosis). Still, this matter will probably not be resolved until two issues are clarified further: whether the 11 Schneiderian symptoms should be construed narrowly or broadly, and whether the 11 Schneiderian symptoms are qualitatively different in persons who have DID (compared with persons who have a psychotic disorder) [10,28,62–64]. The DSM-IV account of DID makes no mention of first-rank symptoms.

Commentary on the literature about the dissociative phenomena of dissociative identity disorder

The preceding 13 sections illustrate the extent to which the empirical literature's picture of DID is strikingly different from the DSM-IV's picture of

DID. Only 2 of the 13 dissociative symptoms in Table 1 are strongly included in the DSM-IV-TR diagnostic criteria for DID: amnesia and objective signs of self-alteration. Of the remaining 11 dissociative symptoms in Table 1, 5 receive no mention whatsoever in the DSM-IV-TR (depersonalization, derealization, awareness of the presence of alters, identity confusion, and first-rank symptoms); 3 are mentioned in the text pertaining to diagnostic features (auditory flashbacks, visual flashbacks, and voices); 2 are listed among the associated descriptive features of DID (conversion and flashbacks); and 1 is mentioned under differential diagnosis (trance).

The "take-home message" is that there is a large difference between the empirical literature's account of the dissociative phenomena of DID and the DSM-IV's account of the dissociative phenomena of DID.

Two major clusters of dissociative phenomena

DID has two major clusters of dissociative phenomena, only one of which is described by DSM-IV: switching from one personality to another with concomitant amnesia. This cluster of dissociative phenomena is, in fact, identical to the DSM-IV model of DID. The second cluster of dissociative phenomena in DID is intrusions into executive functioning and sense of self by alter personalities.[3]

The remaining 11 of the 13 well-replicated dissociative symptoms of DID in Table 1 are intrusions by alter personalities. Strictly speaking, identity confusion is not a dissociative intrusion. Rather, identity confusion is the result of recurrent dissociative intrusions. The DSM-IV makes no mention of intrusions.

The first cluster of dissociative phenomena in DID—switching from one personality to another with concomitant amnesia—is known almost universally, even by the general public. Conversely, the second cluster of dissociative phenomena in DID—intrusion into executive functioning and sense of self by alter personalities—is largely unknown.

For several reasons, even clinicians who treat DID tend to have only a partial awareness or understanding of dissociative intrusions. First, the term *intrusion* has generally not been used to describe DID. That is, clinicians who treat DID readily use the term *intrusion* to refer to criterion B PTSD symptoms [1] (eg, intrusive memories, dreams, flashbacks), but not dissociative symptoms. Second, the notion that dissociative symptoms are intrusive is intuitively recognized by clinicians who treat DID, but not in a focal way. Third, clinicians who treat DID tend to think of these symptoms under a different rubric from intrusion. They think of these symptoms in terms of passive-influence phenomena (Schneiderian first-rank symptoms).

---

[3] I have argued elsewhere that switching with concomitant amnesia is actually a special case of dissociative intrusion. Thus, I contend that the subjective phenomenology of dissociative symptoms is always one of intrusion into executive functioning or sense of self.

More than 20 publications have reported that patients who have DID routinely experience one or more of the eight passive-influence phenomena. These eight Schneiderian first-rank symptoms are experienced as autonomous intrusions into a person's executive functioning and sense of self. In schizophrenia, these intrusions take a psychotic form. That is, the patient gives the intrusion a delusional explanation (eg, "Marilyn Monroe is controlling my thoughts"). In DID, these intrusions take a nonpsychotic form; they are noted and described by the patient, but they are not given a delusional explanation (eg, "I know this sounds crazy, but sudden strong thoughts come into my mind and they feel like they are not mine").

The subjective/phenomenological model of pathological dissociation

The subjective/phenomenological model of pathological dissociation[4] is actually a generalized formulation of the eight Schneiderian passive-influence experiences. According to the subjective/phenomenological model of pathological dissociation, the phenomena of pathological dissociation are recurrent, jarring intrusions into executive functioning and sense of self by self-states or alter personalities. Such dissociative phenomena are startling, alien invasions of one's mind, functioning, and experience. These intrusions are always confusing [65–67] and often frightening. They frequently cause persons who are dissociative to fear for their sanity. The subjective/phenomenological model of pathological dissociation has four corollaries.

Pathological dissociation can affect every aspect of human experience

No aspect of human experience is immune to invasion by dissociative symptoms. Dissociative intrusions can affect one's conscious awareness and one's experience of one's body, world, self, mind, agency, intentionality, thinking, believing, knowing, recognizing, remembering, feeling, wanting, speaking, acting, seeing, hearing, smelling, tasting, and touching.

Most phenomena of pathological dissociation are subjective and invisible

The overwhelming majority of dissociative phenomena are subjective and invisible, rather than objective and visible [4]. Relatively few objective signs of dissociation exist, and the few objective signs that do exist are unreliably discerned, even by well-trained observers [68].

There are two major kinds of pathological dissociation: intrusions and amnesias

Two major kinds of pathological dissociation exist: dissociative symptoms that are partially dissociated from consciousness (intrusions), and

---

[4] Strictly speaking, identity confusion is not a dissociative intrusion. Rather, identity confusion is the *result* of undergoing recurrent dissociative intrusions.

dissociative symptoms that are fully dissociated from consciousness (amnesias). When a dissociative symptom is partially dissociated from consciousness, the individual is contemporaneously (and disturbingly) aware of the jarring, alien intrusions into his or her executive functioning and sense of self. In contrast, when a dissociative event is fully dissociated from conscious awareness (ie, when amnesia occurs), the person has no awareness whatsoever of that occurrence.

Most dissociative symptoms are not fully dissociated from consciousness

With the exception of amnesia, dissociative individuals have contemporaneous, conscious awareness of all other dissociative intrusions (eg, depersonalization, derealization, voices, intrusive thoughts, "made" actions). Thus, with the exception of amnesia, all dissociative events are partially conscious.

A major shortcoming of the DSM-IV is encountered here. DSM-IV's classic picture of DID embraces full dissociation (ie, amnesia), but omits partial dissociation. This omission is a problem because incidents of partial dissociation are vastly more common than incidents of switching-accompanied-by-amnesia [4].

A new model of the dissociative phenomena of dissociative identity disorder

In 2001 [2], I proposed an expanded view of the dissociative phenomena of DID, outlined in Box 1. I believe that this expanded view of DID is more accurate because, unlike DSM-IV, it delineates the predominance of intrusions in the dissociative symptoms of DID. The predominance of dissociative intrusions in DID is predicted by the subjective/phenomenological model of pathological dissociation [4] and supported by the decisive preponderance of intrusions among the 13 well-replicated dissociative symptoms of DID (Table 1).

According to the subjective/phenomenological model of pathological dissociation, the domain of pathological dissociation (ie, intrusions into every aspect of human experience) directly specifies the dissociative symptom-domain of DID [4]. Box 1 is an effort to operationalize this conjecture; it implicitly delineates (1) the entire domain of human experience, (2) the corresponding dissociative intrusions to which each aspect of that domain is subject, (3) the symptom-domain of DID, and (4) the subjective/phenomenological domain of pathological dissociation.[5]

---

[5] Although not identified as such in Box 1, both criterion A (general dissociative symptoms) and criterion B (partially-dissociated intrusions of another self-state) are considered to be partially dissociated intrusions. Criterion A is grouped separately from criterion B because it contains dissociative symptoms that often occur in nondissociative disorders (eg, PTSD, panic disorder, borderline personality disorder, schizotypal personality, major depressive disorder, somatization disorder).

Box 1. The subjective/phenomenological model of dissociative identity disorder

General dissociative symptoms (4 of 6 required)
- Memory problems
- Depersonalization
- Derealization
- Posttraumatic flashbacks
- Somatoform symptoms
- Trance

Evidence of the partially dissociated intrusions of another self-state, as indicated by either 1 or 2:
1. Clinician observation of a self-state that claims (or appears) to be someone other than the person being interviewed, as indicated by the person's
   - Co-conscious awareness of the activities of the self-state; and
   - Remembering what the self-state said and did
   - Experiencing the self-state as "other."
2. At least 6 of the following 11 symptoms of intrusion by a partially dissociated self-state:
   - Child voices
   - Internal struggle, conversation, or argument
   - Persecutory voices that comment harshly, make threats, or command self-destructive acts
   - Speech insertion (unintentional or disowned utterances)
   - Thought insertion or withdrawal
   - "Made" or intrusive feelings and emotions
   - "Made" or intrusive impulses
   - "Made" or intrusive actions
   - Temporary loss of well-rehearsed knowledge or skills
   - Disconcerting experiences of self-alteration
   - Self-puzzlement

Evidence of the fully dissociated intrusions of another self-state (ie, amnesia), as indicated by either 1 or 2:
1. Clinician observation of a self-state that claims (or seems) to be someone other than the person being interviewed, followed by the person's subsequent amnesia for the clinician's encounter with the self-state.
2. Recurrent amnesia, as indicated by the person's report of multiple incidents of at least two of the following:
   - Time loss
   - "Coming to"
   - Fugues
   - Being told of disremembered actions
   - Finding objects among one's possessions
   - Finding evidence of one's recent actions

Before proceeding further, the new model of DID [4] must be distinguished from the diagnostic criteria that reflect that model [2]. Box 1 does not draw a distinction between the model and its diagnostic criteria. In fact, Box 1 explicates the model through a set of diagnostic criteria. Obviously, the new model of DID and diagnostic criteria that reflect that model cannot be completely separated from one another. Still, I am not proposing that the DSM-V diagnostic criteria for DID should include all 25 of the dissociative symptoms in Box 1. Even though I believe that these 25 symptoms routinely characterize DID, the issue of which (and how many) of those symptoms should be used in a new set of diagnostic criteria for DID is a pragmatic and empirical question that remains unanswered.

The present study is not meant to assess a new set of diagnostic criteria for DID; instead, this study assesses the degree to which the subjective/phenomenological model of DID (see Box 1) accurately describes a large sample of DID cases. To the extent that the dissociative symptoms of these persons with DID conform to Box 1, then, to that same extent, the DSM-IV model of DID is deficient.

Testing the subjective/phenomenological model of dissociative identity disorder

Because no instrument comprehensively measured the hypothesized dissociative symptom-domain of DID, it was necessary to develop the Multidimensional Inventory of Dissociation (MID) [65]. The MID has 23 dissociation scales that assess the subjective/phenomenological domain of pathological dissociation and the hypothesized dissociative symptom-domain of DID (see Box 1).[6]

The internal consistency of the MID's 23 dissociation diagnostic scales was good-to-excellent in a large clinical sample (range of Cronbach α = 0.84 to 0.96; median α = 0.91) and had good-to-excellent temporal stability over a 4- to 8-week test–retest interval (range of temporal stability coefficients = 0.82 to 0.97; median coefficient = 0.92) [65]. These results were replicated in Israel with the Hebrew MID (H-MID) [69] and in Germany with the German MID (G-MID) [70]. Each of the 23 dissociation diagnostic scales of the H-MID had good-to-excellent internal consistency (range of Cronbach α = 0.81 to 0.97; median α = 0.93). Each of the 23 dissociation

---

[6] Although the following seven paragraphs about the psychometrics of the MID could be placed in the section on "Methods," they are described here for an important reason. The MID was designed to comprehensively assess the subjective/phenomenological domain of dissociation. Accordingly, the validity and reliability of the MID simultaneously assess three other issues: (1) the validity of the subjective/phenomenological model of dissociation, (2) the validity of the subjective/phenomenological domain of dissociation, and (3) the validity of the subjective/phenomenological model of DID.

diagnostic scales of the G-MID had good-to-excellent internal consistency (range of Cronbach α = 0.80 to 0.96; median α = 0.90).

The MID's convergent validity was demonstrated by the instrument's high correlations with four other measures of dissociation [65]: the DES [54] (r = 0.90), the Dissociation Questionnaire (DIS-Q) [71] (r = 0.83), the SCID-D [33] (r = 0.78), Questionnaire of Experiences of Dissociation (QED) [72] (r = 0.75), and the Somatoform Dissociation Questionnaire-20 (SDQ) [39] (r = 0.75). The convergent validity of the MID was replicated in Israel; the H-MID correlated 0.91 with the Hebrew-DES and 0.89 with the Hebrew-SCID-D. The convergent validity of the MID was also replicated in Germany; the G-MID correlated 0.93 with the German-DES and 0.85 with the German-SCID-D.

Four studies have supported the discriminant validity of the MID's scales [3,65,66,70]. MID scores significantly discriminated among four groups: DID, dissociative disorder not otherwise specified (DDNOS)-1, mixed psychiatric, and nonclinical adults [3,65].[7]

In Germany, G-MID scores significantly discriminated among the same four groups [70]. Finally, various combinations of the 12 MID factor scales significantly discriminated among three patient groups: DID, DDNOS, and mixed psychiatric [66].

The structural validity of the MID was strongly supported by two exploratory factor analyses of the MID's 168 dissociation items [66]. These analyses extracted 12 factors. Confirmatory factor analyses of two independent samples tested a one-factor model of these 12-factor scales; the model explained 96% of the variance in the 12 factors. Thus, the MID's 12-factor scales are robustly explained by a single, overarching construct—pathological dissociation.

The present study

The present study assesses whether the subjective/phenomenological domain of pathological dissociation accurately predicts the dissociative symptoms of persons who have DID. A pilot study found that the incidence of 22 subjective/phenomenological dissociative symptoms in 34 patients who had DID ranged from 74% to 100%, with a median frequency of 91% [14].

The present study analyzed the MID data of 220 clinically-diagnosed cases of DID; a subset of these clinically-diagnosed cases was confirmed with the SCID-D-R (n = 41). The specific purpose of the study was to assess whether DID is characterized by the 23 subjective/phenomenological dissociative symptoms that are measured by the MID (see Box 1).

---

[7] DDNOS-1 is the first example of DDNOS in DSM-IV: "Clinical presentations similar to Dissociative Identity Disorder that fail to meet full criteria for this disorder. Examples include presentations in which a) there are not two or more distinct personality states, or b) amnesia for important personal information does not occur" [37].

Method

Participants

The study comprised 220 persons who had DID diagnoses. All were undergoing active psychotherapy and had received a clinical diagnosis of DSM-IV DID from their therapists. A subset of the sample (n = 41) were administered the SCID-D-R, which confirmed their DID diagnoses. The participants had a mean age of 41 years (SD = 8.8 years) and a mean educational level of 14.6 years (SD = 2.7 years). The sample comprised 90% women (n = 199) and 9% men (n = 20); the gender of one participant was unrecorded. Of these participants, 89% (n = 195) were Caucasian, 4% (n = 8) were Hispanic, 3% (n = 7) were African-American, one participant was Native American, one participant was from the Pacific Islands, and one participant was of mixed racial origin. The race of 3% (n = 7) of the participants was not recorded. The participants comprised 26% inpatients (n = 57) and 73% (n = 161) outpatients; the status of two participants was not known. Participants came from outpatient settings throughout the United States and Canada, and from five inpatient settings in California, Texas, Massachusetts, Canada, and Australia.

Materials

Multidimensional Inventory of Dissociation. The MID is a Likert-format 11-point (0–10, anchored by Never and Always) self-report instrument with 168 dissociation items and 50 validity items. The instructions are: "How often do you have the following experiences when you are **not under the influence of alcohol or drugs**? Please circle the number that best describes you. Circle a '0' if the experience never happens to you; circle a '10' if it is always happening to you. If it happens sometimes, but not all the time, circle a number between 1 and 9 that best describes how often it happens to you." The MID has a Flesch-Kincaid Grade Level of 7.1 [65].

The MID has two scoring systems: mean scores and severe dissociation scores. Severe dissociation scores are based on empirically-determined pass/fail cutoff scores for each item and scale. The cutoff scores maximize the discrimination between persons who have and don't have a severe dissociative disorder. MID severe dissociation scores range from 0 to 168.

The MID has 23 dissociation diagnostic scales that vary in length from 3 to 12 items (Table 2). Seven of these scales are identical to their counterpart in the 14 primary scales. The MID has 50 validity items and 5 validity scales: defensiveness, rare symptoms, attention-seeking behavior, factitious behavior, and emotional suffering. The validity scales were designed to detect two response sets: defensive minimization and exaggerated responding. The present study does not present data from the MID's validity scales; that will be the topic of another publication. Validity data did not alter the substance or meaning of the findings reported here.

Table 2
Incidence of 23 dissociative symptoms in 220 persons who have dissociative identity disorder

MID scale	SCID-D n = 41	Total sample n = 220	Outpatients n = 161	Inpatients n = 57
Mean number of symptoms	19.7	20.2	19.9	21.3
SD	4.7	4.5	4.8	3.2
Percent incidence of each symptom				
General dissociative symptoms:				
Memory problems (5/12)[a]	100	94	93	98
Depersonalization (4/12)	95	95	94	98
Derealization (4/12)	93	92	89	98
Posttraumatic flashbacks (5/12)	93	92	90	96
Somatoform symptoms (4/12)	83	83	81	88
Trance (5/12)	88	87	84	96
Partially-dissociated intrusions				
Child voices (1/3)	95	95	94	95
Internal struggle (3/9)	100	96	95	98
Persecutory voices (2/5)	88	90	87	96
Speech insertion (2/3)	85	83	81	86
Thought insertion/withdrawal (3/5)	93	91	90	95
"Made"/intrusive emotions (4/7)	95	91	90	96
"Made"/intrusive impulses (2/3)	85	89	87	93
"Made"/intrusive actions (4/9)	98	95	93	98
Temp loss of knowledge (2/5)	90	82	80	91
Self-alteration (4/12)	98	95	94	98
Self-puzzlement (3/8)	98	95	93	98
Fully-dissociated intrusions (ie, amnesia)				
Time Loss (2/4)	88	88	87	89
"Coming to" (2/4)	78	79	75	88
Fugues (2/5)	83	75	71	86
Being told of actions (2/4)	85	86	85	88
Finding objects (2/4)	61	74	72	77
Evidence of actions (2/5)	71	77	76	81

Abbreviations: MID = multidimensional inventory of dissociation; SCID-D, Structured Clinical Interview for DSM-IV Dissociative Disorders-Revised; Temp loss of knowledge, temporary loss of well-rehearsed knowledge or skills; Self-alteration, experiences of self-alteration; Being told of actions, being told of disremembered actions; Finding objects, finding objects among one's possessions; Evidence of actions, finding evidence of ones recent actions.

[a] The first numeral is the number of items that must receive a clinically-significant rating by the test-taker for that symptom to be considered present; the second numeral is the number of items on that scale.

The present study used a 259-item precursor of the final version of the MID. The final version of the MID was created by deleting 41 items from the 259-item version. All MID data presented below are based on the final MID (ie, a 218-item scoring of the data from the 259 items). The present study's findings were not used to decide which items to delete from the MID to create the final, 218-item MID.

Structured Clinical Interview for DSM-IV Dissociative Disorders–Revised. The SCID-D-R [33,73,74] is a 277-item semistructured interview that rates five dissociative symptoms (amnesia, depersonalization, derealization, identity confusion, and identity alteration) and diagnoses the five DSM-IV dissociative disorders. The SCID-D-R has good-to-excellent reliability and validity for each of the five dissociative symptoms and the five dissociative disorders. The total SCID-D-R score correlates 0.78 with the DES [9] and 0.78 with the MID [65].

Procedures
During the development of the MID, the members of a dissociation discussion list on the Internet were invited to enlist patients to participate in this study. Therapists were sent a brief analysis of their patient's MID scores. All participants were recruited by their therapists. Participants either completed the MID at their therapist's office or at home between sessions. Forty-one individuals also agreed to participate in a SCID-D-R interview.

Results
Incidence of the 23 dissociative symptoms in 220 clinically-diagnosed cases of dissociative identity disorder. The median incidence of the 23 dissociative symptoms was 90% (range, 74%–96%; see Table 2). The 220 DID cases and the 41 SCID-D-R-diagnosed DID cases had means of 20.2 and 19.7 for dissociative symptoms, respectively.

Mean scores for the 23 dissociation scales. Mean scores on the 23 dissociation scales were virtually identical for the 220 clinically-diagnosed DID cases and the 41 SCID-D-R-diagnosed DID cases (see Fig. 1).
Inpatients who had DID had significantly higher scores on eight dissociation scales than did outpatients who had DID, including flashbacks, trance, persecutory voices, coming to, fugues, being told of recent actions, finding evidence of one's recent actions, and critical items (Table 3).

Internal consistency of the 23 dissociative symptoms. Scores on the 23 dissociation scales had a Cronbach α coefficient of 0.98. Thus, these 23 symptoms constitute a tightly-organized, unitary concept: DID.

Schneiderian first-rank symptoms: the eight passive influence experiences. The 220 patients who had DID had a mean of 7.24 (SD = 1.56) of the 8 predicted first-rank symptoms. The incidence of each symptom was high; 89% experienced voices arguing, 95% experienced voices commenting, 94% experienced "made"/intrusive feelings, 89% experienced "made"/intrusive impulses, 88% experienced "made"/intrusive actions, 94% experienced influences playing on the body, 83% experienced thought withdrawal, and 93% experienced thought insertion.

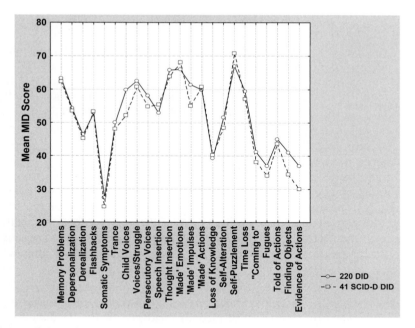

Fig. 1. Multidimensional inventory of dissociation scale scores of 220 persons who were clinically diagnosed with DID and 41 who were diagnosed using the SCID-D-R.

Diagnostic accuracy of the 23 dissociative symptoms. The 23 symptoms were
sorted into three criteria (see Box 1): (A) general dissociative symptoms (4 of
6 symptoms are required), (B) partially-dissociated intrusions (6 of 11 symptoms are required), and (C) fully-dissociated actions (2 of 6 symptoms are
required). To receive a diagnosis of DID, all three criteria must be met:
93% of the DID patients met criterion A; 93% met criterion B; 90% met
criterion C; and 84% met all three criteria. When alternate criterion C
was used (ie, criterion C plus temporary loss of knowledge/skill), 94%
met this criterion and 87% met all three criteria for DID (Table 4).

Discussion

The findings of this study strongly support the subjective/phenomenolog-
ical model of DID. The 23 subjective/phenomenological dissociative symptoms that are measured by the MID had a median incidence of 90% in this
study's 220 DID cases. The average patient who had DID had 20.2 of the 23
symptoms. Thus, as predicted, patients who have DID recurrently undergo
an array of consciously experienced dissociative intrusions into their executive functioning and sense of self. These intrusive phenomena are well-documented in the empirical literature, but are oddly absent from DSM-IV's
account of DID.

Table 3

Mean scores of 23 dissociative symptoms in 220 persons who have dissociative identity disorder

MID symptom-scale	Mean score							
	SCID-D n = 41		Total sample n = 220		Outpatients n = 161		Inpatients n = 57	
	Mean	SD	Mean	SD	Mean	SD	Mean	SD
Mean MID score	50.6	19.6	52.4	19.6	50.2	19.7	59.2**	18.2
Severe dissociation score	124.0	29.1	128.4	32.1	124.4	33.6	139.8**	24.9
General dissociative symptoms								
Memory problems	62.3	19.7	63.6	21.7	61.4	22.3	69.8*	19.4
Depersonalization	53.4	21.0	54.3	21.6	52.6	22.7	58.7	17.3
Derealization	45.2	22.8	46.3	23.0	44.2	23.5	52.3*	20.6
Posttraumatic flashbacks	53.3	26.8	52.8	27.0	49.4	26.3	63.0***	26.5
Somatoform symptoms	24.7	18.8	27.3	17.4	26.2	17.6	30.4	16.5
Trance	48.0	23.2	50.0	23.7	47.0	23.8	59.0***	20.9
Partially-dissociated intrusions								
Child voices	52.2	30.6	59.8	30.2	57.3	30.1	67.4*	29.8
Internal struggle	60.7	26.0	62.6	25.6	60.5	25.8	69.0*	24.5
Persecutory voices	54.8	32.3	58.0	30.6	53.5	31.5	71.5***	23.7
Speech insertion	55.4	26.7	52.9	28.4	51.5	28.8	56.7	27.6
"Made"/intrusive thoughts	63.9	25.7	65.8	23.6	63.8	24.4	71.7*	19.7
"Made"/intrusive emotions	68.1	23.2	66.0	22.9	64.8	23.7	69.8	19.5
"Made"/intrusive impulses	55.0	28.8	61.4	26.9	58.8	27.1	69.2*	25.3
"Made"/intrusive actions	60.8	22.9	59.9	23.0	58.0	23.7	65.3*	20.5
Temp loss of knowledge	40.2	22.8	39.3	25.9	36.8	25.5	47.1*	25.5
Self-alteration	48.5	23.2	51.5	22.6	49.7	22.6	56.9*	22.2
Self-puzzlement	70.8	22.1	67.0	23.7	65.8	24.4	70.7	21.1
Fully-dissociated actions								
Time loss	57.1	28.8	59.5	27.9	56.6	27.9	67.3*	27.1
"Coming to"	38.1	28.5	41.2	29.6	37.0	28.3	53.0***	30.8
Fugues	34.1	25.9	37.0	29.1	33.3	27.9	47.5***	30.3
Being told of actions	43.7	23.7	45.0	26.1	41.6	25.3	53.9***	26.8
Finding objects	34.5	30.8	41.0	30.1	38.0	29.3	48.9*	31.5
Evidence of actions	30.1	25.0	36.9	27.9	33.3	26.3	47.1***	30.3

Comparisons test only the difference between inpatients and outpatients. Bonferroni corrected significance level for 31 comparisons is $P < .016$.

Abbreviations: MID, multidimensional inventory of dissociation; SCID-D, Structured Clinical Interview for DSM-IV Dissociative Disorders-Revised; Temp loss of knowledge, temporary loss of well-rehearsed knowledge or skills; Self-alteration, experiences of self-alteration; Being told of actions, being told of disremembered actions; Finding objects, finding objects among one's possessions; Evidence of actions, finding evidence of one's recent actions.

* $P < .05$; ** $P < .01$; *** $P < .016$.

Implications of the present study for DSM-IV's classic model of dissociative identity disorder

If the 23 subjective/phenomenological dissociative symptoms routinely occur in DID patients (see Table 2), then DSM-IV's model of classic DID must be deficient because it narrowly portrays DID as just an alter disorder. At best, the DSM-IV model of DID can account for only 8 of the 23

Table 4

Diagnostic accuracy of the 23 dissociative symptoms among 220 persons who had dissociative
identity disorder

Proposed diagnostic criteria	Percent who met the criterion			
	SCID-D n = 41	Total Sample N = 220	Outpatients n = 161	Inpatients n = 57
Criterion A: general dissociative symptoms (4 of 6)	95	93	92	96
Criterion B: partially-dissociated intrusions (6 of 11)	98	93	92	98
Criterion C: fully-dissociated intrusions (2 of 6)	93	90	90	91
Alternate Criterion C: C + temporary loss of well-rehearsed knowledge or skills (2 of 7)	95	94	93	96
DID = A + B + C	85	84	82	88
DID = A + B + Alternate C	88	87	85	93

Abbreviations: MID, multidimensional inventory of dissociation; SCID-D, Structured Clinical Interview for DSM-IV Dissociative Disorders-Revised.

dissociative symptoms listed in Box 1: temporary loss of well-rehearsed knowledge or skills; disconcerting experiences of self-alteration; time loss; "coming to"; fugues; being told of disremembered actions; finding objects among one's possessions; and finding evidence of one's recent actions. Thus, DSM-IV provides a very incomplete picture of the dissociative phenomena of DID.

Also, most dissociative symptoms of DID are subjective and invisible (rather than objective and visible). Of the 25 dissociative symptoms in Box 1, 23 are subjective. Because the patients who had DID in this study experienced a mean of 20.2 of those 23 subjective symptoms, subjective dissociative symptoms are clearly pervasive in DID. In contrast, the DSM-IV focuses on a single, objective, diagnostic sign of DID: switching from one personality to another. This diagnostic sign occurs infrequently [4,75] and is usually difficult to discern [4,75]. Because it bases the diagnosis of DID solely on this infrequent objective sign, the DSM-IV has made DID unnecessarily difficult to detect, provided clinicians with a one-sided picture of the disorder, and thereby contributed to the skepticism that has beset this disorder.

Implications of the present study for the sociocognitive model of dissociative identity disorder

For the last decade, proponents of the sociocognitive model [76–82] have argued that DID is caused by social influence:

DID is a socially constructed condition that results from inadvertent therapist cueing (eg, suggestive questioning regarding the existence of possible alters), media influences (eg, film and television portrayals of DID), and broader sociocultural expectations regarding the presumed clinical features of DID. For example, proponents of the sociocognitive model believe that the release of the book and film *Sybil* in the 1970s played a substantial role in shaping conceptions of DID in the minds of the general public and psychotherapists [77].

The sociocognitive model of DID is necessarily wed to the DSM-IV's model of classic DID. Why? Because the general culture's model of DID is classic DID. Classic DID is clearly reflected in *Sybil*. Classic DID has also been reflected in countless portrayals of DID in contemporary films and television programs. In short, the DSM-IV's essential phenomena of classic DID (ie, multiple personalities + switching + amnesia) are very familiar to the general culture.

Although not intended as such, the present findings refute the sociocognitive model of DID because 15 of the 23 subjective dissociative symptoms that were measured (the criterion A symptoms except for trance and the criterion B symptoms except for self-alteration; see Box 1) are invisible (ie, completely experiential), unknown to the media, unknown to the general public, and largely unknown to the mental health field. Nevertheless, these 15 subjective dissociative symptoms occurred in 83% to 95% of persons who had DID (Table 2). The pervasive presence of these symptoms cannot be explained (away) by the sociocognitive model's "usual suspects"—therapist cueing, media influences, and sociocultural expectations regarding the clinical features of DID. There can be no therapist cueing, media influences, or sociocultural expectations about dissociative symptoms that are invisible, unknown to the media, unknown to the culture, and largely unknown to the mental health field.

The sociocognitive model explains and predicts the classic signs of DID, but the sociocognitive model neither predicts nor can explain (1) most of the empirical literature's well-replicated dissociative symptoms of DID (Table 1), (2) most of the subjective/phenomenological dissociative symptoms of DID (Box 1), or (3) most of the findings of the present study. In contrast, the subjective/phenomenological model of DID predicts and explains all of the symptoms of classic DID, all 13 of the well-replicated empirical findings about DID (Table 1), all 23 of the subjective/phenomenological dissociative symptoms in Box 1, and all 23 of the dissociative findings of the present study (Table 2).

On the grounds of greater verisimilitude—most importantly, its ability to predict a large number of dissociative phenomena that cannot be predicted by either the DSM-IV model of DID or the sociocognitive model of DID—the subjective/phenomenological model of DID should be considered superior, and the sociocognitive model of DID must be judged to be refuted.

Limitations

The strength of the present study is limited by two aspects of its methodology. First, the study is primarily based on a clinically-diagnosed sample of DID cases (rather than a sample of DID cases that were diagnosed with a structured interview such as the SCID-D-R). Fig. 1, however, demonstrates that there is a remarkable resemblance between the 220 patients who had DID who were clinically diagnosed and the 41 who were diagnosed by the SCID-D-R. Still, the SCID-D-R was administered in a clinical setting by therapists who were not blind to the patients' presenting symptoms, and was not subject to reliability checks across raters. Second, the present study did not employ SCID-D-R-diagnosed comparison groups (eg, general psychiatric patients, nonclinical adults, patients who had other dissociative disorders). Gast and colleagues [70], however, did use SCID-D-R-diagnosed comparison groups in their investigation of the diagnostic efficiency of the German MID. Their results replicated those of the present study. In a sample comprised of patients who had DID, patients who had DDNOS-1, general psychiatric patients, and nonclinical adults, Gast and colleagues reported that the dissociative symptoms in Box 1 (as assessed by the G-MID) had a positive predictive power of 0.93, a negative predictive power of 0.84, and an overall predictive power of 0.89 for major dissociative disorder (DID or DDNOS-1).

Why the subjective/phenomenological model of dissociative identity disorder is important

Is it important that DID patients report all of these dissociative symptoms? Does it really matter? Yes, these dissociative symptoms are important not only because of what they say about DID but also because of what they imply about the nature of pathological dissociation itself.

Despite over a century of research, no generally accepted definition of *dissociation* or *pathological dissociation* exists. The DSM-IV and ICD-10 do not agree about which phenomena represent pathological dissociation and which do not. Moreover, although they tend to be interpreted otherwise, neither the American Psychiatric Association (APA) nor the World Health Organization (WHO) has attempted to define dissociation. True to their nature as systems of classification, the DSM and ICD have characterized the dissociative disorders, not dissociation. Starting with the clinical entities that each deems to be dissociative, the APA and WHO have simply described the essential features that dissociative disorders hold in common. Thus, the DSM-IV-TR states that "the essential feature of the Dissociative Disorders is a disruption in the usually integrated functions of consciousness, memory, identity, or perception" [1]. Similarly, ICD-10 states that "the common theme shared by dissociative (or conversion) disorders is a partial or complete loss of the normal integration between memories of the past, awareness of identity and immediate sensations, and control of bodily movements" [52].

These common, essential features do not define dissociation, but researchers almost routinely treat them as if they do. In the United States, almost every article on dissociation quotes the DSM statement about the essential features of the dissociative disorders and then treats that statement as if it were a definition of dissociation; however, it is not. Moreover, not only is it not a definition of dissociation, it is a partisan claim, because the APA and the WHO have competing systems of classification and disagree on the matter. For these reasons, I contend that the DSM-IV-TR description of the essential features of the dissociative disorders is a long way from being an acceptable definition of dissociation.

This issue (how to define dissociation) is where the larger importance of the subjective/phenomenological model of DID emerges. This model of DID arose from a process that was diametrically opposite to the process through which the DSM-IV and ICD-10 arrived at their statements about the essential features of the dissociative disorders. The new model of DID arose from two conjectures about the nature of pathological dissociation, whereas the "definitions": of dissociation in the DSM and ICD are merely semantic conveniences that rationalize their respective sets of diagnoses and criteria.

The subjective/phenomenological model of DID is a direct consequence of two conjectures: that the phenomena of pathological dissociation are recurrent, jarring intrusions into executive functioning and sense of self, and that pathological dissociative phenomena affect every aspect of human experience. The MID was developed to test these conjectures. Through 23 dissociative symptoms, the MID attempts to tap every aspect of human experience, and the dissociative events that can befall each aspect of human experience [65]. The MID research program has sought to corroborate (or refute) these conjectures about the nature and domain of pathological dissociation.

The conjecture that every aspect of human experience is subject to dissociative intrusion has a corollary: that very different phenomena from very different domains of human functioning and human experience "go together" (eg, amnesia, depersonalization, derealization, trances, conversion symptoms, flashbacks, hearing the voice of a child, hearing persecutory voices, self-confusion, experiences of self-alteration, "made" speech, "made" thoughts, "made" impulses, "made" actions). This corollary is an improbable prediction. Virtually no one outside the dissociative disorders field would predict that these strikingly different clinical phenomena belong together. This conjecture can be tested statistically by calculating the internal consistency and factor structure of the MID's 23 dissociative symptoms. These particular statistical analyses subject the conjecture to what Popper [83–85] would call "grave danger of refutation." That is, unless the MID's 23 symptoms "go together" (ie, unless they have a very high α coefficient), the conjecture and its corollary will be refuted. Similarly, unless confirmatory factor analysis shows that the MID's 23 dissociative symptoms have a robust unifactorial solution, the conjecture and its corollary will be refuted.

Not only did the corollary survive these tests, but it did so repeatedly. In 15 different clinical and nonclinical samples, in five countries and five languages, the α coefficient of the MID's 23 dissociative symptoms has been 0.96 or higher (P.F. Dell, unpublished data, 2004). In two large samples from multiple countries, two independent confirmatory factor analyses have shown that the unifactorial model of the MID's 12-factor scales has a comparative fit index (CFI) of 0.96 [66]. Thus, the unifactorial model of pathological dissociation explained 96% of the variance in subjects' scores on the 12-factor scales. These findings provide powerful corroboration for the subjective/phenomenological model of pathological dissociation. The phenomena that are specified by the subjective/phenomenological model of dissociation do "go together."

The subjective/phenomenological model of dissociative identity disorder

This model of DID was deduced from two conjectures. If both are true (if pathological dissociative intrusions can affect every aspect of human experience, and if those pathological dissociative intrusions group together), then it seems likely that persons who have been diagnosed with the prototypical form of dissociative psychopathology (ie, DID) would be characterized by dissociative intrusions in every domain of their experience. This deduction can be tested statistically by determining whether persons who have DID manifest all 23 dissociative symptoms that are measured by the MID. The present study showed that 220 persons who had DID had a mean of 20.2 of the 23 dissociative symptoms. Two other studies have also demonstrated that patients who have DID are characterized by these 23 dissociative symptoms [14,70].

Summary

Data from 220 persons who had DID were used to compare three models of DID: the DSM-IV's classic model of DID (ie, multiple personalities + switching + amnesia), the subjective/phenomenological model of DID (Box 1), and the sociocognitive model of DID. The DSM-IV narrowly portrays DID as an alter disorder; the subjective/phenomenological model portrays DID as a far more complex dissociative disorder. The data indicate that the subjective/phenomenological model of DID is a superior predictor of the dissociative phenomena of DID. The three studies [14,70] that corroborate the subjective/phenomenological model of DID are important. They show that the subjective/phenomenological model of DID is more comprehensive and more accurate than the DSM-IV's classic model of DID. They also refute the sociocognitive model of DID. The subjective/phenomenological model of DID was deduced from a novel, empirically supported model of pathological dissociation [4]; that model fully explains the empirical literature on DID, whereas the DSM-IV model of DID can account for little of that literature.

Acknowledgements

This paper is the culmination of a project that has consumed me for 5 years. I gratefully acknowledge the patience and support of my wife, Sue Crommelin, who had to live with me and my obsession. I am also grateful to clinicians far and wide who helped me to collect these data, especially Marcia Cotton, Don Fridley, Jack Howley, Richard Hicks, Martin Dorahy, and my colleagues at Psychotherapy Resources of Norfolk, Elizabeth Gay, Alexandra Kedrock, Sandy Lane, and Laura Thom. This paper benefited considerably from the critical input of John O'Neil, Donald Beere, Stephen Braude, Elizabeth Howell, and Ruth Blizard.

References

[1] American Psychiatric Association. Diagnostic and statistical manual of mental disorder. 4th edition, text revision. Washington (DC): American Psychiatric Association; 2000.

[2] Dell PF. Why the diagnostic criteria for dissociative identity disorder should be changed. J Trauma Dissociation 2001;2(1):7–37.

[3] Dell PF. Dissociative phenomenology of dissociative identity disorder. J Nerv Ment Dis 2002;190(1):10–5.

[4] Dell PF. The subjective/phenomenological view of pathological dissociation. In: Dell PF, O'Neil JA, editors. Dissociation and the dissociative disorders: DSM-V and beyond, in press.

[5] Berger D, Ono Y, Nakajima K, et al. Dissociative symptoms in Japan. Am J Psychiatry 1994; 151:148–9.

[6] Bliss EL. Multiple personalities: a report of 14 cases with implications for schizophrenia and hysteria. Arch Gen Psychiatry 1980;37:1388–97.

[7] Bliss EL. Multiple personalities, allied disorders and hypnosis. New York: Oxford University Press; 1986.

[8] Boon S, Draijer N. Diagnosing dissociative disorders in The Netherlands: a pilot study with the Structured Clinical Interview for DSM-III-R Dissociative Disorders. Am J Psychiatry 1991;148:458–62.

[9] Boon S, Draijer N. Multiple personality disorder in The Netherlands: a clinical investigation of 71 patients. Am J Psychiatry 1993;150:489–94.

[10] Boon S, Draijer N. Multiple personality disorder in the Netherlands: a study on reliability and validity of the diagnosis. Amsterdam: Swets & Zeitlinger; 1993.

[11] Coons PM. Clinical phenomenology of 25 children and adolescents with dissociative disorders. Child Adolesc Psychiatr Clin N Am 1996;5(2):361–73.

[12] Coons PM, Bowman ES, Kluft RP, et al. The cross-cultural occurrence of MPD: additional cases from a recent survey. Dissociation 1991;4(3):124–8.

[13] Coons PM, Bowman ES, Milstein V. Multiple personality disorder: a clinical investigation of 50 cases. J Nerv Ment Dis 1988;176:519–27.

[14] Dell PF. Should the dissociative disorders field choose its own diagnostic criteria for dissociative identity disorder? Reply to Cardeña, Coons, Putnam, Spiegel, and Steinberg. J Trauma Dissociation 2001;2(1):65–72.

[15] Dell PF, Eisenhower JW. Adolescent multiple personality disorder: a preliminary study of eleven cases. J Am Acad Child Adolesc Psychiatry 1990;29(3):359–66.

[16] Fagan J, McMahon PP. Incipient multiple personality in children: four cases. J Nerv Ment Dis 1984;172(1):26–36.

[17] Goodwin J. Childhood DID: the male population. In: Silberg JL, editor. The dissociative child: diagnosis, treatment, and management. Lutherville (MD): Sidran Press; 1996. p. 69–84.

[18] Hornstein NL, Putnam FW. Clinical phenomenology of child and adolescent dissociative disorders. J Am Acad Child Adolesc Psychiatry 1992;31(6):1077–85.

[19] Kluft RP. Childhood multiple personality disorder: predictors, clinical findings, and treatment. In: Kluft RP, editor. Childhood antecedents of multiple personality. Washington (DC): American Psychiatric Press; 1985. p. 168–96.

[20] Lewis DO, Yeager CA, Swica Y, et al. Objective documentation of child abuse and dissociation in 12 murderers with dissociative identity disorder. Am J Psychiatry 1997;154(12): 1703–10.

[21] Loewenstein RJ, Putnam FW. The clinical phenomenology of males with multiple personality disorder: a report of 21 cases. Dissociation 1990;3(3):135–43.

[22] Martinez-Taboas A. Multiple personality in Puerto Rico: analysis of fifteen cases. Dissociation 1991;4(4):189–92.

[23] McCallum KE, Lock J, Kulla M, et al. Dissociative symptoms and disorders in patients with eating disorders. Dissociation 1992;5(4):227–35.

[24] Middleton W, Butler J. Dissociative identity disorder: an Australian series. Aust N Z J Psychiatry 1998;32:794–804.

[25] Putnam FW, Helmers K, Trickett PK. Development, reliability, and validity of a child dissociation scale. Child Abuse Negl 1993;17:731–41.

[26] Ross CA, Miller SD, Reagor P, et al. Schneiderian symptoms in multiple personality disorder and schizophrenia. Compr Psychiatry 1990;31(2):111–8.

[27] Ross CA, Miller SD, Reagor P, et al. Structured interview data on 102 cases of multiple personality disorder from four centers. Am J Psychiatry 1990;147:596–601.

[28] Ross CA, Joshi S. Schneiderian symptoms and childhood trauma in the general population. Compr Psychiatry 1992;33:269–73.

[29] Ross CA, Anderson G, Heber S, et al. Dissociation and abuse among multiple personality patients, prostitutes, and exotic dancers. Hosp Community Psychiatry 1990;41(3):328–30.

[30] Ross CA, Heber S, Norton GR, et al. Differences between multiple personality disorder and other diagnostic groups on structured interview. J Nerv Ment Dis 1989;179(8):487–91.

[31] Ross CA, Norton GR, Wozney K. Multiple personality disorder: an analysis of 236 cases. Can J Psychiatry 1989;34:413–7.

[32] Sar V, Yargic LI, Tutkun H. Structured interview data on 35 cases of dissociative identity disorder. Am J Psychiatry 1996;153:1329–33.

[33] Steinberg M, Rounsaville B, Cicchetti D. The structured clinical interview for DSM-III-R dissociative disorders: preliminary report on a new diagnostic instrument. Am J Psychiatry 1990;147:76–81.

[34] Steinberg M, Steinberg A. Systematic assessment of dissociative identity disorder in adolescents using the SCID-D: three case studies. Bull Menninger Clin 1995;59:221–31.

[35] Zoroglu S, Yargic LI, Tutkun H, et al. Dissociative identity disorder in childhood: five Turkish cases. Dissociation 1996;9(4):253–60.

[36] Putnam FW, Guroff JJ, Silberman EK, et al. The clinical phenomenology of multiple personality disorder: review of 100 recent cases. J Clin Psychiatry 1986;47:285–93.

[37] American Psychiatric Association. Diagnostic and statistical manual of mental disorders. 4th edition. Washington (DC): American Psychiatric Association; 1994.

[38] Fink D, Golinkoff M. MPD, borderline personality disorder and schizophrenia: a comparative study of clinical features. Dissociation 1990;3:127–34.

[39] Nijenhuis ER, Spinhoven P, Van Dyck R, et al. The development and the psychometric characteristics of the Somatoform Dissociation Questionnaire (SDQ-20). J Nerv Ment Dis 1996; 184:688–94.

[40] Nijenhuis ERS, Spinhoven P, Van Dyck R, et al. The development of the Somatoform Dissociation Questionnaire (SDQ-5) as a screening instrument for the dissociative disorders. Acta Psychiat Scand 1997;96:311–8.
[41] Nijenhuis ERS, Spinhoven P, Van Dyck R, et al. Psychometric characteristics of the Somatoform Dissociation Questionnaire: a replication study. Psychother Psychosom 1998;67: 17–23.
[42] Ross CA, Heber S, Norton GR, et al. Somatic symptoms in multiple personality disorder. Psychosomatics 1989;30(2):154–60.
[43] Ross CA, Anderson G, Fraser GA, et al. Differentiating multiple personality disorder and dissociative disorder not otherwise specified. Dissociation 1992;5:88–91.
[44] Sar V, Kundakci T, Kiziltan E, et al. Differentiating dissociative disorders from other diagnostic groups through somatoform dissociation in Turkey. J Trauma Dissociation 2000;1(4): 67–80.
[45] Saxe GN, Chinman G, Berkowitz MD, et al. Somatization in patients with dissociative disorders. Am J Psychiatry 1994;151:1329–34.
[46] Janet P. L'Automatisme Psychologique: Essai de Psychologie Expérimentale sur les Formes Inférieures de l'Activité Humaine. Paris (France): Félix Alcan; 1889.
[47] Kihlstrom JF. One hundred years of hysteria. In: Lynn SJ, Rhue JW, editors. Dissociation: clinical and theoretical perspectives. New York: Guilford Press; 1994. p. 80–93.
[48] Laria AJ, Lewis-Fernández R. The professional fragmentation of experience in the study of dissociation, somatization, and culture. J Trauma Dissociation 2001;2(3):17–48.
[49] Nemiah JC. Dissociation, conversion, and somatization. Annu Rev Psychiatry 1991;10: 248–60.
[50] Nijenhuis ERS. Somatoform dissociation: phenomena, measurement, and theoretical issues. Assen (The Netherlands): Van Gorcum; 1999.
[51] Nijenhuis ERS. Somatoform dissociation: major symptoms of dissociative disorders. J Trauma Dissociation 2000;1(4):7–29.
[52] World Health Organization. The ICD-10 classification of mental and behavioural disorders: clinical descriptions and diagnostic guidelines. Geneva: World Health Organization; 1992.
[53] Kluft RP. First-rank symptoms as a diagnostic clue to multiple personality disorder. Am J Psychiatr 1987;144(3):293–8.
[54] Bernstein EM, Putnam FW. Development, reliability, and validity of a dissociation scale. J Nerv Ment Dis 1986;174:727–35.
[55] Waller NG, Putnam FW, Carlson EB. Types of dissociation and dissociative types: a taxometric analysis of dissociative experiences. Psychol Methods 1996;1:300–21.
[56] Kluft RP. The phenomenology and treatment of extremely complex multiple personality disorder. Dissociation 1988;1:47–58.
[57] Rivera M. Multiple personality disorder and the social systems: 185 cases. Dissociation 1991; 4(2):79–82.
[58] Van der Hart O, Witztum E, Friedman B. From hysterical psychosis to reactive dissociative psychosis. J Trauma Stress 1993;6:43–64.
[59] Schneider K. Clinical psychopathology. New York: Grune & Stratton; 1959.
[60] Kluft RP. Making the diagnosis of multiple personality disorder (MPD). Directions in Psychiatry 1985;5(23):3–10.
[61] Yargic LI, Sar V, Tutkun H, et al. Comparison of dissociative identity disorder with other diagnostic groups using a structured interview in Turkey. Compr Psychiatry 1998;39(6): 345–51.
[62] Kluft RP. Schneider's first-rank symptoms. Dr. Kluft replies. Am J Psychiatry 1987;144(10): 1378.
[63] Koehler K. First rank symptoms of schizophrenia: questions concerning clinical boundaries. Br J Psychiatry 1979;134:236–48.

[64] Ross CA. Dissociative identity disorder: diagnosis, clinical features, and treatment of multiple personality disorder. 2nd edition. New York: John Wiley & Sons; 1997.

[65] Dell PF. Multidimensional Inventory of Dissociation (MID): a comprehensive self-report instrument for pathological dissociation. J Trauma Dissociation, in press.

[66] Dell PF, Lawson D. Investigating the domain of pathological dissociation with the Multidimensional Inventory of Dissociation (MID). Submitted for publication; 2006.

[67] Jaspers K. General psychopathology, vol. I. 7th edition. In: Hoenig J, Hamilton MW, editors. translators. Baltimore (MD): Johns Hopkins University Press; 1997.

[68] Bremner JD, Krystal JH, Putnam FW, et al. Measurement of dissociative states with the Clinician-Administered Dissociative States Scale (CADSS). J Trauma Stress 1998;11: 125–36.

[69] Somer E, Dell PF. The development and psychometric characteristics of the Hebrew version of the Multidimensional Inventory of Dissociation (H-MID): a valid and reliable measure of dissociation. J Trauma Dissociation 2005;6(1):31–53.

[70] Gast U, Rodewald F, Dehner-Rau C, et al. Validation of the German version of the Multidimensional Inventory of Dissociation (MID-d). Presented at the 20th fall conference of the International Society for the Study of Dissociation. Chicago, November 2–4, 2003.

[71] Vanderlinden J, van Dyck R, Vandereycken W, et al. The Dissociation Questionnaire (DIS-Q): Development and characteristics of a new self-report questionnaire. Clin Psychol Psychother 1993;1:21–7.

[72] Riley KC. Measurement of dissociation. J Nerv Ment Dis 1988;176:449–50.

[73] Steinberg M. Structured Clinical Interview for DSM-IV Dissociative Disorders (SCID-D), Revised. Washington (DC): American Psychiatric Press; 1994.

[74] Steinberg M. Handbook for the assessment of dissociation. Washington (DC): American Psychiatric Press; 1995.

[75] Kluft RP. The natural history of multiple personality disorder. In: Kluft RP, editor. Childhood antecedents of multiple personality. Washington (DC): American Psychiatric Press; 1985. p. 197–238.

[76] Lilienfeld SO, Kirsch I, Sarbin TR, et al. Dissociative identity disorder and the sociocognitive model: recalling the lessons of the past. Psychol Bull 1999;125(5):507–23.

[77] Lilienfeld SO, Lynn SJ. Dissociative identity disorder: multiple personalities, multiple controversies. In: Lilienfeld SO, Lynn SJ, Lohr JM, editors. Science and pseudoscience in clinical psychology. New York: Guilford Press; 2003. p. 109–42.

[78] McHugh PR. Resolved: multiple personality disorder is an individually and socially created artifact. Affirmative. J Am Acad Child Adolesc Psychiatry 1995;34:957–9.

[79] Merskey H. The manufacture of personalities: the production of multiple personality disorder. Br J Psychiatry 1992;160:327–40.

[80] Sarbin TR. On the belief that one body may be host to two or more personalities. Int J Clin Exp Hypn 1995;43:163–83.

[81] Spanos NP. Multiple identity enactments and multiple personality disorder: a sociocognitive perspective. Psychol Bull 1994;116:145–65.

[82] Spanos NP. Multiple identities & false memories: a sociocognitive perspective. Washington (DC): American Psychological Association; 1996.

[83] Popper KR. The logic of scientific discovery. London: Routledge Classics; 2002.

[84] Popper KR. Conjectures and refutations: the growth of scientific knowledge. New York: Harper; 1965.

[85] Popper KR. Objective knowledge: an evolutionary approach. Revised edition. Oxford (United Kingdom): Oxford University Press; 1979.

**PSYCHIATRIC
CLINICS**
OF NORTH AMERICA

ELSEVIER
SAUNDERS

Psychiatr Clin N Am 29 (2006) 27–43

How Metaphors Shape the Concept and Treatment of Dissociation

Karen G. Way, PhD[a,b]

[a]Private Practice, 320 Raritan Avenue, Highland Park, NJ 08904, USA
[b]Raritan Bay Mental Health Center, Perth Amboy, NJ, USA

There has been a growing understanding over the last few decades that metaphors act as organizers of experience. Starting with Pepper's [1] article, "The Root Metaphor Theory of Metaphysics," and coming of age in Lakoff and Johnson's [2] *Metaphors We Live By*, the study of metaphors has expanded exponentially. Once dismissed as disposable verbal decorations, metaphors explain one thing in terms of another without making an explicit comparison. Sometimes the metaphors are presented directly, as in "My love is a rose." More often they appear indirectly, partly submerged beneath the flow of speech, as in "She blooms when I touch her." In this indirect form, a metaphoric proposition can become part of a deep layer of cultural assumptions, serving as "multidimensional structures [that] characterize experiential gestalts, which are ways of organizing experiences into structured wholes" [2]. Such metaphors may be called "root," or "generative," or "concept" metaphors, and they frame cultural perception.

Metaphors operate not just as comparisons, but as connections between that which is understood well (body, earth, sensory information, common experience) and that which is hard to understand (abstractions, nonsensory phenomena, uncommon experience). The connection works both ways. "The unfamiliar is illuminated by the familiar. But usually there is more to it. Apart from an illustrative and heuristic function, a metaphor has a constitutive one: it changes the context in which it occurs and is itself changed by it" [3]. Such a claim can be put more even more broadly: "discourses changed by metaphor reorganize reality" [3].

Metaphor analysis has addressed the verbal reorganization of reality in many areas of the social sciences, as described in Leary's classic article [4] on the history of metaphor in psychology. Leary cites examples of how metaphors for self and mind "have directed the gaze—not to mention the

---

E-mail address: kway@optonline.net

doi:10.1016/j.psc.2005.10.006   *psych.theclinics.com*

theoretical and practical activities—of researchers to different parts of the nervous system." In this sense, metaphors can be said to set the problem of the phenomena they illustrate. Schön [5] describes how problem-setting metaphors operate in social policy. As an example, he notes that social services are often said to be "fragmented." Fragmentation implies an original whole, an esteemed quality in most cultures, which leads policy makers to add more layers of bureaucracy to help coordinate the fragments back into a whole. In actuality, social services are never originally whole but tend to grow individually, and the addition of extra layers to create a metaphor-mandated unity only makes coordination more difficult. Similarly, slums can be defined by metaphor as "festering," as sources of physical, economic, and social disease (in which case they must be eradicated), or they can be seen as natural, not-yet-successful communities (in which case they must be nourished and preserved). Schön [5] demonstrates that analyzing these problem-setting, "generative" metaphors can help align effort and result. "We can spell out the metaphor, elaborate the assumptions that flow from it, and examine their appropriateness in the present situation" [5].

The same kind of analysis can be applied to metaphors that set problems in psychotherapy. By "identifying metaphors and unpacking their assumptions and entailments" [6], it is possible to understand better which problem-setting metaphors compel which solutions. Attention to metaphors in the psychotherapeutic setting is not new; many have noticed how a metaphor can be read as a clue to unsaid meaning, as "an outcropping of unconscious fantasy," or as a buffer of indirection, offering the patient "the necessary, the safe distance from content" [7]. Used consciously by the therapist, metaphors have a stealth capacity, making possible "an indirect form of treatment. Like other forms of indirection, therapeutic metaphors do not engender the kind of resistance to considering new ideas that direct suggestions often can" [8].

Because of their indirection, stealth, and evocativeness, metaphors are particularly powerful in setting the clinical problem of trauma. As poets know, metaphors can gesture at topics too large or strange for speech, pointing at realities outside the culturally constructed frame of the normal. For victims of trauma, particularly the interpersonal trauma most likely to cause severe dissociative symptoms [9], metaphors can say the unsayable, can reach across gaps in memory, or permit expression where speech has been directly or indirectly forbidden. Both clinicians and patients reach for metaphor to explain and contain the aftereffects of unconstruable experience. In trying to conceptualize posttraumatic dissociation, mental health professionals have created several metaphoric domains.

This article examines some of dissociation's most common metaphors to see how they set the clinical problem of dissociation, particularly the problem of dissociative identity disorder (DID) caused by interpersonal trauma. Because metaphors are inexact, nonlinear, and culturally resonant, they do not fit well into simple lists. Nevertheless, it is possible to assemble two meta-categories of metaphors of dissociation.

In the first category, the self is a thing that is changed and damaged by its encounter with trauma. This can happen through division (the self shatters, divides, grows separate, is compartmentalized); through multiplication (the self wishes for reinforcements and gets them); and through subtraction (the self is perforated by trauma, leaving gaps, black holes, silence). Agency in this category belongs to the situation that acts on the self—whether it be the sheer force of trauma, the triggering of protective mechanisms of the mind, or external others who intend to provoke dissociative processes in their victim.

In the second category, the self is its own agent, and dissociation is an automatic but potentially governable action. Dissociation in this category is often pictured as a redistribution of attention, by narrowing focus or turning the mind's gaze away from real relationships in the present, toward interior replication or fog.

Both categories speak to the experience of interpersonal malevolence. In both, a metaphor for self underlies the metaphor for dissociation of self. The most important difference in the examples that follow is between noun-based metaphors that feature the self as a passive item on which trauma has acted, versus verb-based metaphors that feature the self as the active subject of a sentence describing the present.

Self as a thing, dissociation as division or multiplication

The metaphor of the self as a thing, as an item naturally possessed by every adult, is so common that it may seem literal. Nevertheless, self is often more accurately understood as a reified idea. Atwood and coworkers [10] group all such reification metaphors together, tracing their dominance back to Descartes:

> When one is regarded as possessing a mind, and this mind in turn is conceived as having an interior that is occupied by conscious (and perhaps unconscious) psychic contents, a structure is being imposed that sharply delineates the boundaries of one's personhood in respect to an objectively real outer world. Such a picture dichotomizes the subjective field into an inside and an outside, reifies and rigidifies the distinction between them, and envisions the resulting structure as constitutive of human existence in general.

Gottlieb [11] identifies the bounded, structured self as a prerequisite for the concept of multiple personality disorder:

> It should be remarked that most currently accepted explanations of [multiple personality disorder's] psychopathogenesis rely on a concretistic conception of the mind whereby quantitative strain is viewed as causing its falling apart into constituent elements, a rending of the mental fabric, a division into parts. This conception of mental functioning is very like the one articulated by Janet (1889) as le désagrégation psychologique.

Whether shattered, falling apart, or failing to come together, the division of the reified self is by far the most common root metaphor for dissociation [12].

Dissociation as division

The most passive version of the brittle self imagines the mind as a container shattered by the impact of trauma. Such metaphors depersonalize both perpetrator and victim, turning the first into an abstract force and the second into an inert target. Generally, the more trauma, the more the self falls apart: "Traumas produce their disintegrating effects in proportion to their intensity, duration, and repetition" [13].

The struck self may fragment into indistinct shards, or may separate at its seams into identifiable components of mind or experience. For example, Barach [14] describes dissociation as "a disjunction of the association between related mental contents." Braun [15] proposes the well-known acronym BASK, standing for the components of traumatic experience most likely to be separated from one another by dissociation: Behavior, Affect, Sensation, and Knowledge. Spiegel and Cardena [16] offer a slightly different array: "Dissociation can be thought of as a structured separation of mental processes (eg, thoughts, emotions, conation, memory, and identity) that are ordinarily integrated." When an identifiable piece of the self is separated, it can undergo a process of personification or at least vivification in "the creation of a new entity by the splitting off or coalescing of energy which forms the nucleus of a separate personality or fragment" [15]. As pieces break off from an imagined center, the logic of the metaphor leads to the idea that the center, or host, becomes depleted [17]. In other versions, split-off parts are imagined as puzzle pieces [18,19] scattered by trauma; without all pieces, the self cannot be whole.

In the developmental version of this metaphor, the normal self does not begin whole but becomes so during childhood. Trauma interrupts the process of consolidation, preventing components from coming together naturally. "DID may originate not with a 'coming apart' process, but with the maintenance of earlier arousal states that have not been integrated normally" [19]. "We are not born into this world with a single, unified personality," says Putnam [20]. Instead we begin as "discrete behavioral states," experiential bundles defined by "affect, arousal and energy level, motor activity, posture and mannerisms, speech (eg, rate, volume, pitch, word choice), cognitive processing (eg, varying degrees of abstract thinking), access to knowledge and autobiographical memory, and sense of self." If some of these states are rendered incompatible by unbearable trauma, they cannot come together during development to form a unitary self.

Computer metaphors add their own vocabulary to the description of how the elements of the self come together. For example, Bucci [21] refers to "subsymbolic processing systems," and Liotti [22] to "interpersonal motivational systems," and "inborn algorithms for the processing of social information." These systems develop (depending on the theory) through the integration of "internal working models ... where expectations about the behaviour of a particular individual towards the self are aggregated" [23]. If some of the internal models are composed of chaotic or traumatic experience, integrating them may not be possible. To preserve daily functioning, incompatible models or subsystems may have to be kept separate, or dissociated.

Metaphors of a more active self imagine trauma as the indirect cause of internal division; the direct cause is self-protective mental mechanisms that segregate traumatic material to protect mental functioning. There are psychoanalytic versions of these mechanisms, specifying the "vertical splitting" of dissociation rather than the "horizontal splitting" of classic repression [24,25], and information processing versions "whereby information—incoming, stored, or out-going—is actively deflected from integration with its usual or expected associations" [18]. The goal of such mechanisms is the protection of the "apparently normal personality" that manages daily life, from the disruptive "emotional personality" that has been infected with trauma [26]. A somewhat less reified version describes the defensive separation of acceptable self-states that can be claimed as "me" from the toxic self-states that are called "not-me" [27].

The concept of the "self-state," an aggregate of attributes that exists only in certain contexts, is connected to metaphors for the natural plurality of the self. If the self is conceptualized as an organized whole made up of lesser wholes, then DID becomes a kind of disharmony in a family or a civil war between self-states [28,29]. In addition to "internal family," other versions of multiple wholes include "orchestra" and "athletic team" [17]. Although plurality is celebrated by such metaphors, cooperative wholeness is valued more.

Dissociation as addition or multiplication

The patient's own experience of multiplicity is less likely to be one of division than of addition; less the feeling of rending apart and more the experience of discovering an internal other. The mechanism of creating new selves is often described as a combination of spontaneous hypnosis and extreme need. Bliss [30] quotes a patient, speaking in third person of herself, "She creates personalities by blocking everything from her head, mentally relaxes, concentrates very hard, and wishes." Fine [31] describes a child's need for reinforcements, "to either have a 'buddy to take the hit,' a 'strong protector,' to mediate with the outside world or a 'friend' with whom to run away." Sometimes beginning as imaginary friends, sometimes modeled on fictional characters and superheroes, alter personalities accrete individual history (and individuality) every time they are "out" to do whatever job made them necessary [18].

In some versions of the creation metaphor, selves generated for a specific crisis are then left behind as time moves on, frozen in an achronic stasis. The metaphor for time is one of steady flowing; the self that will not grow older is left behind as other selves age. Sinason [25] describes the dramatic thawing of a left-behind self: "Instantly, to aid the woman, out of cold storage came the brave 6-year-old friend. Frozen in a terrible state of now-ness that had not changed for over 30 years, she emerged."

Some metaphors of self-multiplication include an internal psychic machine to do the job, such as Gottlieb's [11] "enabling fantasy," or Brenner's [32] "pathognomonic psychic structure at the core of DID, whose function is not only to disown intolerable memories, affects, and drives, but to personify these conflicts through the creation of so-called 'alter personalities.'" These metaphorical constructs, whose intentionality is part of their invention, have real-life counterparts in the external perpetrators and abusers who consciously create altered states, and even alters in their victims. Such an idea does not require the existence of secret international conspiracies. The physical preparation for possession trance, the desensitization training of military recruits, the intimate "grooming" of victims by sexual predators, and the well-publicized techniques of interrogators and torturers are all based on knowledge of how to "break" a mind and create a new, biddable self. When imagining the mechanisms of DID, it is important to keep in mind that the agent of intentional multiplication need not be metaphorical at all.

Treatment metaphors: many into one

If the self is a passive thing that is split by trauma, or a clever thing that segregates the material of trauma, or a generative thing that multiplies itself to create allies in a crisis, then how can it be made whole again in a clinical setting? Some of the simpler, less personified variations suggest their own solutions. The disassembled puzzle should be reassembled [19,20]. Information that was refused or partitioned must be discovered and accepted. As Sinason [25] says, "To heal, you have to finally 'take in' all the words you heard." Janet popularized the idea that traumatic memories become "unconscious 'fixed ideas' that must be 'liquidated'" by translating them "into a personal narrative" [33]. Another version of equalizing information across barriers is implicit in the BASK acronym: if the mind has separated behavior, affect, sensation, and knowledge about a given experience, then a therapist can work "to equalize the BASKs of cooperative personalities and promote spontaneous integration of increasingly like-minded personalities" [31].

The metaphor of the plural self simplifies the problem of many-into-one. Instead of aiming for one, the clinician aims for a better organization of many. For example, Fraser [34] urges clinicians to "engage all the personalities in the therapeutic process and form them into a new team." Kluft [35] quotes Caul's comment describing a business version of the goal: "It seems to me that after treatment you want to end up with a functional unit, be it a corporation, a partnership. Or a one-owner business." By making metaphors of internal community more concrete rather than less, therapists can exploit the potential of cooperation such metaphors carry. Fraser [34] encourages patients to imagine an internal conference room where each alter gets a chance to speak, learn about other alters, and make decisions. Krakauer [36] uses similar imagery to propose "visualized internal structures" to the lightly hypnotized patient, establishing, for example, "the hall of safety, the conference or meeting room, and the theater." Shirar [19] helps dissociative children imagine an entire neighborhood with separate houses, connecting walkways, individual rooms, "telephones in every house, and an intercom system inside the house with a speaker in every room."

Clinicians who believe that plurality is not only undesirable but is the essence of the problem of DID are likely to emphasize the root metaphor of part and whole. "The global message from the therapist should always be that all of the alters constitute a whole person" [18]. Ross [37] delivers similar advice: "The most important thing to understand is that alter personalities are not people.... They are fragmented parts of one person: There is only one person." This message is delivered in the clinician's terminology: "I try to avoid using the word 'personality'.... I initially stick to descriptions such as 'part,' 'side,' 'aspect,' or 'facet' because this is one of the major themes of the treatment approach—namely, that the personalities are a 'part' of a whole person" [18]. Children understand quickly: "Using puppets or doll figures, I explain parts as something we all have.... 'I have a Happy part, and a part of me that feels Scared sometimes, and a Mad part. I feel sad sometimes, so of course I have a Sad part" [19]. Even the word "part," used without any explicit reference to the whole, carries the clear implication that there is, was, or will be a whole, and that each part belongs to it. Such parts cannot be erased, exiled, or miniaturized without confusing implications about the resulting wholeness of the whole. Worse, once a relational matrix develops between alters within a patient, any action taken against an alter can (and is likely to) be seen as a reenactment of the original abuse. Breaking a habit is hard enough; when the habit has become a person, the metaphor of breaking suggests an attack.

Ideally, as segregated information and affects are shared across dissociated parts of the mind, the need for division decreases and "part-people" lose the distinctness that makes their existence possible. The part-whole metaphor is then dropped, and a new whole is greeted. In less ideal cases, the therapist may resort to rituals of magic or spiritual transformation, searching for an image that allows the patient to picture the merging of people. A more efficient solution may be to depersonify (or rereify) the parts of the unitary self. Through ceremony or suggestion, internal personalities are reimagined as some form of matter that is physically capable of blending, merging, or flowing. Kluft [35] offers an example of helping a patient visualize alters turning into separate streams of light and then joining into one stream. Metaphors of fluidity (water, paint, flowing colors) show up frequently in prescriptions for integration [18]. However much the container metaphor of the Cartesian mind is offered as a refuge from chaos, fluidity remains the metaphor of health.

The self as a thing, dissociation as gap, hole, no-thing

The metaphors of division and multiplication serve to convey the clinician's overwhelming impression of "too many" (too many attitudes, schemas, incompatible emotions, interests, names, presentations, and so on) for one patient. The observer's natural impulse is to name these manifestations, to count and categorize what there is too much of. It is a much harder task to see what there is none of, to name what is missing, to become aware of the spaces around and between the contending selves. There are persistent metaphors for dissociation that are images of loss, gaps, holes, and silence. For example: "The character structures of many survivors show a surprising mosaic of areas of high level psychologic functioning coexisting with the potential for severe regression. It is as though we see 'black holes' in an otherwise throbbing, pulsating, and alive galaxy" [38]. Van der Kolk and coworkers [39] also write about "the black hole of trauma," and quote Krystal [40] on the reactions of some Holocaust survivors: "no trace of registration of any kind is left in the psyche; instead, a void, a hole, is found."

Within the black hole of dissociated trauma, language fails. Laub [41] quotes the child of Holocaust survivors, who refers to the "then" of her parents' unspoken past: "Before that 'then' was the gaping vertiginous black hole of the unmentionable years." Throughout Western trauma literature since 1980, the Holocaust acts as a singularity, as the historical trauma that other traumas might somewhat resemble [42], but that in its totality resembles none. Lanzmann [43] describes the unknowability of the Holocaust story as an unbridgeable gap: "Between all these conditions—which were necessary conditions maybe, but they were not sufficient—between all those conditions and the gassing of three thousand persons, men, women, children, in a gas chamber, all together, there is an unbreachable discrepancy. It is simply not possible to engender one out of the other. There are no solutions of continuity between the two; there is rather a gap, an abyss, and this abyss will never be bridged." The abyss of dissociated trauma can expand and replicate into human evil: "Malevolence is inextricably linked to a relational system in which there is a continuous 'retrospective falsification of the past' [44] and a continuous erasure of the present" [45]. "The evil act is therefore internally obscured and interpersonally obscuring; the perpetrator's relational field is infected with the disappearance of history" [45].

At the very center of trauma, metaphor itself fails. In the most extreme cases, trauma writers point to a failure of signification: "the collapse of the imaginative capacity to visualize atrocity" [41]. Boulanger [46] writes of how "the real resists being colonized by the symbolic." Des Pres [47] talks about the "fact of trauma and its resistance to symbolization and fantasy," describing the conditions in which "metaphors tend to actualize, the word becomes flesh." Austrian philosopher Jean Amery, a survivor of Auschwitz, writes [48]:

> It would be totally senseless to try and describe here the pain that was inflicted on me. Was it "like a red-hot iron in my shoulders," and was another "like a dull wooden stake that had been driven into the back of my head?" One comparison would only stand for the other, and in the end we would be hoaxed by turn on the hopeless merry-go-round of figurative speech. The pain was what it was. Beyond that there is nothing to say.... If someone wanted to impart his physical pain, he would be forced to inflict it and thereby become a torturer himself.

In these metaphors, pathologic dissociation is a silence that testifies to topics for which no metaphoric vehicle can be found, experiences that cannot be linked, even by comparison, to any cultural norms.

Treatment metaphors: crossing the gap

The treatment options for the conditions defined by such metaphors are profoundly existential. Loss is loss; there is no filling the abyss. But the speechlessness and isolation that mark such experiences can be addressed. Sometimes the clinician's willingness to witness loss can begin a dialog that reestablishes relationality [45,49]. When the "the abandonment and isolation wrought by these traumas" becomes a topic in therapy, both grieving and human connection become possible [50].

Furthermore, the metaphor of dissociation as a gap (in history, self, or language) carries the associated possibility of a gap bridged. Bromberg [51] describes the isolation of the patient, existing as "an island of tortured affect," searching for "some way of processing demonic internal reality through a human relationship, but there are no thoughts that bridge past and present." Likewise, Grand [45] cites Benjamin's [52] metaphor of swimming across a gap: "Because that traumatized self is defined by solitude, the survivor's resurrection requires that she be known by another in this solitude, for, as Benjamin notes, 'The sea of death can be crossed only by reaching the other.'"

These metaphors of island and sea are linked to the deeper conceptual metaphor of mental health as fluidity and flowing. Boulanger, criticizing psychoanalytic metaphors of the rigidly structured self, proposes instead the metaphors of recent theorists who "view personality as a fluid entity, a river rather than a building, which in its ebb and flow is constantly subject to the exigencies of experience" [53]. Among those theorists is Mitchell [54], who proposes a flowing river as a metaphor for the self in time, to be held in continuous counterpoint to the spatial metaphors of the self fixed to the moment.

The fixed, rigid, solid self is a prerequisite for metaphors of fragmentation and gap. When the self is fragmented, it must be reassembled. When it is perforated or hollowed, forever lacking certain parts, the loss must be mourned within human connection. In all these scenarios, the path to mercy seems to travel through metaphors of liquidity, melting what was rigidly separate into a new whole.

Self as an agent who dissociates

The metaphor of the self as dissociating agent has an unfortunate history in the treatment of dissociation. The idea that a patient has any agency in the process of dissociation was seized in the 1990s by the False Memory Syndrome Foundation as proof that both the dissociation and the causative trauma were fake, manufactured by the patient or induced by the therapy [55]. Even Segall [56], who fortifies his excellent essay on "metaphors of agency and mechanism in dissociation" with statements of support for dissociative patients, assumes that agency means performance and malingering. It has seemed better to many writers to emphasize the passivity of the trauma-struck individual and leave agency aside. To give up the metaphors of agency, however, is to give up the best chance of understanding and treating dissociation. None of these metaphor categories is sufficient alone, but the category of action metaphors is particularly important in understanding the experience, as opposed to the appearance, of dissociation.

The primary metaphors of agency in conceptualizing dissociation are metaphors of perception and attention. To dissociate is to reduce or reallocate mental vision, which in turn reduces what can be known. For example, Spiegel [57] uses a camera metaphor to describe the dissociative action of hypnosis:

> Hypnosis is a state of aroused, attentive focal concentration with a relative suspension of peripheral awareness. This state involves a narrowing of the focus of attention. Hypnotic concentration differs from ordinary concentration in somewhat the same way a telephoto lens in a camera differs from a wide-angle lens. A hypnotized individual focuses on one perception, image, or idea with great intensity at the expense of peripheral awareness.... The more intensely one focuses on one aspect of experience, the more the remaining peripheral awareness is dissociated and unconscious.

Krueger [58] uses a similar metaphor: "Within a particular state of mind the focal length is frozen, making it difficult to reflect or observe." Chefetz [59] refers to filters: "Not all minds have the same perceptual filters. These filters are an implicit factor in the experience of knowing." Bucci [21] writes of how dissociation reduces the areas where vision is allowed: "The zones that must be avoided proliferate, leading to the tunnel vision of neurotic life." Bromberg [60] describes how dissociation "reduces what is in front of someone's eyes to a narrow band of perceptual reality," with particular limits on self-awareness. "Dissociation as a defense, even in a relatively normal personality structure, limits self-reflection to what is secure or needed for survival of selfhood" [61].

A related metaphor of agency imagines dissociated attention as scattered. Goldberg [62,63] describes how the mind can avoid authenticity by refusing to focus: "It is as if the senses themselves are distracted so that the mind remains unassailable. One may also observe a peculiar quality of *attention* in dissociating individuals: attention fixes on the sensory surround, focusing the individual on peripheral physical and mental operations (thereby distracting from the worlds of internal and external reality)" [63]. In Goldberg's complex description, the DID patient both creates and sequesters the world he or she sees [63]:

> Actual contact, by which I mean reciprocal communication between actual subjects (or emotional intercourse between whole objects), is obstructed by this invisible sensory cocoon wall and, in the place of a world of subjects, is constructed a world of omnipotently created part objects—a narcissistic world in which the type of communication and emotional reality are authored and controlled by the patient alone. This is a world that makes intercourse with other people both redundant and impossible.

The pathology of such agency does not lie in the invention of traumas, but in the desperate invention of a sensory-rich intrapersonal life that fills the patient's field of vision, blocking out actual life.

Treatment metaphors: widening perception

When the clinical problem is defined as an action (in this case, the pathologic misallocation of attention) then treatment is drawn toward activity. Instead of static inventories of alters and puzzle pieces, the focus of therapy becomes a series of actions: perception, emotional reaction, inquiry, revelation, and intersubjective experiencing. Boulanger [46,53] urges more attention to the flow of experience and less to the delineation of rigid psychic structure. Chefetz [59], staying as close to verbs as possible, uses the phase "different ways of being" instead of parts and alters. Here as elsewhere, health is found in moving away from fixity and toward fluidity, what Goldberg calls "the pluralistic, fluid qualities of integrated self-experience" [63].

Verbal metaphors of seeing and knowing are not just valuable for being fluid, but for being inhabited metaphors in an inhabited world. The metaphors of the fragmented or multiple self encourage the clinical focus on the patient as "done-to," as a passive target struck by a traumatic force as quantifiable and inhuman as a volt. Yet interpersonal trauma requires two people in the moment of experience, one knowing the feeling of doing, one perceiving (learning, receiving) the doing of the other, even in the moment of victimization. The patient overcomes an important restriction on focus when he or she can imagine the doing of the other, be it the therapist, the indifferent witness, or the perpetrator. Chefetz recounts the moment when his patient finally gains what D.J. Siegel calls "mindsight" [64], the ability to encompass the mind of the other in a relational moment: "You know, like it is bad enough that he raped me, but then to humiliate me? Can you imagine what was in his mind? Like, what could he have been thinking about" [59]? With agency comes admission to a world of genuine others, some good, some bad, and a genuine self, even in the experience of catastrophe.

In Segall's comparison of metaphors of agency (fantasizing) with metaphors of mechanism (splitting), he finishes by recommending a mix of both: "Therapists do best when they understand the advantages and weaknesses of each of these metaphors, and strive towards a middle path, understanding the client as both process and person, object and agent, fragmented, and yet, ultimately whole" [56]. Such a conclusion is inarguable, yet remains stuck in the metaphoric frame of the expert who examines a phenomenon. The recovered patient is not just whole, but acts from within his or her wholeness, interacting in human complexity with the therapist. Just as dissociation can be learned from the skewed attention of the abusive other, so too can connection be learned from therapy where people pay attention to each other as agents responsible for their actions.

Conclusions

In the two meta-categories of metaphors for dissociation (the self as a thing fragmented by trauma, multiplied by trauma, or eviscerated by trauma; and the self as an agent narrowing its range of interpersonal perception to avoid trauma) the problem is solved according to how the problem is set metaphorically.

If the self is a thing, and dissociation is the splitting or multiplication of the thing in response to trauma, then both patient and clinician can expect a multitude of countable things: selves, states, roles, attitudes, and presentations. The deep metaphor shared by both association and dissociation guarantees there will be more than one of whatever is being counted, because two are needed to move together or apart. For the patient, snarled in the chaos and dysfunction of discontinuous living, there may be some fleeting consolation in the possession of "manyness." Although self-fragments are an involuntary testimony of disaster, there is a temptation for both patient and clinician to marvel at the intricacy and number of parts. They offer the patient denial of the damage of trauma, a way to say, "I, who have lost so much, have all these." In the therapy of parts, the patient is invited to stand with the clinician and gain mastery by observing the system. Treatment involves metaphors of reassembly and merger. Personification is turned back into reification so that images of blending, melting, flowing, and joining can describe the return to unitary wholeness.

If the self is a thing, and dissociation is the gap, the destroyed sectors left by trauma, then the clinician and patient face a stark existential task.

Admitting out loud that words do not suffice is itself a kind of testimony. The metaphors of negation complement the metaphors of fragmented manyness. Neither are voluntary creations of the patient, but both invite the patient to stare in horror at the effects of trauma. Both also present a contagious fascination to the clinician.

If the self is seen as a relational agent, apparent actor in a relational world, and dissociation is an interpersonal, behavioral option learned from the other during trauma, then the clinician and patient can both expect to act out dissociative scenarios in treatment. The dissociating self avoids danger by narrowing vision to a fragment of time, by refusing to focus in from the periphery, or by staring obsessively at internal fantasy. Metaphors for treatment use verbs (perceiving, evading) rather than the configurations of nouns (parts, holes), encouraging the patient to move away from stasis and toward fluidity. The abusive other appears in treatment not as an introjected ghost, but as a series of relational options constantly offered (withdraw, pretend, project, deny, enjoy pain) and often taken by both patient and clinician. Eventually, some degree of shared humanity returns, not just to the clinical scenario, but also to the original traumatic scenario.

All these metaphor categories are accessed during most treatments of dissociative disorders, with differing emphasis. Interestingly, the conceptualization of recovery in each of these categories carries images of fluidity: melting the alters into one another; swimming across the sea of death to the island of the relational other; learning fluid verbs instead of fixed avoidance, movement instead of stasis. The advantage of putting more emphasis on the self as agent is that images of fluidity are conveyed from the beginning, without the attractive distraction of counting up parts.

By working toward metaphors of process rather than thing, the clinician has more opportunity to stand inside dissociative process with the patient, rather than inviting the patient to stand safely outside the relational field as the clinical observer. The outsider's view offers detachment and potential control to a patient who may feel agonizingly out of control. But detachment is a bit like dissociation. Detachment reinforces skills learned during trauma. In contrast, the verbal metaphors of perception draw attention to the immediacy of perceiving, to actions for which both clinician and patient are accountable.

Metaphors that encourage the outsider's point of view also support a sense of a more (more parts, more holes, more layers of known or unknown history), but the daily experience from the patient's point of view is not so much the richness of invented variety as the persistent experience of less. The dissociating self, minute by minute, sees only a fragment of the world, instead of the large visual field of the healthier person who can tolerate more things in the view at once. Able to bear only one unconflicted fraction at a time, the dissociated patient is sole viewer of disconnected vistas that are alternately vivid and lost, producing an experience of loneliness, power, and a nagging sense of missing something. Pizer [65] recounts a therapeutic use of metaphor that captures the poignancy and loneliness of such a constricted view:

> In my work with Donald, I had recurrently noted his distance or abstractness and had developed with him a language for our noting together his cognitive and communicative style that resulted from splitting and dissociation: he described how initially he had only seen fragments of my office, never putting the whole picture together; I introduced the image of his looking out at the world through holes cut in a cardboard box, turning his head to see unconnected, discontinuous images; and I described his style of associations as island enshrouded in fog, kept separate and isolated, awaiting the lifting of the fog to reveal one vast, continuous inner landscape.

Once the problem is identified as constriction rather than manyness, the clinical task changes from assembling puzzles to widening the holes in the box.

The most important clinical difference between metaphors of self as a multiplied and fragmented thing and metaphors of self as a seeing person is the location of the "I" of the patient. In the first case, the faceless action of dissociation has broken what should be whole. In the phrase, "Trauma broke his mind," both abuser and victim are depersonalized, the abuser into a force, the victim into a breakable target. In the second case, where metaphors describe the self's actions, the interpersonal transaction is harder to reduce. The victim learns at the hands of another the art of seeing the world in pieces. To make the victim whole, the world must be made whole, which requires restoring selfhood to both sides of the malevolent exchange. The clinical challenge of trauma-born dissociation can be thought of as a shift of metaphors: How to change the self from an it to an I, from passive noun to active pronoun, on both sides of a world-breaking interpersonal catastrophe.

The good news is that every word carries the potential of relationality: A "word is a two-sided act. It is determined equally by whose word it is and for whom it is meant ... Each and every word expresses the 'one' in relation to the "other" [66]. Metaphors add an extra dimension, expressing abstraction in relation to body and ground. "The important thing," says Bucci [67], "is to get the symbolizing process going, get some referential connections operating." If trauma freezes language, "referential connections" unfreeze it, opening the possibility of fluid change. Clinicians can exploit this possibility by emphasizing metaphors of agency even while respecting the witness of parts, enlisting the patient in the universal project of imagining a culture that can address all human experience.

Summary

The clinical metaphors that set the problem of pathologic dissociation can be categorized in two groups: noun-based metaphors that represent the self as a thing that is divided, multiplied, or perforated by trauma;

and verb-based metaphors that represent the self as an agent who reduces perception and redirects attention. Although both metaphor groups have their uses, verb-based metaphors help lead away from dissociative disconnection and toward responsibility, interactive relationality, and the recovery of human meaning in trauma.

References

[1] Pepper S. The root metaphor theory of metaphysics. J Philos 1935;32:365–74.
[2] Lakoff G, Johnson M. Metaphors we live by. Chicago: University of Chicago Press; 1980.
[3] Maasen S, Weingart P. Metaphors and the dynamics of knowledge. New York: Routledge; 2000.
[4] Leary DE. Psyche's muse: the role of metaphor in the history of psychology. In: Leary DE, editor. Metaphors in the history of psychology. New York: Cambridge University Press; 1990. p. 1–78.
[5] Schön DS. Generative metaphor: a perspective on problem-setting in social policy. In: Ortney A, editor. Metaphor and thought. 2nd edition. New York: Cambridge University Press; 1993. p. 137–63.
[6] Deignan A. Corpus-based research into metaphor. In: Cameron L, Low G, editors. Researching and applying metaphor. New York: Cambridge University Press; 1999. p. 170–99.
[7] Arlow JA. Metaphor and the psychoanalytic situation. Psychoanal Q 1979;48:363–85.
[8] Lankton C, Lankton SR. Tales of enchantment: goal-oriented metaphors for adults and children in therapy. New York: Brunner/Mazel; 1989.
[9] American Psychiatric Association. Diagnostic and statistical manual of mental disorders, revised. 4th edition. Washington: American Psychiatric Association; 2000.
[10] Atwood GE, Orange DM, Stolorow RD. Shattered world/psychotic states: a post-Cartesian view of the experience of personal annihilation. Psychoanal Psychol 2002;19:281–306.
[11] Gottlieb RM. Does the mind fall apart in multiple personality disorder? Some proposals based on a psychoanalytic case. J Am Psychoanal Assoc 1997;45:907–32.
[12] Way K. The grammar of trauma: how psychologists' metaphors construct the dissociative response to interpersonal trauma. Fielding Graduate University; unpublished dissertation 2005.
[13] van der Kolk BA, van der Hart O. Pierre Janet and the breakdown of adaptation in psychological trauma. Am J Psychiatry 1989;146:1530–40.
[14] Barach PM. Multiple personality disorder as an attachment disorder. Dissociation 1991;4: 117–23.
[15] Braun BG, editor. Treatment of multiple personality disorder. Washington: American Psychiatric Press; 1986.
[16] Spiegel D, Cardena E. Disintegrated experience: the dissociative disorders revisited. J Abnorm Psychol 1991;100:366–78.
[17] Braude SE. First person plural: multiple personality and the philosophy of mind. Revised edition. Lanham (MD): Rowman & Littlefield; 1995.
[18] Putnam FW. Diagnosis and treatment of multiple personality disorder. New York: Guilford Press; 1989.
[19] Shirar L. Dissociative children: bridging the inner and outer worlds. New York: WW Norton; 1996.
[20] Putnam FW. Discussion: are alter personalities fragments or figments? Psychoanal Inquiry 1992;12:95–111.
[21] Bucci W. Psychoanalysis and cognitive science: a multiple code theory. New York: Guilford; 1997.
[22] Liotti G. Understanding the dissociative processes: the contribution of attachment theory. Psychoanal Inquiry 1999;19:757–83.

[23] Fonagy P. Multiple voices versus meta-cognition: an attachment theory perspective. In: Sinason V, editor. Attachment, trauma and multiplicity: working with dissociative identity disorder. New York: Taylor & Francis; 2002. p. 71–85.

[24] Foote B. Dissociative identity disorder and pseudo-hysteria. Am J Psychother 1999;53: 320–44.

[25] Sinason V. Introduction. In: Sinason V, editor. Attachment, trauma and multiplicity: working with dissociative identity disorder. New York: Taylor & Francis; 2002. p. 3–20.

[26] Nijenhuis ERS, Van der Hart O, Steele K. Trauma-related structural dissociation of the personality. Trauma Information Pages. Available at: http://www.trauma-pages.com/nijenhuis-2004.htm. Accessed June 2, 2005.

[27] Chefetz RA, Bromberg P. Talking with "me" and "not-me." Contemp Psychoanal 2004;40: 409–64.

[28] Ross CA. Subpersonalities and multiple personalities: a dissociative continuum. In: Rowan J, Cooper M, editors. Subpersonalities: the people inside us. Florence (KY): Taylor & Francis; 1999. p. 183–97.

[29] Schwartz RC. The internal family systems model. In: Rowan J, Cooper M, editors. The plural self: multiplicity in everyday life. Thousand Oaks (CA): Sage; 1999. p. 238–53.

[30] Bliss EL. Multiple personality, allied disorders, and hypnosis. New York: Oxford University Press; 1986.

[31] Fine CG. The tactical-integration model for treatment of dissociative identity disorder and allied dissociative disorders. Am J Psychother 1999;53:361–76.

[32] Brenner I. Deconstructing DID. Am J Psychother 1999;53:344–61.

[33] van der Kolk BA, Weisaeth L, van der Hart O. History of trauma in psychiatry. In: van der Kolk BA, McFarlane AC, Weisaeth L, editors. Traumatic stress: the effects of overwhelming experience on mind, body, and society. New York: Guilford; 1996. p. 47–74.

[34] Fraser GA. Fraser's "dissociative table technique" revisited, revised: a strategy for working with ego states in dissociative disorders and ego-state therapy. Journal of Trauma and Dissociation 2003;4:5–28.

[35] Kluft RP. Clinical approaches to the integration of personalities. In: Kluft RP, Fine CG, editors. Clinical perspectives on multiple personality disorder. Washington: American Psychiatric Press; 1993. p. 101–33.

[36] Krakauer SY. Treating dissociative identity disorder: the power of the collective heart. Philadelphia: Brunner-Routledge; 2001.

[37] Ross CA. Multiple personality disorder: diagnosis, clinical features, and treatment. New York: John Wiley; 1989.

[38] Laub D, Auerhahn N. Failed empathy: a central theme in the survivor's Holocaust experiences. Psychoanal Psychol 1989;6:377–400.

[39] van der Kolk BA, McFarlane AC, Weisaeth L. Traumatic stress: the effects of overwhelming experience on mind, body, and society. New York: Guilford; 1996.

[40] Krystal H, editor. Massive psychic trauma. New York: International Universities Press; 1968.

[41] Laub D. The empty circle: children of survivors and the limits of reconstruction. J Am Psychoanal Assoc 1998;46:507–29.

[42] Bujak MJ. Concentration camp imagery as a psychic organizer in dissociative identity disorder individuals: review of literature and construction of a theoretical explanation (UMI No. 9984971). Diss Abstr Intl 2000;61(9B):4973.

[43] Lanzmann C. The obscenity of understanding: an evening with Claude Lanzmann. In: Caruth C, editor. Trauma: explorations in memory. Baltimore: Johns Hopkins Press; 1995. p. 200–20.

[44] Bromberg PM. "Speak! That I may see you": some reflections on dissociation, reality, and psychoanalytic listening. Contemp Psychoanal 1994;4:517–49.

[45] Grand S. The reproduction of evil: a clinical and cultural perspective. Hillsdale (NJ): Analytic Press; 2000.

[46] Boulanger G. Wounded by reality: the collapse of the self in adult onset trauma. Contemp Psychoanal 2002;38:45–76.

[47] Des Pres T. The survivor: an anatomy of life in the death camps. New York: Oxford University Press; 1976.

[48] Amery J. At the mind's limits. New York: Schocken Books; 1986.

[49] Herman JL. Trauma and recovery. New York: Basic Books; 1992.

[50] Roth S. Discussion: a psychoanalyst's perspective on multiple personality disorder. Psychoanal Inquiry 1992;12:112–23.

[51] Bromberg PM. On knowing one's patient inside out: the aesthetics of unconscious communication. Psychoanal Dialogues 1991;1:399–422.

[52] Benjamin J. Like subjects, love objects: essays on recognition and sexual difference. New Haven (CT): Yale University Press; 1995.

[53] Boulanger G. The cost of survival: psychoanalysis and adult onset trauma. Contemp Psychoanal 2002;38:17–44.

[54] Mitchell S. Hope and dread in psychoanalysis. New York: Basic Books; 1993.

[55] Hacking I. Rewriting the soul: multiple personality and the sciences of memory. Princeton (NJ): Princeton University Press; 1995.

[56] Segall SR. Metaphors of agency and mechanism in dissociation. Dissociation 1996;9:154–68.

[57] Spiegel D. Trauma, dissociation, and hypnosis. In: Kluft RP, editor. Incest-related syndromes of adult psychopathology. Washington: American Psychiatric Press; 1990. p. 247–61.

[58] Krueger DW. Integrating body self and psychological self: creating a new story in psychoanalysis and psychotherapy. New York: Brunner-Routledge; 2002.

[59] Chefetz RA. I wish I didn't know now what I didn't know then: longing for a coherent mind: Interpreting implicit processes in the psychoanalytic exploration of mind. In: Longing: psychoanalytic musings on desire. Presented at the William Alanson White Institute. New York; October 23–24, 2004.

[60] Bromberg PM. Something wicked this way comes: trauma, dissociation, and conflict. The space where psychoanalysis, cognitive science, and neuroscience overlap. Psychoanal Psychol 2003;20:558–74.

[61] Bromberg PM. Standing in the spaces: essays on clinical process, trauma, and dissociation. Hillsdale (NJ): Analytic Press; 1998.

[62] Goldberg P. The role of distractions in the maintenance of dissociative mental states. Int J Psychoanal 1987;68:511–24.

[63] Goldberg P. Successful dissociation, pseudovitality, and inauthentic use of the senses. Psychoanal Dialogues 1995;5:493–510.

[64] Siegel DJ. Toward an interpersonal neurobiology of the developing mind: attachment relationships, "mindsight, " and neural integration. Infant Ment Health J 2001;22:67–94.

[65] Pizer SA. Negotiating potential space: illusion, play, metaphor, and the subjunctive. Psychoanal Dialogues 1996;6:689–712.

[66] Shotter J. Life inside dialogically structured mentalities: Bakhtin's and Voloshinov's account of our mental activities as out in the world between us. In: Rowan J, Cooper M, editors. The plural self: multiplicity in everyday life. Thousand Oaks (CA): Sage; 1999. p. 71–92.

[67] Bucci W. Varieties of dissociative experiences: a multiple code account and a discussion of Bromberg's case of "William." Psychoanal Psychol 2003;20:542–57.

ELSEVIER
SAUNDERS

Psychiatr Clin N Am 29 (2006) 45–62

PSYCHIATRIC
CLINICS
OF NORTH AMERICA

Normative Dissociation

Lisa D. Butler, PhD

*Department of Psychiatry & Behavioral Sciences, Stanford University School of Medicine,
401 Quarry Road, #2320, Stanford, CA 94035-5718, USA*

The stream of consciousness—that flow of perceptions, purposeful thoughts, fragmentary images, distant recollections, bodily sensations, emotions, plans, wishes, and impossible fantasies—is our experience of life, our own personal life, from its beginning to its end. As scientists, we may approach the subject for the joy of discovering how it works. As clinicians, therapists, and social engineers, we may study it to reduce human suffering. But simply as people, we are drawn to it precisely because it is that portion of our being at once most familiar and most mysterious.

Pope KS, Singer JL, editors. *The stream of consciousness—scientific investigations into the flow of human experience, p. 1.*

Although the literature corresponding to the study of dissociation is concerned primarily with pathology, most dissociative experiences are not pathological—a large proportion of the stream of consciousness is taken up with normative dissociative experiences. In the dissociation literature, these experiences, which include daydreaming, fantasy, and absorption in everyday experiences, among others, fall under the rubric of *nonpathological dissociation*. The term implies a change in the state of consciousness that is not induced organically, does not occur as part of a psychiatric disorder, and involves the temporary alteration or separation of what are normally experienced as integrated mental processes [1].

Two elements seem to be common to nonpathological and pathological dissociative experiences, nonetheless. Specifically, both involve a telescoping of the attentional field to concentrate on a narrow range of experience and the concomitant exclusion of other material (internal or external) from awareness and, to some degree, from accessibility, which may result in a temporary lack of reflective consciousness [2,3], among other experiential changes.

Fantasy, daydreaming, and absorption in daily activities (in particular recreational activities) are considered by many dissociation theorists to be

E-mail address: butler@psych.stanford.edu

doi:10.1016/j.psc.2005.10.004

instantiations of nonpathological dissociation [1,4,5]; and because they are associated with dissociative pathology, items representing each are included in the most widely used measure of dissociation, the Dissociative Experiences Scale (DES) [6,7]. Additionally, there is little disagreement that formal and self-hypnotic states are dissociative in nature [2,8–10], and many theorists view night dreams as meaningfully related to daydreams in underlying process [11–14], with some noting their overlap with dissociative states [15,16]. Similarly, many other altered states of consciousness, such as meditation or religious trance, seem to involve dissociative elements [17,18]. Research examining college and general populations establishes that the prevalence of dissociative experiences is greater than previously understood [19,20] and that the nonpathological subset of dissociative experiences (the absorption-imaginative involvement factor in the DES) are the most common [19–21, reviewed in 7,22], although derealization and depersonalization experiences also are prominent in college samples.

The primacy and ubiquity of dissociation in normal human experience are not well appreciated, however. Because pathological dissociation likely represents, at least in part, a disorder of ordinary dissociative processes [1], I use the term *normative dissociation*, instead of nonpathological dissociation (with a few exceptions), to describe the presence of normal dissociative process. In this article, I briefly examine the literature concerning the four most common normative dissociative experiences (absorption in daily activities, daydreaming, fantasy, and night dreaming) and outline some functions that normative dissociation may serve in everyday life and how they may be distorted or hijacked in pathological dissociative states. I also discuss some of the implications of these findings for the putative dissociative continuum. By considering the nature and functions of the ordered normative process, the character of the disordered pathological process may be better understood.

The dissociations of everyday life

The heart of the normative dissociative process would seem to be *absorption*—intense focal concentration and cognitive involvement in one or more aspects of conscious awareness [23,24]. As is the case in dissociative symptoms and hypnotic states, in normative dissociation, the narrowing of focus and commitment of cognitive resources to the attentional object result in the exclusion of other *content* from the phenomenal field and, at times, consequent alteration of the *context* in which the attentional object is experienced [2]. The excluded content may include sensations, perceptions, thoughts, feelings, or memories. The altered context may involve, for example, changes in feelings of relatedness to self or the world, a diminished sense of volition, or loss of self-awareness and reflection (metacognition), as many people experience—or come to realize they have experienced—on a long-distance drive or when watching an engrossing film. Typically these changed aspects are noticed in retrospect; they come into awareness once self-reflection is re-engaged. In everyday life, such dissociative experiences include absorption in daydreaming, imaginative productions, meditation, and pastimes that capture attention and dislodge self-awareness, such as reading an enthralling book.

The relationship between narrowing of attention and dissociative experience was first observed a century ago by Janet [25], who noted that the absorption found in dissociated states represented a "retraction in the field of consciousness" [26, p. 331]. The construct of absorption, however, came to prominence in research seeking to outline the dispositional characteristics related to hypnotic susceptibility. In this pursuit, Tellegen and Atkinson [23,24] identified a group of items that compose a factor they term "openness to absorbing or self-altering experience," or *absorption*, for short, which involves "a state of 'total attention' during which the available representational apparatus seems to be entirely dedicated to experiencing and modeling the attentional object, be it a landscape, a human being, a sound, a remembered incident, or an aspect of one's self" [23, p. 274]. Further, Tellegen and Atkinson [23] note that once this sharply focused attentional process is achieved, several additional experiential features arise: a heightened sense of reality of the attentional object, an imperviousness to normally distracting events, and an altered sense of reality in general and in the self in particular—elements all recognizable in dissociative states, including those that are normative. It is perhaps not surprising, therefore, that absorption is correlated with hypnotic susceptibility, and even more strongly associated with dissociativity, fantasy proneness, and daydreaming [23,27–31].

The differences between attention and absorption are important to this discussion, because these states differ not only in their intensity of focus but also in their attendant qualities. With attention, material is forefront in phenomenal awareness, but the surround remains, or is readily accessible, and attention is immediately subject to volition. In absorption, the focus of attention is more concentrated and stable, and environmental and personal contexts may be diminished or lost, including higher order intrapsychic cognitive structures and processes, such as self-reflection and feelings of volition. As Kihlstrom [15, see also 4] notes, awareness and voluntary control are key elements to consciousness; when there are disruptions in one or both of these processes, dissociation may be present.

Another clue to the difference between attention and absorption may be in the phenomenology of these experiences: the former feels like *observation*, whereas the latter feels more like complete involvement or *engagement*. But, why do humans have this capacity to engage so fully when they simply could observe? It seems reasonable to speculate that full engagement and the qualities associated with it afford benefits or enable functions not available with mere attention. As the following discussion of normative dissociative experiences makes clear, each appears to depend on one or more of the properties of the highly absorbed (or dissociated) condition: maximal commitment of cognitive resources, a decrease in susceptibility to external cues and distractions, suspension of reality constraints and critical judgment, loss of self-reference (and associations to it), and reductions in self-consciousness and self-evaluation.

In general, it is academic psychologists who have documented the frequency, forms, and character of the most common manifestations of dissociation, whereas researchers in clinical psychology or psychiatry have been concerned with manifestations of dissociation in disordered states. Consequently, it is the former literature that is principally described in this article.

Absorption in everyday activities

Many people experience absorption when engaged in everyday activities. Some become engrossed in recreational pastimes, others become immersed in work. Whether one is reading a murder mystery or drafting a manuscript, absorption in the activity reduces the potential for distraction, increases the allocation of necessary cognitive resources, and allows for full engagement with the attentional object.

Absorption also may be the process that underlies the human capacity to enjoy, and even the motivation to engage in, many of those activities. For example, filmmakers intentionally seek to induce an altered state of consciousness in their audience, one in which viewers are so captivated by the narrative on the screen that they lose track of where (and who) they are, suspend their critical faculties, and become enthralled by the alternate universe in the film [32,33]. Filmmakers see this state of absorption and suspension of judgment, which parallels other nonpathological dissociative experiences, such as hypnotic states [2,32], as essential to the pleasurable film-going experience [33]. Presumably, it contributes to the enjoyment of other visual and dramatic arts, fiction, and perhaps music, as well.

Taking it further, Butler and Palesh [32, see also 1] propose that the choice to watch a film, video, or television—indeed, to partake in any activity in which intense absorption and other dissociative aspects inhere (such as loss of awareness of surroundings, suspension of self-awareness or critical faculties, and time distortion) may be viewed as a deliberate engagement in dissociative experience. Consider also that the amount of time and effort people devote to these pastimes represents a considerable share of daily life. Apparently, intentional normative dissociative episodes are numerous and widespread.

Although engrossing recreational pursuits, such as reading for pleasure, listening to music, and watching artistic performances, share the property of absorption with activities such as daydreaming and imaginative involvement, they differ in two important respects: the deliberateness with which they are engaged and the source of their absorbing subject matter. In the former cases, the material is imported into consciousness from the outside world, whereas in daydreams, the content arises spontaneously as an individual's own deliberative or fantasy material. Other activities, such as meditation, religious trance, exercise (when *the zone* is achieved), or long-distance driving that results in *highway hypnosis* (the "spacing out" and loss of awareness of self, time, and the task at hand), also may involve absorption in private productions.

A less investigated form of normative dissociation is identified by Pica and Beere [34] in the *positive dissociative experiences* often found to accompany events and activities of personal significance (such as engaging in sports, sex, hobbies, or prayer; anticipating or hearing good news; having contact with nature; and performing and listening to music). Such experiences involve absorption and alterations in the experience of self, body, or world, reminiscent of experiences of depersonalization and, in particular, derealization, but with a positive affect tone [1]. These experiences seem to overlap conceptually and phenomenologically with the common psychological event of *flow* [35,36] and the less familiar *peak* experience [37]. (As with other normative dissociative experiences, flow and peak experiences are not conceptualized as dissociative experiences in their respective literatures [1,34].)

Flow states (or optimal experiences) are described as a function of a dynamic interplay between challenges and skills, wherein the perceived challenge neither overmatches nor underuses existing skills. When this state is achieved, there is a merging of action and awareness such that attention is completely absorbed in the activity, reflective self-consciousness is lost, and time sense is distorted [35,36]. The feelings of self-efficacy and intrinsic reward associated with the activity are what distinguish flow from other dissociative experiences [1].

In his early theorizing related to the construct of flow, Csikszentmihalyi [38] observes that "every time people enjoy what they are doing, or in any way transcend ordinary states of existence, they report specific changes in the attentional process" [p. 342]. Further, he suggests that "the exercise of voluntary attention has a positive survival value, and therefore concentration has been selected out (*sic*) through evolution by becoming associated with pleasurable activities" [p. 344]. As Csikszentmihalyi's later research on flow indicates, "concentration," in the context of optimal experience, denotes marked absorption and its attendant effects on other aspects of experience, including a complete and highly focused commitment of cognitive resources. These observations highlight what may be one reason that dissociation of this sort is such a central aspect of human experience: absorption is necessary for the accomplishment of some activities of import.

Daydreaming and fantasizing

Most dissociations of everyday life occur in a private world—an interior universe of reverie and fantasy about which few people speak. Nonetheless, in his seminal book on the topic, Jerome Singer [12] describes his own history of daydreaming. He describes two major forms. One involves "the ongoing stream of associations, interior monologues, and occasional elaborated fantasies of a spontaneous nature associated with particular problems or chains of thought" [p. 16]. The second involves repeated, complex fantasies involving self-created, colorful characters that he refers to by name, who act out evolving story lines. These fantasies are typically engaged in volitionally (under particular circumstances, such as boredom), and Singer reports that they have been a part of his conscious life since childhood.

In general, these two types of experiences map onto what commonly is meant by the terms, daydreaming and fantasy: the typical daydream begins spontaneously, is experienced as an ongoing series of brief associated thoughts or images triggered by internal or external stimuli or cues [12,39–42], and deals most often with current life concerns [14,41]. In contrast, the development of a fantasy may be an elected pastime; it is more elaborate and continuous, composed of more pure imagination (rather than, for example, memory), and directed at self-amusement, pleasure, distraction, or escape [12,14,41].

Because definitional distinctions between these phenomena are not always consistent, Klinger [14] suggests that it is more helpful to think of daydreams (including fantasies) as presenting in different forms that are reflected in distinctive dimensions. As Klinger puts it, thoughts may be "more or less fanciful, more or less spontaneous, and more or less removed from the here or now" [p. 83]. In short, some daydreams are more like fantasies, whereas in others the mind spontaneously veers off task (often described as distractibility or *mindwandering*) or flows to other concerns in other times. As an example of the last form, Singer [42] has observed "I think I can confidently predict that anyone reading this article will at some point drift away, hopefully only momentarily, to thoughts of forthcoming rendezvous, anticipated dinners, delightful summer vacations, or clever bits of revenge on political opponents in their psychology departments" [p. 729]. In general, when the term daydreaming is used in the literature, it subsumes fantasies and mindwandering, as it does for much of what is discussed in this section.

"Daydreaming is both one of the most common and one of the most private things we do" [14, p. xii]. Overall, research indicates that the majority of individuals—more than 9 in 10—report being aware of daydreaming in some form on a daily basis [43], and laboratory and field studies (using thought sampling) suggest that a significant proportion of mental activity—up to half—is spent in some form of daydreaming [14,39,40], although daydreaming frequency and intensity generally decrease with age through adulthood [44].

The structure of daydreams also has been studied widely. Assessments of thousands of subjects with Singer and Antrobus' Imaginal Processes Inventory [45] indicate a typical three-factor structure: a positive orientation to daydreaming associated with frequent, vivid, and deeply absorbing visual and auditory imagery and constructive problem solving; daydreams of a generally negative emotional tone, often involving aversive affects, such as fear, regret, or guilt, and that also may involve highly vivid and real-feeling fantasies of daring personal heroism and achievement; and the propensity to mindwandering and cognitive distraction, which is associated with anxiety and self-doubt, less clear and more fragmentary daydreams, and tendencies to boredom and difficulties in concentrating [42,45]. Individual daydreaming styles relate to idiosyncratic levels of each of these factors.

Daydreaming occurs chiefly when alone and in the absence of diverting external stimuli or cognitively demanding tasks, such as when sitting quietly gazing out a window or drifting into sleep, when bored, or during routinized physical activities, such as driving, showering, jogging, or playing simple computer games [12,14,39,42]. A typical lapse into daydreaming is spontaneous and the experience fleeting. Their automaticity and evanescence, and the characteristic lack of self-awareness during them, mean that most daydreams pass relatively unnoted [1,12,14].

The reveries that accompany such activities involve absorption in the internal world of perception, thought, imagination, or memory, along with the contemporaneous loss of awareness of self, place, behavior, and passage of time. (See Singer and Pope [27] regarding the similarities between self-hypnosis and daydreaming.) Nonetheless, upon introspection (or retrospection) regarding the contents of awareness during such episodes, typically one observes a phenomenal field devoted to activity—musing over past events, imagining future conversations or activities, problem solving, judgment making, and planning. In short, the mind is at work, milling the grist of daily life [1,14,39,41]. Absorption, in the case of daydreaming, may allow for the assignment of cognitive resources to these issues, less encumbered by reality constraints, critical judgment, and confining habits of thought that might limit the associations made. It is possible that daydreaming provides a complement to the strategies of regular conscious cognition, in that it may arrive at solutions to problems that cannot be resolved with more routinized, self-conscious, goal-directed, or logical thinking.

In daydreaming, absorption engages persistent concerns or unaddressed challenges, with opportunities for examination and resolution arising in part through the flow of less restricted associations and in part through the trial and error and rehearsal of alternatives afforded by imagination [14,39]. In fantasy, absorption and the imaginal process are merged to allow for exploration of what "might be" or "might have been" without the nagging constraints of convention or current reality. Daydreams and fantasy may also be used to engage intuition, creativity, or other unconscious processes, allowing the nondirective contemplation of material that might be less suited to conscious reflection [1,12,14,27,41].

In Singer's [42] view, mental life is a continuous effort at tracking sensory inputs, cognitively organizing experiences, re-examining memories, and monitoring "a continuous set of plans and anticipations and a variety of unfinished businesses which compete for our limited attentional capacities with the demands of steering our selves through a physical and social world" [p. 729]. In challenging and complex circumstances, cognitive resources are spent attending to immediate and pressing demands; daydreams tend to arise when other more intentional or situationally required cognitive operations subside, much as how background processing in a computer resumes once the processor is relatively idle.

One additional finding is worth considering. Several studies have found that some individuals spend an extraordinarily large part of their lives in deep and elaborate fantasy production. Wilson and Barber [46,47, see also 48] identified such a group, which they labeled *fantasy-prone personalities*, among a sample of highly hypnotizable, nonclinical female subjects. (The investigators [46] estimate that such personalities compose up to 4% of the population.) These individuals reported fantasizing a large part of the time (in most cases, more than 50% of the time), and many of these fantasies had a hallucinatory quality that felt "as real as real," making them difficult at times to distinguish from reality [cf. 48]. Although the women studied were well educated and most were relatively well adjusted [cf. 48], virtually all of them also reported other less common dissociation-spectrum experiences, including intense fantasies that affected them physically; vivid hypnagogic imagery and reliving of personal memories; out-of-body experiences; automatic writing; and beliefs that they had psychic experiences, religious visions, or healing powers. In short, these women appear to constitute a group that has extraordinary dissociative capacities in the absence of frank dissociative pathology, and this finding may be seen as evidence consistent with a continuity between normative and pathological dissociation.

Dreaming

"The world of dreams is our real world whilst sleeping, because our attention then lapses from the sensible world. Conversely, when we wake the attention usually lapses from the dream-world and that becomes unreal" [49, p. 294]. Many observers have remarked on the apparent continuity between the dreams of day and night [4,13–16,42,49,50]. For example, Singer [12] observes, "it seems likely that dreams and daydreams represent different points along a common continuum of ongoing cerebral activity" [p. 51]. Similarly, Klinger [14] notes, "our thoughts flow through the day and continue into sleep, and then with perhaps occasional breaks, through sleep and back into wakefulness" [p. 24]. Evidence consistent with these assertions comes from findings that there seems to be a 90-minute cyclicity to dreams and daydreams [51] that continues throughout the 24-hour day and that subjects scoring highly on the daydreaming factors described previously report equivalent forms and contents in their night dreaming material [50].

The contents of dreams also underscore the latter's essential connection with the waking state. Night dreaming has long been thought to provide an opportunity to grapple with current concerns and unfinished business from waking experience [11]; and it may offer unique resources to this effort because the constraints imposed by waking consciousness, with its values, biases, and superordinate structures of evaluation, may be suspended.

In short, the dreams of night seem to share form, content, and purpose with the reveries of day. But are they dissociative? Kihlstrom [15] notes that the mental activity during sleep "qualifies as dissociated because it is not under voluntary control, and because it is not represented in memories accessible to the person during the normal waking state" [p. 175]. Additionally, if night dreams are akin to daydreams in their function, then the difference between them may not be one of process, but simply one of context (awake versus asleep). As Freud observed, "at bottom, dreams are nothing other than a particular form of thinking, made possible by the conditions of the state of sleep. It is the dream-work that creates that form...the fact that dreams concern themselves with attempts at solving the problem by which our mental life is faced is no more strange than that our conscious waking life should do so" [cited in 13, p. 314]. It is not clear, however, whether the construct of absorption—as delineated by Tellegen and colleagues [23,24] and used in this article—is applicable to the sleep state.

A goal of this article is to broaden views on dissociation from a concentration on pathology to an outlook that includes everyday experience. This expansion of focus seems warranted because the evidence suggests that normative dissociative experiences are not only common, but pervasive; they are not simply a diversion from everyday experience, but a central feature of it; and they are not incidental in the stream of consciousness, but integral to it. To elaborate the point that normative dissociation is embedded in and essential to daily functioning, the following section enumerates some possible functions of dissociation including, but not limited to, those that are defensive. By examining the ubiquity and utility of the dissociations of everyday life, disorders of dissociation may come to seem a little less mysterious and improbable and their phenomenology less alien.

Proposed functions of normative dissociation and some parallels in dissociative pathology

The previous discussion indicates that normative dissociative experiences are experiences that almost all persons have and that make up a substantial proportion of cognitive activity; however, the roles or *functions* that they serve—why evolution selected them for the cognitive repertoire—have received less attention [1,52]. Commentators who have a clinical orientation [9,10,52–54] understandably emphasize the defensive value of dissociation in protecting the individual from overwhelming experience. Those who have the capacity to dissociate can evade awareness of aversive perceptual, emotional, or behavioral inputs; menacing meanings, associations, and preoccupations; past traumas that would otherwise haunt their memories; and the weight of choices made. In other words, the exercise of this capacity may allow individuals to psychologically survive traumatic circumstance.

Nonetheless, even though dissociation may be put to the purpose of psychological defense, it does not (necessarily) follow that that is the sole—or even the primary—function that determined its natural selection. The successful psychological navigation of traumatic situations was only one type of selection pressure on which the evolving cognitive apparatus was tested. For example, Ludwig [52] outlines seven possible functions of dissociation (broadly defined) that cover more psychological ground: automatization of behaviors, economy and efficiency of effort, resolution of irreconcilable conflicts, escape from the constraints of reality, isolation of catastrophic experiences, cathartic discharge of feelings, and enhancement of the herd sense. Although he argues for several of these from a clinical perspective—demonstrating their utility in coping with extreme experience—they may be applied equally to more normative life events.

Additionally, it is important to bear in mind that the "disorder" in the disorders that include severe and longstanding dissociative symptoms—dissociative amnesia, dissociative fugue, dissociative identity disorder, and in some cases, posttraumatic stress disorder (PTSD)—is neither in the fact that dissociation per se is present, nor that it was deployed in the face of trauma as a tactic (or reflex) of immediate survival, but rather that severe dissociation and its psychological fallout continue in the absence of such conditions. In short, the process itself becomes disordered in some manner or its functions are recruited to purposes that are maladaptive.

So, what are the functions of normative dissociation? Why is it that humans daydream, fantasize, choose activities that supplant thoughts with extraneous recreational material, or experience profound moments of positive feeling in some altered mental states? Elsewhere I have proposed [1] three general adaptive functions that normative dissociations may serve and highlight some correspondences between them and manifestations in dissociative pathology; these are outlined briefly in this section.

Normative dissociation, in the form of daydreaming, is used for mental processing

Evidence suggests that although some daydreams are fanciful, most are concerned with what Klinger [14,41] terms, "current concerns." In daydreams, people anticipate, rehearse, create, and plan; revisit what they have done and said; remember things they have forgotten; imagine how to do things differently; and address immediate practical problems that press for attention. In short, daydreaming enables processing and working through. Given that so much of waking mental activity is spent in some form of daydreaming state—not to mention the time spent dreaming during sleep—it seems clear that this capacity confers a significant benefit: it advances resolution of the myriad issues and challenges of daily lives.

The pathological counterpart to the normative "dreaming" of day and night may be, therefore, the processing failure indicated by the unbidden and repetitive intrusive thoughts, flashbacks, and nightmares of traumatic re-experiencing [55]. In Horowitz's model of the cognitive processing of discrepant experience, intrusion symptoms are a signal that normal processing is incomplete. The information (ie, the traumatic experience and its meanings) is discrepant with existing mental structures, and efforts to assimilate or accommodate the material have been short-circuited due to the painful negative affects it evokes. Additionally, the maladaptive daydreams of dissociative patients [56] and the ruminative preoccupations associated with depression and PTSD [55,57] may be examples of the hijacking of this processing by pathological or unintegrated affect.

Normative dissociation in the form of cognitive involvement
in absorbing activities (or elaborate fantasies) is used for escape

As described previously, much of what is done for recreation involves activities that fill up conscious awareness with fantasy provided from without, and in doing so a concomitant loss of awareness of self, place, behavior, and passage of time is experienced. (For some people this also may be achieved through the construction of vivid personal fantasies.) In seeking out and engaging in such activities, self-awareness can be reduced and personal concerns thereby dislocated, at least temporarily [see also 58]. In this way, dissociation may act as a psychological clutch allowing the individual to disengage from aversive or wearisome experience (R.W. Garlan, PhD, personal communication, July 8, 2003). Or as Singer suggests, "flights into escapist behaviors ... (may) reflect the painfulness of having to be continuously aware of the variety of unfinished businesses in one's life which cannot be acted upon relatively quickly" [42, p. 734, see also 58].

The adaptive benefit of absorption in externally derived (or internally generated, directed fantasy) material is that it relieves one, at least temporarily, of contemplating one's own more spontaneous internal productions. Such activities, precisely because of their dissociation-inducing aspects, can provide distraction, diversion, or escape [see also 27,52,59], thereby potentially reducing stress and improving mood. (This is similar to the therapeutic uses to which hypnosis often is put, such as managing distress and pain [60,61].) Given that such activities are sought out and engaged in voluntarily, this can be viewed as an instrumental use of normative dissociation for healthy escape that can provide both psychic respite and an opportunity for rejuvenation.

This instrumental use of dissociation is reminiscent of pathological states where maladaptive behaviors are enacted to deploy dissociation to manage affective states, such as when engaging in self-cutting [62] or binge eating [58] to dispel dysphoria [see also 56]. Using dissociation to escape unpleasant or intolerable experiences is a defensive function bridging ordinary and extraordinary experiences. Additionally, the involuntary immersion into a flashback in PTSD or the identity and amnesia of a given alter in dissociative identity disorder may be seen as pathological parallels to the alternate phenomenal reality voluntarily entered into in many recreational or imaginal activities.

Normative dissociation, in the form of positive dissociative or flow experiences, reinforces worthy activities

As discussed previously, there seems to be a third class of normative dissociative experiences, which are characterized by aspects of depersonalization and derealization (including time distortion), but that are unique in their association with distinctively positive affect that arises secondary to personally significant or challenging life experiences. The benefit of dissociating, particularly in the case of flow experiences, is that absorption allows for the full commitment of attention to the activity and a reduction in distractibility and self-consciousness and may, therefore, enhance performance in skilled activities (such as sports or performing) or enhance the flow of creativity. Additionally, the strong positive affect may make these experiences highly positively reinforcing—perhaps signaling the organism that the activities associated with them are life-affirming and worth repeating. Consequently, flow researchers have suggested that these experiences may play a role in the progress and transmission of culture [63].

The benign derealization and marked positive affect of positive dissociative and flow states are a striking counterpoint to the bewildering and incapacitating peritraumatic dissociative symptoms and terror many people endure in the face of trauma. In peritraumatic dissociation, personal significance also is high (as a result of threat) but the experience is aversive because the challenge or danger exceeds or overwhelms existing resources and capabilities. Additionally, Watkins and Watkins [64] have noted the negatively reinforcing effects of dissociation in dissociated states. "If the defensive operation of displacing pain to an 'unconscious' alter is successful, it is reinforced by a lowering of tension. A reinforced process is self-perpetuating" [p. 3].

The potential reinforcing effects of dissociative experiences—reducing boredom, stress, or distress or enhancing mood—would seem to apply equally well to all types of dissociation. To the extent that such experiences yield psychological benefits, they would be sought out either actively or unconsciously. Moreover, this discussion of functions suggests how readily dissociative processes can be recruited to serve a variety of purposes—adaptive or maladaptive. If successful human adaptation and advancement was facilitated by the myriad of opportunities for processing, respite, and pleasurable engagement afforded by normative dissociative experiences, those humans who engaged in them surely had an advantage in the contest for survival.

Otherwise, the tendency for humans to lapse into dissociative experiences of daydreams or fantasy most assuredly would have favored the tiger!

The notion of a dissociative continuum

Theorists observe that dissociative experiences appear to manifest in minor and major forms, falling along a continuum [4,6,52,53,65] that ranges from transient commonplace events involving absorption to more chronic and relatively rare conditions characterized by dissociative pathology. These descriptions imply that experiences sampled at different points on the continuum would be expected to differ on one or a variety of dimensions, including duration and severity, the extent of impact on functioning, the conditions that precipitate them (such as stress or trauma), and their incidence over a lifetime or in the population at large [1].

With reference to these dimensions, everyday dissociative experiences are brief and mild; they do not impair functioning (rather, they seem integral to it); they are not associated with trauma (although other environmental conditions may precipitate them); and they are quotidian and unremarkable experiences for most people. Severe dissociative pathologies, in contrast, may be chronic, severe, and debilitating; are typically associated with tremendously difficult life experiences or histories; and are relatively rare.

The continuum may be illusory, however, because clinical characteristics and prevalence aspects are not the features to which the continuum notion intuitively applies. The invocation of a continuum suggests a *common process*, a meaningful seamlessness between nonpathological and pathological dissociation in that regard; and it also implies *variability* in levels—that experiences at the "major" end presumably have more of whatever the experiences at the "minor" end have [6,66]. And although there is evidence of common process, specifically absorption, in findings that Dalenberg [67] has assembled from her research and that of others that show absorption to be associated strongly with both nonpathological and pathological dissociation, it is not clear that the ends of the continuum differ meaningfully with respect to the level or amount of that process. Indeed, Putnam and colleagues [68] examined whether or not the previously observed "steady progression" [6, p. 730] of DES scores from normal subjects to patients who have dissociative identity disorder represent true differences in DES scores across groups or if, instead, the mean scores were skewed by the proportion of high dissociators within given diagnostic groups. Their analyses indicated the latter: higher average scores within the dissociative disorder and PTSD groups reflected a greater share of highly dissociative individuals in these groups. A different way to consider the issue is to note that nonclinical groups primarily endorse dissociative experiences of absorption and imaginative involvement but are much less likely to endorse items associated more closely with dissociative disorders (eg, memory and identity disturbance items), whereas dissociative patients tend to endorse both [5,7,20,22,67].

Waller and colleagues [5] also revisited the continuum concept and demonstrated that for severe dissociative pathology (such as in DID), the continuum metaphor breaks down and a taxon—or unique type—stands apart. They conclude, "we have discovered that markers of nonpathological dissociation—such as indicators of absorption and imaginative involvement—measure a dimensional construct, whereas markers of pathological dissociation—such as indicators of amnesia for dissociative states, derealization, depersonalization, and identity alteration—measure a latent class or typological construct" [p. 315].

These findings suggest that factors in addition to the basic processes of dissociation are at work in the creation of dissociative syndromes, and one obvious candidate is traumatic experience, particularly in a developmental context. In other words, traumatic experience—perhaps interacting with other factors, such as inadequate developmental environments [9,69]—may distort, constrain, or hijack the fundamental (and normally adaptive) dissociative trait, much as the biology of a bipolar syndrome may be viewed as hijacking the normal trait of affect balance.

Additionally, as Gold [70] observed recently, perhaps the relationship of nonpathological to pathological dissociative phenomena should be likened to the changes that occur in compounds under different conditions. Consider the effects of temperature on water: the liquid form can freeze and become a solid or boil and become a gas. Each arises in a different environmental condition, and each of these phase changes introduces a new state with its own emergent characteristics. By analogy, the syndrome state of a given psychological trait—the apparent "break" in the continuum—represents the psychological equivalent of a phase change. The syndrome of dissociativity—the taxon—that can develop under conditions of traumatic stress may, therefore, encompass both the essential normative dissociativity from which the shift ensues and unique properties of the new state that are determined by the interaction of dissociation with other factors, generating characteristics that cannot be described fully, or perhaps even predicted directly, from the manifestation in normal circumstances.

Summary

Cardeña [71] has advised that, "To be useful as a concept, dissociation should not be applied to ordinary instances of less-than-full engagement with one's surrounding, experiences, and actions. Rather, it should pertain to qualitative departures from one's ordinary modes of experiencing, wherein an unusual disconnection or disengagement from the self or the surrounding occurs as a central aspect of the experience" [p. 23]. Bearing this admonition in mind, it seems reasonable to assert that the utility of the term depends on its ability to capture a distinct, and therefore meaningful, aspect of experience. It does not follow, however, that theorizing necessarily proceed from the premise that what is called dissociation must be by definition unusual and not ordinary.

In this article I have endeavored to make the case for the primacy and ubiquity of dissociation in normal human experience. In most cases, the manifestations of normative dissociation may be understood as instantiations of absorption (and concomitant phenomena) as they operate in different arenas of mental activity. When absorbed in everyday activities, the material or task captures the phenomenological field, allowing for healthy temporary escape into alternate universes or a level of engagement that promotes optimal performance. In daydreaming, absorption engages persistent concerns or unaddressed challenges, with opportunities for resolution arising in part through the flow of wider associations and in part through testing and rehearsal of alternatives in fantasy. In pure fantasy, absorption and the imaginal process are merged to allow for fanciful explorations unconstrained by convention or reality. In dreaming, we may identify dissociation in its involuntariness and memory deficits and in the discontinuity of its phenomenology with the waking state. In most cases the normative dissociative experience is an admixture of absorption and its object, with intense focal concentration and suspension of contextual features—such as self-awareness and reflection, feelings of relatedness to self or the world, constraints of normal thinking, or awareness of volition—which allow for the conditions necessary to the achievement of its benefits. The fact of the pervasiveness of such experiences does not disqualify their essentially dissociative nature.

I have also argued that pathological dissociation represents, at least in part, a disorder of normative dissociative processes by examining the forms (absorption in activities, daydreams, fantasies, and dreams) and functions (processing, escape, and reinforcement) of dissociation in daily life. Additionally, I have discussed some of the implications of these findings for the putative dissociative continuum. By appreciating the pervasiveness, mechanisms, and utility of the dissociations of everyday life, we illuminate one "portion of our being at once most familiar and most mysterious" [72, p. 1] and perhaps, also, gain a fresh vantage point from which to consider the impressive clinical and empirical knowledge base that has accrued in the study of the dissociative disorders.

Acknowledgments

The author thanks Richard A. Chefetz for this opportunity, for his tremendously constructive critiques of and suggestions for this manuscript, and for the good fortune of his graciousness; Robert W. Garlan, as always, for his invaluable observations regarding and contributions to this manuscript; and Xin-Hua Chen for her help in preparing the manuscript.

References

[1] Butler LD. The dissociations of everyday life [editorial]. J Trauma Dissociation 2004;5:1–11.

[2] Butler LD, Duran REF, Jasiukaitis P, et al. Hypnotizability and traumatic experience: a diathesis-stress model of dissociative symptomatology. Am J Psychiatry 1996;153:7, 42–63.

[3] Spiegel DS, Cardeña E. New uses of hypnosis in the treatment of posttraumatic stress disorder. J Clin Psychiatry 1990;51(Oct Suppl):39–43.

[4] Hilgard ER. Divided consciousness: multiple controls in human thought and action. New York: John Wiley & Sons; 1977.

[5] Waller NG, Putnam FW, Carlson EB. Types of dissociation and dissociative types: a taxometric analysis of dissociative experiences. Psychol Methods 1996;1:300–21.

[6] Bernstein EM, Putnam FW. Development, reliability, and validity of a dissociation scale. J Nerv Ment Dis 1986;174:727–35.

[7] Carlson EB, Putnam FW. An update on the Dissociative Experiences Scale. Dissociation 1993;5:16–25.

[8] Hilgard ER. Hypnotic susceptibility. New York: Harcourt Brace Jovanovich; 1965.

[9] Kluft RP. Treatment of multiple personality—a study of 33 cases. Psychiatr Clin North Am 1984;7:9–29.

[10] Spiegel D, Cardeña E. Disintegrated experience: the dissociative disorders revisited. J Abnorm Psychol 1991;100:366–78.

[11] Freud S. The interpretation of dreams. New York: Basic Books; 1965.

[12] Singer JL. Daydreaming—an introduction to the experimental study of inner experience. New York: Random House; 1966. p. 16, 51.

[13] Starker S. Dreams and waking fantasy. In: Pope KS, Singer JL, editors. The stream of consciousness—scientific investigations into the flow of human experience. New York: Plenum Press; 1978. p. 301–19.

[14] Klinger E. Daydreaming. Los Angeles: Jeremy P. Tarcher; 1990. p. xii, 24, 83.

[15] Kihlstrom JF. Conscious, subconscious, unconscious: a cognitive perspective. In: Bowers KS, Meichenbaum D, editors. The unconscious reconsidered. New York: John Wiley & Sons; 1984. p. 149–211.

[16] Barrett DL. The dream character as a prototype for the multiple personality "alter." In: Lynn JS, Rhue JW, editors. Dissociation. Washington, DC: American Psychological Association Press; 1994. p. 123–35.

[17] Castillo RJ. Depersonalization and meditation. Psychiatry. J Study Interpersonal Process 1990;53:158–68.

[18] Luhrmann TM. Yearning for God: trance as a culturally specific practice and its implications for understanding dissociative disorders. J Trauma Dissociation 2004;5:101–29.

[19] Ray WJ, Faith M. Dissociative experiences in a college age population: follow-up with 1190 subjects. Person Individ Diff 1995;18:223–30.

[20] Ross CA, Joshi S, Currie R. Dissociative experiences in the general population. Am J Psychiatry 1990;147:1547–52.

[21] Ross CA, Joshi S, Currie R. Dissociative experiences in the general population: a factor analysis. Hosp Community Psychiatry 1991;42:297–301.

[22] Ray WJ. Dissociation in normal populations. In: Michelson LK, Ray WJ, editors. Handbook of dissociation—theoretical, empirical, and clinical perspectives. New York: Plenum Press; 1996. p. 51–66.

[23] Tellegen A, Atkinson G. Openness to absorbing and self-altering experiences ("absorption"), a trait related to hypnotic susceptibility. J Abnorm Psychol 1974;83:268–77.

[24] Tellegen A. Practicing the two disciplines for relaxation and enlightenment: comment on Qualls and Sheehan. J Exp Psychol 1981;110:217–26.

[25] van der Hart O, Horst R. The dissociation theory of Pierre Janet. J Trauma Stress 1989;2:397–412.

[26] Janet P. The major symptoms of hysteria. London: MacMillan; 1907.

[27] Singer JL, Pope KS. Daydreaming and imagery skills as predisposing capacities for self-hypnosis. Int J Clin Exp Hypn 1981;29:271–81.

[28] Frischholz EJ, Braun BG, Sachs RG, et al. Construct validity of the Dissociative Experiences Scale (DES): I. the relation between the DES and other self-report measures of dissociation. Dissociation 1991;4:185–8.

[29] Frischholz EJ, Lipman LS, Braun BG, et al. Psychopathology, hypnotizability, and dissociation. Am J Psychiatry 1992;149:1521–5.

[30] Rhue JW, Lynn SJ. Fantasy proneness, hypnotizability, and absorption—a re-examination: a brief communication. Int J Clin Exp Hypn 1989;37:100–6.

[31] Kihlstrom JF, Glisky ML, Angiulo MJ. Dissociative tendencies and dissociative disorders. J Abnorm Psychol 1994;103:117–24.

[32] Butler LD, Palesh O. Spellbound: dissociation in the movies. J Trauma Dissociation 2004;5: 63–88.

[33] Silverman K. The subject of semiotics: on suture. In: Brady L, Cohen M, editors. Film theory and criticism. New York: Oxford University Press; 1998. p. 137–47.

[34] Pica M, Beere D. Dissociation during positive situations. Dissociation 1995;8:241–6.

[35] Csikszentmihalyi M. Flow: the psychology of optimal experience. New York: HarperCollins; 1990.

[36] Nakamura J, Csikszentmihalyi M. The concept of flow. In: Snyder CR, Lopez SJ, editors. Handbook of positive psychology. London: Oxford Press; 2002. p. 89–105.

[37] Maslow A. The farther reaches of human nature. New York: Viking; 1971.

[38] Csikszentmihalyi M. Attention and the holistic approach to behavior. In: Pope KS, Singer JL, editors. The stream of consciousness—scientific investigations into the flow of human experience. New York: Plenum Press; 1978. p. 335–58.

[39] Klinger E. Modes of normal conscious flow. In: Pope KS, Singer JL, editors. The stream of consciousness—scientific investigations into the flow of human experience. New York: Plenum Press; 1978. p. 225–58.

[40] Singer JL. Experimental studies of daydreaming and the stream of thought. In: Pope KS, Singer JL, editors. The stream of consciousness—scientific investigations into the flow of human experience. New York: Plenum Press; 1978. p. 187–223.

[41] Klinger E. Structure and functions of fantasy. New York: John Wiley; 1971.

[42] Singer JL. Navigating the stream of consciousness: research in daydreaming and related inner experience. Am Psychol 1975;30:727–38.

[43] Singer JL, McCraven V. Some characteristics of adult daydreaming. J Psychol 1961;51: 151–64.

[44] Giambra LM. Frequency and intensity of daydreaming: age changes and age differences from late adolescent to the old-old. Imagination Cognition Personality 1999–2000;19: 229–67.

[45] Singer JL, Antrobus JS. Daydreaming, imaginal processes, and personality: a normative study. In: Sheehan PW, editor. The function and nature of imagery. New York: Academic Press; 1972. p. 175–202.

[46] Wilson SC, Barber TX. Vivid fantasy and hallucinatory abilities in the life histories of excellent hypnotic subjects ("somnambules"): preliminary report with female subjects. In: Klinger E, editor. Imagery, vol. 2, Concepts, results, and applications. New York: Plenum; 1981. p. 158–72.

[47] Wilson SC, Barber TX. The fantasy-prone personality: implications for understanding imagery, hypnosis, and parapsychological phenomena. In: Sheikh AA, editor. Imagery: current theory, research, and application. New York: Wiley; 1983. p. 340–87.

[48] Lynn SJ, Rhue JW. Fantasy proneness: hypnosis, developmental antecedents, and psychopathology. Am Psychol 1988;43:35–44.

[49] James W. The principles of psychology. New York: Dover; 1950.

[50] Starker S. Daydreaming styles and nocturnal dreaming. J Abnorm Psychol 1974;83:52–5.

[51] Kripke DF, Sonneschein D. A biological rhythm in waking fantasy. In: Pope KS, Singer JL, editors. The stream of consciousness—scientific investigations into the flow of human experience. New York: Plenum Press; 1978. p. 321–32.

[52] Ludwig AM. The psychobiological functions of dissociation. Am J Clin Hypn 1983;26: 93–9.

[53] Putnam FW. The diagnosis and treatment of multiple personality disorder. New York: Guilford; 1989.

[54] Spiegel D. Multiple personality as a post-traumatic stress disorder. Psychiatr Clin North Am 1984;7:101–10.

[55] Horowitz MJ. Stress response syndromes. Northvale (NJ): Aronson; 1986.

[56] Somer E. Maladaptive daydreaming: a qualitative inquiry. J Contemp Psychother 2002;32: 197–212.

[57] Reynolds M, Brewin C. Intrusive memories in depression and posttraumatic stress disorder. Behav Res Ther 1999;37:201–15.

[58] Baumeister RF. Escaping the self: alcoholism, spirituality, masochism and other flights from the burden of selfhood. New York: Basic Books; 1991.

[59] Hilgard JR. Personality and hypnosis: a study of imaginative involvement. Chicago: University of Chicago Press; 1970.

[60] Hilgard ER, Hilgard JR. Hypnosis in the relief of pain. Los Altos, CA: William Kauffman; 1975.

[61] Spiegel H, Spiegel D. Trance and treatment: clinical uses of hypnosis. New York: Basic Books; 2004.

[62] Gardner DL, Cowdry RW. Suicidal and parasuicidal behavior in borderline personality disorder. Psychiatr Clin North Am 1985;8:389–403.

[63] Massimini F, Delle Fave A. Individual development in a bio-cultural perspective. Am Psychol 2000;55:24–33.

[64] Watkins JG, Watkins HH. Ego states—theory and therapy. New York: W.W. Norton; 1997.

[65] Nemiah JC. Dissociative disorders. In: Kaplan HI, Sadock BJ, editors. Comprehensive textbook of psychiatry. 5th edition. Baltimore: Williams & Wilkins; 1981. p. 1028–44.

[66] Taylor WS, Martin MF. Multiple personality. J Abnorm Soc Psychol 1944;39:281–300.

[67] Dalenberg CJ. What is normal about normal and pathological dissociation? The dissociative continuum: views from the nonpathological end. Presented at the Annual Meeting of the International Society for the Study of Dissociation. New Orleans, LA; November 2004.

[68] Putnam FW, Carlson EB, Ross CA, et al. Patterns of dissociation in clinical and nonclinical samples. J Nerv Ment Dis 1996;184:673–9.

[69] Gold SN. Not trauma alone: therapy for child abuse survivors in family and social context. New York: Brunner-Routledge; 2000.

[70] Gold SN, discussant. The dissociative continuum: views from the nonpathological end. Presented at the Annual Meeting of the International Society for the Study of Dissociation. New Orleans, LA; November 2004.

[71] Cardeña E. The domain of dissociation. In: Lynn JS, Rhue JW, editors. Dissociation. Washington, DC: American Psychological Association Press; 1994. p. 1–31.

[72] Pope KS, Singer JL. Introduction: the flow of human experience. In: Pope KS, Singer JL, editors. The stream of consciousness—scientific investigations into the flow of human experience. New York: Plenum Press; 1978. p. 1–6.

ELSEVIER
SAUNDERS

PSYCHIATRIC
CLINICS
OF NORTH AMERICA

Psychiatr Clin N Am 29 (2006) 63–86

From Infant Attachment Disorganization to Adult Dissociation: Relational Adaptations or Traumatic Experiences?

Karlen Lyons-Ruth, PhD[a],*, Lissa Dutra, EdM, MA[b],
Michelle R. Schuder, PhD[a], Ilaria Bianchi, MA[c]

[a]Harvard Medical School, Cambridge Hospital, Department of Psychiatry,
1493 Cambridge Street, Cambridge, MA 02139, USA
[b]Department of Psychology, Boston University, 648 Beacon Street, 4th Floor,
Boston, MA 02215, USA
[c]Department of Psychology, Catholic University of the Sacred Heart,
Largo Gemelli 1, 20123 Milan, Italy

In 1997, Putnam [1] pointed out that relatively little was known about the etiology and development of dissociation other than the presumed etiologic role of trauma; however, the fact that nontraumatized individuals sometimes demonstrated dissociation and that not all trauma survivors dissociate suggested that there may be more to the etiology and development of dissociation than trauma alone. Putnam [1] explored the role of various potential moderating variables including age, sex, culture, genetic factors, and education/intelligence in the development of dissociation, and although moderating trends were found for some of these variables, existing research has not convincingly demonstrated that any of these variables significantly influence dissociation.

Family environmental factors, however, are the one set of factors that have been most consistently related to dissociation. Factors such as inconsistent parenting or disciplining, [2–4] level of family risk [5], and parental dissociation, as measured by the Dissociative Experiences Scale [6], have been shown to be associated significantly with higher levels of dissociation in adulthood. Most available research on dissociation, however, has focused on trauma, leaving many unanswered questions regarding how other family

* Corresponding author.
E-mail address: klruth@hms.harvard.edu (K. Lyons-Ruth).

0193-953X/06/$ - see front matter © 2005 Elsevier Inc. All rights reserved.
doi:10.1016/j.psc.2005.10.011

factors intersect with familial abuse in the developmental trajectories leading to dissociative disorders.

Barach [7] was one of the first theorists to connect dissociation with attachment theory. In his article, Barach [7] suggested that multiple personality disorder (now known as dissociative identity disorder) was a variant of an "attachment disorder." He pointed out that individuals who had this disorder tended to demonstrate the extreme detachment, or emotional unresponsiveness, experienced by children faced with a loss of their primary caretaker, as described by Bowlby [8]. Barach [7] further suggested that children of unresponsive caretakers were also likely to engage in dissociative or "detached" behaviors. As one offshoot of attachment studies, developmental theorists and researchers have begun to explore the role of early childhood attachment and parenting in the etiology and development of dissociative symptomatology.

Liotti's [9] theorizing has more specifically implicated disorganized patterns of infant attachment behavior as potential precursors to the development of dissociation later in life. He pointed out that there are parallels between infant disorganization and dissociation. Both phenomena reflect a pervasive lack of behavioral or mental integration. This primary failure of integration in infancy may result in vulnerability to dissociative organization of mental life in the developing child and grown adult. Liotti's view might be best conceptualized as a vulnerability model in which early dyadic processes lead to a "primary breakdown" or lack of integration of a coherent sense of self. Liotti's model offers an alternative to the theory that the primary function and etiology of dissociation is as a defense against trauma. Although Liotti [9] did not suggest that disorganized attachment is the only etiologic factor in dissociation, he hypothesized that disorganized attachment patterns constitute an initial step in the developmental trajectories that leave an individual vulnerable to developing dissociation in response to later experiences of trauma.

Bowlby [8] first suggested that infants may internalize unintegrated internal working models of their relationships with primary caregivers and of themselves in relation to those caregivers. Main and Hesse [10] further hypothesized that parents of disorganized infants may engage in frightened or frightening interactions with their children, thereby presenting the infant with the paradox that the parent is a source of threat and a source of protection. Under these paradoxic conditions, during times of stress when the attachment system is activated, contradictory internal working models of self and other may become evident. These seemingly incompatible models of the parent as a source of fear and a source of protection from fear are similar to Barach's [7] model of an abusive parent causing a child to be faced with the incompatible notion that his parent is his protector and his persecutor.

Main and Hesse [10] further theorized that when the parent appears frightened in his or her interactions with the infant, the infant may infer that there is something threatening in the environment that should be feared. Although such a perceived environmental threat would lead a securely attached infant to approach his parent for protection, a frightened parent may communicate apprehension to the child. Under these conditions, the infant may sense the helplessness of the parent in the face of threat and demonstrate conflict about approaching him or her for protection by displaying contradictory simultaneous or sequential approach-avoidance behaviors typical of disorganized detachment. Alternatively, the parent's frightened stance may cause the child to infer that he, himself, is frightening the parent, again leading to conflict in approaching and further threatening an already frightened parent. Lyons-Ruth and colleagues [11,12] demonstrated that parental withdrawal from the infant's attachment overtures at times of infant arousal is also associated with infant disorganization, whether or not the parent's behavior is directly frightened or frightening to the infant. Thus, the infant's internalization of contradictory models of the self as frightened or threatening and of the parent as hostile or helpless/withdrawing can be conceptualized in terms of contradictory models that generate incompatible behavioral and mental tendencies. This primary lack of integration around basic strategies for seeking comfort and protection under stress is what Liotti [9] suggested may confer vulnerability to dissociative processes later in life.

Liotti [9] further speculated that there are three pathways that disorganized infants might take toward (or away from) the development of dissociative symptomatology. In the first pathway, there is no further trauma, and interactions with the parent become less fear imbued and more consistent over the childhood years. Regardless of whether this consistency is positive or negative, Liotti [9] posited that this would result in the child's eventually choosing one of the available incompatible working models of attachment relationships and developing in accordance with that working model. The second pathway, in which parent-child interactions continue to be inconsistent and contradictory but the child does not encounter severe trauma, would lead to infrequent dissociation during times of extreme stress. In this scenario, although the child is viewed as vulnerable to the development of dissociative symptoms, there are not sufficient environmental stressors to potentiate this vulnerability, leaving the child asymptomatic or displaying only mild or fleeting dissociative symptoms. In the third pathway, the disorganized/disoriented infant is predisposed to dissociation, has ongoing severe stressors, and vulnerability is potentiated. Here, the child experiences continued reinforcement of increasingly unintegrated simultaneous/ sequential contradictory internal working models of self-other relatedness and repetitive severe trauma. This child is likely to move toward the extreme of developing dissociative identity disorder.

Liotti's model of early difficulties in achieving an integrated set of behavioral and mental responses to fear or threat offers a strong hypothesis for why it is that some people exposed to trauma develop dissociation, whereas others do not. This model suggests that disorganized attachment negatively impacts the onset of early individually based processes of mental integration that become the basis for later dissociation. Although Liotti's model sets forth the notion that infant disorganization lays the groundwork and acts as a key precursor for the development of dissociation, experiences of significant trauma remain an important and necessary factor in this diathesis-stress model.

Does infant attachment disorganization contribute to the development of adult dissociative symptoms?

Aspects of Liotti's model have recently been empirically supported by longitudinal studies. Ogawa and colleagues [13] tested Liotti's model in a sample of 126 children from low-income environments followed from birth to age 19 years. Dissociative symptoms were assessed at age 19 years with the standard Dissociative Experiences Scale [14]. From a trauma-based model of the etiology of dissociation, one might expect trauma to be the strongest predictor of adult dissociative symptoms—and trauma did correlate with later symptoms. Specifically, chronicity of abuse, severity of abuse, and age of onset of abuse were highly intercorrelated, and prediction from overall chronicity, severity, and age of onset of abuse to clinical levels of dissociation at age 19 years (Dissociative Experiences Scale–taxon scale) was modest (canonic $r = 0.25$; 6% variance explained). Prediction from maternal psychologic unavailability and disorganized attachment in the first 24 months of life, however, was much stronger (canonic $r = 0.58$; 34% variance explained). In addition and most important, trauma history did not significantly add to the prediction of dissociation in young adulthood after accounting for maternal psychologic unavailability and disorganized attachment in the first 24 months of life. Although concurrent abuse made a contribution to the prediction of dissociation-like behaviors judged by teachers during the school years, even at this age, the effects of early care and attachment continued to be independent predictors of dissociation, unmediated by concurrent abuse.

A secondary but less powerful analysis was also reported by Ogawa and colleagues [13] that appeared to establish a role for traumatic events in potentiating the relationship between disorganized attachment and later dissociation. The independent influence of early caregiving on dissociation was not included in that analysis, however, making it difficult to integrate that partial analysis with the results of the more powerful and inclusive multivariate regression analysis also presented.

These findings support the conceptualization of disorganized attachment as one key precursor in the development of dissociation; however, contrary to Liotti's model, the findings also suggest that disorganization of attachment may be more central to the development of dissociation than the trauma itself. Furthermore, infant disorganized attachment behaviors and parental emotional unavailability made separate and independent contributions to prediction. Therefore, Ogawa and colleagues [13] study also demonstrated that parental factors beyond those that overlapped with disorganized attachment in infancy predispose children to the development of dissociation; however, the measure of parental emotional unavailability used in the study was based on global clinical ratings and has not been further defined or replicated outside the original laboratory [15]. Further, the evidence indicates that such parent-child communication processes may produce dissociative symptoms even when the infant's attachment strategies are not disorganized during the first 2 years of life, suggesting that infant disorganization may be a sufficient but not necessary component in the development of dissociation. Instead, something in the parent-infant dialog itself may independently influence the development of dissociation. The word *dialogue* is used here in the broadest sense to encompass all meaningful verbal and affective communications between the child and the parent because early in life, the parent-infant dialog primarily involves exchange of affective signals.

Dutra and Lyons-Ruth [16] also investigated the association between infant attachment and the later development of dissociative symptoms in a second prospective longitudinal sample of 56 infants at social risk followed from birth to age 19 years. Participants were low–socioeconomic status, at-risk families and, as in the Ogawa and colleagues' [13] study, adolescent dissociative symptomatology was measured by the Dissociative Experiences Scale [14] at age 19 years. Results of this second longitudinal study confirm and extend Ogawa and colleagues' [13] findings. Analyses indicated that five measures of infant, childhood, and adolescent maltreatment failed to predict adolescent dissociative symptomatology. Maternal post-traumatic stress disorder, depressive symptoms, and depressive and anxiety disorders also failed to predict adolescent dissociation. Only concurrent maternal dissociative symptoms were related to dissociative symptoms in the adolescent. In contrast, infant disorganization, maternal lack of involvement with the infant at home at 12 months, and disrupted maternal affective communication in the laboratory at 18 months contributed significantly to the prediction of dissociative symptoms at age 19 years.

As in the Ogawa and colleagues' [13] study, when all predictors were considered together, only the measures of early care were independent predictors of later symptoms. In contrast to the Ogawa and colleagues' [13] study, however, and somewhat in contrast to the Liotti hypothesis, the maternal care measures were stronger predictors of dissociation at age 19 years than the measure of infant disorganization itself. When the quality of early caregiving was accounted for, infant disorganization no longer added to the prediction of dissociation. The difference between these results and those of Ogawa and colleagues' [13] is likely due to the more comprehensive measures of maternal care in infancy that were included in these analyses. The pathway toward adult dissociative symptoms seems more heavily influenced by the potentially enduring context of disrupted forms of parent-child communication than by the early vulnerability to mental segregation in-dexed by the infant's disorganized attachment behaviors.

These two sets of findings indicate that the pathways from infant disor-ganization to adult dissociation may be more dynamic and complex than they seem at first glance. Liotti's "first pathway" of development represents disorganized infants who experience more stability with their parent later in life and manage to "escape" becoming vulnerable to dissociation by settling on one of their contradictory models of self and other. This pathway offers a model for why not all disorganized infants develop dissociative symptom-atology later in life. Disorganized infants who later show dissociative symp-toms may be on a different pathway, however, in that the continuation of what Liotti termed "inconsistent interactions with their parents" may serve to reinforce or crystallize their vulnerability to developing dissociation in the face of stressors. In fact, the Ogawa and colleagues' [13] study indicated that deviant parenting may lead to the experience of serious dissociative symp-toms (taxon symptoms on the standard questionnaire [14]), even in the ab-sence of traumatic stressors. This population, however, is under-represented in inpatient settings and neglected in dissociation research. Thus, a more nuanced exploration is warranted of enduring patterns of disrupted par-ent-child communication processes, processes that may act to continually reinforce the child's segregated and contradictory mental processes. Such ex-ploration might facilitate a better understanding of the population of non-abused individuals who have serious dissociative symptoms and help fill in some of the theoretic gaps inherent in the models of dissociation that have been reviewed thus far.

These results also begin to offer hypotheses regarding the specific aspects of the parent-infant dialog that may be linked to later dissociation. Liotti [9] posited a link between infant disorganization and later dissociation based on the concept of multiple, unintegrated working models of the parent. This hy-pothesis, however, mostly stems from the contradictory behavioral tenden-cies observed in the disorganized infant, not from theory regarding parental characteristics. In contrast, the parental behaviors hypothesized to relate to infant disorganization have been parental behaviors that are frightened, frightening, or disrupted in overall affective communication patterns. Paren-tal inconsistency per se has not been a part of the theorizing regarding pre-dictors of infant disorganization. Instead, parental inconsistency has been linked in earlier theory to organized but ambivalent/resistant infant attach-ment strategies. Lyons-Ruth and colleagues [12] hypothesized that hostile/frightening and helpless/fearful parenting stances are alternate aspects of a single hostile/helpless internal working model, but to date no study has at-tempted to isolate the role of contradiction in maternal behavior compared with consistent frightening or other disrupted behavior patterns in the etiol-ogy of infant disorganization or later dissociation.

The caregiving predictors related to later dissociation in these two longi-tudinal studies converge in underscoring aspects of the mother's unavailability to respond to the infant's attachment cues as key precursors to dissociative symptoms. Although Ogawa and colleagues [13] did not examine a variety of features of the early parent-infant dialog, their analysis highlighted one aspect that they termed "psychologic unavailability." In addition, neglect in the first 2 years of life contributed to clinically significant dissociative symptoms at some ages in that study. In the Dutra and Lyons-Ruth [16] study, a similar measure of lack of responsive involvement with the infant was the strongest predictor among the four dimensions of maternal home behavior coded from videotapes.

Maternal hostile/frightening behavior was another dimension that was expected to relate to dissociation because of the central role of maternal frightening behavior in theories of infant disorganization and the central role of abuse in theories of dissociation. Maternal hostile or intrusive behaviors coded at home or in the laboratory, however, were one of the weakest predictors, even though these hostile behavior codes included codes for frightening maternal behaviors and were related to other negative child outcomes in the study. Therefore, the "quieter" caregiving deviations such as withdrawing from emotional contact, being unresponsive to the child's overtures, or displaying contradictory, role-reversed, or disoriented responses when the infant's attachment needs are heightened appear to be the maternal responses most implicated in pathways toward dissociation.

It is important to note that both of these studies examined the relative influence of infant disorganization and maternal care with respect to moderate levels of dissociation. These data do not rule out the possibility that traumatic experiences are influential in the genesis of the more severe forms of dissociation captured by the diagnosis of dissociative identity disorder. These findings suggest that the caregiving context is likely to play more of a major role in all forms of dissociation than previously thought and needs to be conceptualized and assessed separately from traumatic events. Accordingly, the potential relative contribution of these variables with respect to the development of dissociative disorders remains an area for future research. In addition, other factors in childhood and adolescence are yet to be examined as mediators of these effects and, thus, it is possible that experiences other than trauma during childhood and adolescence, such as the development of behavior problems or the quality of later parent-child interaction, may be critical in mediating the association between early deviations in care and later dissociation. The existence of such later mediators, however, do not discount the importance of the finding that pathways to dissociation begin in infancy and are grounded in aspects of parent-infant interaction.

Redefining stress and trauma in infancy: the hypothesis of hidden trauma

As discussed by Schuder and Lyons-Ruth [17], the traditional perspective on trauma views trauma from the perspective of the traumatic event and its characteristics. According to the *Diagnostic and Statistical Manual of*

Mental Disorders, Fourth Edition [18], a traumatic event involves threat to the physical integrity of oneself or another person. In human infancy, however, experienced threat is closely related to the caregiver's affective signals and availability rather than to the actual degree of physical or survival threat inherent in the event itself. Equipped with limited behavioral and cognitive coping capacities, the infant cannot gauge the actual degree of threat. Instead, primary experiences of threat in infancy include the threat of separation from the caregiver and the threat of having little caregiver response to the infant's signals of distress.

Thus, the relevant traumas of infancy most often result from the "hidden traumas" of caregiver unavailablity and interactive dysregulation. These hidden traumas are woven into the fabric of interaction between caregiver and infant and do not necessarily stand out as salient events to the observer. Physiologic evidence reviewed later reveals that these more subtle traumatic events during infancy engender physiologic consequences similar to threat events salient for older children and adults. Hidden traumas of infancy seem to contribute to the early hyper- or hyporegulation of stress responses mediated through the limbic hypothalamic-pituitary-adrenocortical (LHPA) axis.

The role of fearful arousal

The attachment system was considered by Bowlby [19] to be a preadapted behavioral system for combating and reducing fearful arousal and maintaining a sense of felt security. Contrary to general clinical usage, from a theoretic perspective, the attachment system is only one of a number of goal-corrected behavioral/motivational systems that operate within relationships, and all or most of the interactions between parents and children are not integral to the attachment system, even in infancy. For example, interactions around play, teaching, or even routine caregiving do not necessarily engage emergency attachment motivations or affects.

Under normal conditions, an adequately functioning attachment relationship in which the infant can openly signal discomfort and receive a sensitive response from the caregiver serves to buffer the infant against extreme levels of fearful arousal. The attachment system itself, however, may also malfunction. Based on accumulated research findings, disorganized and controlling forms of attachment behavior are now thought to represent a malfunction of the attachment relational system in infancy and childhood that exposes the infant to excessive unmodulated stress [20,21]. In addition, sometime between age 18 months and 6 years, with the cognitive developments of the preschool period, many formerly disorganized infants reorganize their attachment behaviors into what are termed "controlling" attachment behaviors toward the parent. These controlling behaviors can take two very different forms: controlling through punitive, hostile, or humiliating behaviors or controlling through more solicitous, directing, caregiving behaviors. These controlling strategies are seen as strategies for maintaining the involvement and attention of the caregiver by organizing or directing the behavior of the parent or by engaging in provocative or hostile behavior that creates parental engagement [20]. There is striking discontinuity in the shift from disorganized behavior in infancy to a controlling strategy in the preschool period, in that the surface behaviors and the apparent emotional tone of the attachment-related interactions become different from the hesitant, apprehensive, or conflicted behaviors observed in infancy. Because extensive longitudinal data have not been available to chart this process of reorganization over time, little is understood about when these changes typically occur, what proportion of disorganized infants are able to make this developmental shift, and what strengths or vulnerabilities are associated with the transition to controlling forms of attachment. Both groups of controlling children, however, show deviations in fantasy play and elevated rates of behavior problems with peers in school [20].

Although the attachment relational system is viewed as only a single circumscribed motivational system among other systems, it is also regarded as pre-emptive when aroused because it mobilizes responses to fear or threat. In that sense, the quality of regulation of fearful affect available in attachment relationships is foundational to the developing child's freedom to turn attention away from issues of threat and security toward other developmental achievements, such as exploration, learning, and play.

A large body of earlier research on fearful arousal has documented the range of individual coping responses to pain or fear, captured by the summary label "fight or flight." In addition, Seligman [22] and others described "freezing" and "learned helplessness" as responses occurring when more active responses are unavailable or ineffective. Recently, Taylor and colleagues [23] advanced an alternative "tend or befriend" hypothesis regarding primary responses to threat among social primates, arguing that fight or flight may be more relevant to male stress responses, whereas various forms of affiliative responses may be more common in female stress responses. From an attachment point of view, however, affiliative responses to threat would be expected to be important to all social primates without regard to sex because it is a basic system for regulation of early arousal, and no major differences between the sexes have emerged in the research literature to date.

This entire array of coping or defensive responses to the arousal of fear appears, in some form, in the behaviors associated with the disorganized/controlling spectrum of attachment behaviors. These behaviors are often brief and seem puzzling or contradictory. It is unfortunate that their significance was not recognized during the first 15 years of attachment research. The formal criteria for defining disorganized behaviors are summarized in Box 1. These sequences of behavior are often considered disorganized when evidence of two or more contradictory behavioral tendencies appear to be competing for expression. This conflict at the level of behavioral

---

Box 1. Indices of disorganized-disoriented infant attachment behavior

1. Sequential display of contradictory behavior patterns, such as strong attachment behavior suddenly followed by avoidance, freezing, or dazed behaviors
2. Simultaneous display of contradictory behaviors, such as strong avoidance with strong contact-seeking, distress, or anger
3. Undirected, misdirected, incomplete, and interrupted movements and expressions; for example, extensive expressions of distress accompanied by movement away from rather than toward the mother
4. Stereotypies, asymmetric movements, mistimed movements, and anomalous postures such as stumbling for no apparent reason and only when the parent is present
5. Freezing, stilling, and slowed "underwater" movements and expressions
6. Direct indices of apprehension regarding the parent, such as hunched shoulders and fearful facial expressions
7. Direct indices of disorganization and disorientation, such as disoriented wandering, confused or dazed expressions, or multiple, rapid changes in affect

---

Adapted from Main M, Solomon J. Procedures for identifying infants as disorganized/disoriented during the Ainsworth strange situation. In: Greenberg M, Cicchetti D, Cummings EM, editors. Attachment in the preschool years: theory, research and intervention. Chicago: University of Chicago Press; 1990. p. 121–60.

---

tendencies in infancy is thought to foreshadow later, more internalized forms of conflict in childhood and adolescence, including dissociative phenomena.

Another form of atypical attachment behavior distinct from disorganization may also be relevant to dissociation. This behavior is the indiscriminate attachment behavior seen among infants reared in institutional settings with very poor care and with no selective attachment figure available [24]. A lack of selectivity in attachment behavior is also noted clinically among high-risk home-reared infants and can be observed in the standard attachment assessment in the infant's tendency to accept comfort from an unfamiliar laboratory assistant even though actively distressed. In recent work, such indiscriminate attachment behavior was also associated with disrupted affective communication between parent and infant, particularly disoriented behaviors on the part of the parent, and strongly predictive of later behavior problems in the child [25,26]. Indiscriminate attachment behavior may also be relevant to later dissociation, given its relation to unresponsive care. This form of attachment behavior has not yet been studied in relation to dissociation.

Attachment quality, the limbic hypothalamic-pituitary-adrenocortical axis, and hidden trauma

A growing body of literature suggests that hypothalamic-pituitary-adrenocortical axis activity in infants and young children varies with characteristics of the caregiving environment and the quality of the child's relationship with the caregiver [27–29]. As noted by Spangler and Schieche [27], research on infant adrenocortical function in response to separation from the parent indicates that infants classified as securely attached do not demonstrate elevations in cortisol levels [21,30]. The pattern typically observed is one of decreasing cortisol levels from the beginning to 30 minutes after the end of the procedure. In contrast, studies examining disorganized patterns of attachment behavior have found that disorganized children produce larger increases in cortisol in response to separation and reunion than children classified as securely or insecurely attached [21,31]. In related work, Ashman and colleagues [28] presented evidence that a mother's depression in the first 2 years of the child's life is the best predictor of cortisol elevations at age 7 years. Similarly, in a study of 282 4.5-year-old children, Essex and colleagues [32] reported that maternal depression beginning in infancy was the most potent predictor of children's cortisol levels at 4.5 years of age.

As is also the case in other species [33,34], it appears that a sensitive and responsive caregiving system can provide an LHPA axis buffer for the human infant and toddler. When the caregiving system functions adequately, the young child appears to be able to experience conditions that elicit behavioral distress and that produce inhibition of approach or fearfulness without producing increases in glucocorticoids. This point is elaborated by Spangler and Grossmann [30] who argued that securely attached infants possess appropriate stress-reducing behavioral strategies in relation to the caregiver and therefore exhibit negligible increases in cortisol levels when aroused.

Other work that may be relevant to the hypothesis of hidden trauma in the early caregiving system, with specific reference to the emotional unavailability of caregivers, are studies of orphanage-reared children. Children reared in orphanages in Romania have been the focus of several studies of the relation between environmental regulation and LHPA axis activity. Ten years ago, Romanian orphanages were described as grossly depriving; that is, lacking in social stimulation, physical stimulation, and opportunities for attachment relationships [35]. Carlson and colleagues [36,37] assessed salivary cortisol levels among toddlers in Romanian orphanages over several days at wakeup, noon, and late afternoon/evening in a group of 2-year-olds who had lived in the orphanage for most of their lives. Compared with home-reared two-year-old Romanian children, the orphanage-reared children showed no evidence of the expectable daily rhythm in cortisol levels (a peak in the morning, at half of morning levels by late afternoon, and negligible levels by midnight) over the daytime hours. Moreover, many of the orphanage-reared children appeared to have lower than expected morning levels of cortisol compared with family-reared children. In addition, as reported by Gunnar and colleagues [29], Russian children under age 4 years living in orphanage settings evidence a similarly absent daily rhythm in cortisol production [38].

These findings from orphanage-rearing studies are consistent with reports of daytime cortisol patterns for neglected infants reared in their families of origin [38] and for preschool-aged children in foster care [39]. Gilles and colleagues [40] investigated daytime cortisol levels in family-reared infants who were characterized as low risk for neglect, high risk for neglect, or neglected. Salivary cortisol was assessed in the morning, at noon, and in the evening. The neglected and high-risk groups had a flatter and lower pattern of daytime cortisol production than the low-risk infants. Neglected infants demonstrated the lowest early morning levels and had the flattest pattern of daytime cortisol production.

In sum, the evidence suggests that the organization of LHPA axis activity during infancy is substantially under the influence of caregiver regulation. The infant whose caregiver has been unable to provide basic regulation around fearful arousal fails to develop a coherent attachment strategy for reducing physiologic arousal in the face of moderate stress, leading to under- or overactivity in the stress-response system.

The disrupted parent-infant dialogue

If disrupted parental affective communication in infancy is one of the most powerful predictors of early disorganization and later dissociative symptoms, what do those responses look like? First, surprisingly, parental behavior that is coded as insensitive, using the standard but very global rating scale for sensitivity, has been only weakly correlated with infant disorganized attachment behavior [41]. This failure of parental sensitivity to relate to disorganization is most likely due to methodologic factors such as the diversity of parental profiles within the disorganized group and the lack of detailed behavioral descriptors in the most widely used scale for rating sensitivity.

Statistically, 15% of infants in relatively advantaged and apparently low-risk samples display disorganized attachment strategies [41]. Given the role of fearful arousal and physiologic stress responses in the theory and data on disorganization, it is tempting to equate disorganized attachment strategies with clearly maltreating relationships because maltreatment is associated with infant disorganization [42]. That criterion for problematic parental behavior, however, is too extreme to account for the range of parental behaviors observed to be associated with disorganized strategies. How, then, do we capture the parental behaviors most important to the infant's stress regulation?

The measure of disrupted affective communication used in the Dutra and Lyons-Ruth [16] study coded five aspects of parental behavior that included all indices of Main and Hesse's frightened or frightening behavior inventory (M. Main and E. Hesse, unpublished data, 1992). These five aspects included (1) a set of responses termed "affective communication errors," which included simultaneous conflicting affective cues to the infant and failures to respond to clear affective signals from the infant; (2) disoriented responses; (3) negative-intrusive responses; (4) role-confused responses; and (5) parental withdrawing responses. All five classes of behavior could be coded reliably; intraclass r values ranged from 0.73 to 0.84. Box 2 gives examples of each type of disrupted communication.

Higher levels of disrupted maternal behavior in the separation procedure were associated with infant disorganized attachment strategies in the laboratory and with increased infant distress at home. It was also important that the infant's sex or cumulative demographic risk was not significantly related to maternal disrupted behavior [11]. Three additional laboratories have applied this coding system to mother-infant cohorts across a broad socioeconomic range outside the separation procedure and replicated the link to infant disorganization [43–45].

Hostile or helpless profiles of parenting

The most clinically interesting and unexpected finding regarding the parental affective communication patterns within the disorganized group was that mothers of disorganized infants were even more different from one another than they were from other mothers whose infants were not disorganized. In other words, two polarized types of behavioral profiles were observed within the group of mothers whose children had been classified as disorganized. The authors assigned the summary labels of "hostile/self-referential" or "helpless/fearful" to these two subgroups of mothers and infants. Elsewhere, Lyons-Ruth and colleagues [12] reasoned that these differing constellations of behavior can be meaningfully explained as alternate behavioral expressions of a single underlying hostile/helpless dyadic internal working model of attachment relationships.

Parents who displayed the parenting profile labeled hostile/self-referential had significantly higher rates of role confusion (self-referential behavior) and negative-intrusive behavior than the helpless/fearful subgroup of mothers. Negative-intrusive and role-confused behaviors were also strongly correlated; these parents displayed a contradictory mix of rejecting behaviors and behaviors that sought attention from their infants. Infants of hostile/self-referential mothers were more likely to show a complex mix of disorganized, avoidant, and resistant behaviors.

Box 2. Dimensions of disrupted maternal affective communication

1. Affective errors
   a. Contradictory cues (eg, invites approach verbally, then distances)
   b. Nonresponse or inappropriate response (eg, does not offer comfort to distressed infant)
2. Disorientation (items from M. Main and E. Hesse, unpublished data, 1992)
   a. Confused or frightened by infant (eg, exhibits frightened expression)
   b. Disorganized or disoriented (eg, sudden loss of affect unrelated to environment)
3. Negative-intrusive behavior (including frightening items from M. Main and E. Hesse, unpublished data, 1992)
   a. Verbal negative-intrusive behavior (eg, mocks or teases infant)
   b. Physical negative-intrusive behavior (eg, pulls infant by the wrist)
4. Role confusion (includes items from Sroufe and colleagues[46]; M. Main and E. Hesse, unpublished data, 1992)
   a. Role reversal (eg, elicits reassurance from infant)
   b. Sexualization (eg, speaks in hushed, intimate tones to infant)
5. Withdrawal
   a. Creates physical distance (eg, holds infant away from body with stiff arms)
   b. Creates verbal distance (eg, does not greet infant after separation)

In contrast, mothers who were labeled helpless/fearful regarding attachment were more fearful, withdrawing, and inhibited and sometimes appeared particularly sweet or fragile. They were unlikely to be overtly hostile or intrusive and usually gave in to the infant's concerted bids for contact; however, they often failed to take the initiative in greeting or approaching the infant and often hesitated, moved away, or tried to deflect the infant's requests for close contact before giving in. Infants of helpless/fearful mothers looked different from infants of hostile/self-referential mothers, in that they continued to express their distress, approach their mothers, and gain some physical contact with them, even though they also displayed disorganized behaviors including signs of conflict, apprehension, uncertainty, helplessness, or dysphoria. In other words, these parents "advertised" some potential for responsive contact, and then often delivered contradictory behaviors.

Given the earlier-reported associations between emotionally unavailable forms of early care and later dissociation, the subtle nature of the helpless/fearful profile of maternal behavior is important to note, as is the subtlety of many of the disorganized behaviors shown by their infants. The hostile/self-referential profile of maternal behaviors and infant behaviors is much easier to identify as maladaptive, yet recent data indicate that a helpless/fearful profile is likely to characterize slightly more than half of all disorganized relationships [47,48].

Although fearful or withdrawn parenting behaviors might seem less problematic than behaviors that are more frightening or hostile, there is repeated evidence that both subgroups of disorganized infants are at risk for a variety of negative outcomes including elevated cortisol secretion in response to mild stressors in infancy, inhibited or chaotic fantasy play in preschool, elevated internalizing and aggressive behaviors toward peers in kindergarten and second grade, and elevated rates of controlling attachment patterns toward parents by age 6 years [20]. In recent work, maternal withdrawing behaviors from the infant were found to be related to the infant's later borderline features in young adulthood [49].

In addition, both subgroups are related to a maternal history of trauma, with different forms of maternal trauma associated with hostile or withdrawing profiles. Mothers who had a history of physical abuse or witnessed violence were more likely to display the hostile profile of behavior at home, whereas mothers who had a history of sexual abuse or parental loss (but not physical abuse) were more likely to withdraw from interaction with their infants. Clinical treatment of sexual abuse survivors clearly reveals the underlying fear and rage of those who have been sexually victimized; however, sexually abused mothers appeared more likely to manage their negative affects by moving away from interaction with the infant, whereas mothers who had witnessed violence or had been physically abused appeared to handle their underlying fear by identifying with an aggressive style of interaction [50].

Longitudinal case illustration

To illustrate the types of early-disrupted mother-infant communication patterns observed in longitudinal research, one of the videotaped mother-infant interactions is described. Afterward, excerpts from the same child's description of his attachment relationships on the adult attachment interview at age 19 years are presented. The implications of these reports are discussed and illustrated by an additional brief vignette of a patient in treatment.

When the child, whom the authors call Justin, was 18 months old, the mother and child were videotaped during a "strange situation" session, an experimental procedure developed by Ainsworth and colleagues [51] to assess infant attachment strategies. Mother and child underwent a sequence of eight 3-minute episodes, involving two mother-infant separations (the first, leaving the child with a stranger and the second, leaving the child alone). The child's reactions to separation and reunion with the mother were used as indices of his/her security of attachment with the mother and served as the basis for classifying the infant into one of four attachment categories: secure, avoidant, ambivalent, or disorganized. Justin was classified as disorganized in infancy and reported high levels of dissociation at age 19 years.

When alone with mother in the first episode, Justin wanders around the room without being able to focus on a toy or initiate focused activity. Watching the video in slow motion, the child's movements appear lost, confused, and aimless—he walks around, turning and turning, briefly touching and then leaving a few objects. The frequency of this behavior increases after his mother's lack of response to his attempt to initiate an interaction by showing her a toy. The child's disoriented behavior dissipates, however, after the mother's departure, when he is given the opportunity to interact with the stranger. His attempt to engage the stranger in a game with the ball is successful and he seems to enjoy the interaction.

After the first reunion, his mother enters the room but neither approaches nor greets Justin. She stands on one leg, the other leg relaxed, with her right hand in her pocket and leans back a bit, without interacting. The child lowers his gaze and moves toward the door, a sign of disorganization in the presence of the parent. Subsequent attempts from the mother to interest him with the toys are not successful. Rather, he attempts to keep his distance by refusing any shared activity with his mother and proceeds to engage in a new sequence of disoriented, aimless behaviors. During the second separation, the child becomes distressed. On reunion, his mother stands hesitantly but does not try to comfort her distressed child. Instead, she asks for a kiss and wants him to tell her about his activities while she was out of the room.

These examples of parent-infant dialog involve subtle movements and slight affective cues that are not apparently traumatizing or even openly conflictual, yet they have a measurable effect on the quality of the dyadic exchange and on the child's subsequent behavioral organization. The authors stress the "dialogic" quality of such disrupted communications because the smallest movements and affective cues reciprocally influence one another and impact the course of the interaction.

The child presented in this vignette endorsed a significant level of dissociative symptoms at age 19 years. On the Dissociative Experiences Scale, for example, Justin endorsed often "finding [himself] someplace and not remembering how [he] got there" and "getting confused about whether [he] has done something or only thought about doing it" as a young adult. The parallels between these experiences and his observed disorientation and aimlessness following his parent's withdrawal in his early interactions are noteworthy. In addition, when administered the Adult Attachment

Interview (AAI), a semistructured interview that evaluates attachment in adulthood, this young man verbally described a sense of disorientation and of being pulled in several directions in his early childhood, which is reminiscent of the disorientation and aimless qualities of the taped interaction. He describes early childhood as follows: "Bounce here, bounce there. Go to court one week for my parents and have to go talk to judges and all this... I really didn't have many friends at the time because I was always...moving from here to there." His disappointment with the lack of stability that characterizes his relationship with his mother is also addressed in the AAI: "Each time I get bounced around it takes me six months to get settled back down and then resentment builds for another while. Every time I try to...finally open up I get moved around and just basically shut down again." Not surprisingly, this young man expresses hope that his relationship with his parents will move toward stability in his adulthood, "and then I can reach a sort of equilibrium around here."

He also describes a role-reversed, caregiving stance toward his parents during the AAI. "From the age of twelve on...I kind of brought myself up...I started becoming an adult at the age of twelve, I think...I consider my mom more of a friend right now than a mom...someone I can go and talk to and hang out with...And I know she's my mother and everything, but I just have this weird feeling about—she's so young." When his mother would cry in front of him after fighting with his father, Justin reports, "I used to stay by her side...and help her out. I'd give her a hug or something...tried to make her laugh." He also describes trying to think of ways to solve his parents' conflicts when he was 6 years old: "[When I heard them fighting] it just made me start thinking—think and think. Think of ways of trying to fix—but could never."

It is notable that the withdrawn and role-reversed nature of the parent's involvement with the child was evident in the second-to-second interactive dialog between mother and infant, after which the child eventually begins to focus on his mother's needs, per her request, rather than attend to his own needs.

Clinical implications

Attachment strategies, including their defensive and conflicted components, are examples of the nonconscious, implicit, behaviorally based representations of how-to-be-with-others that are developed in infancy before the explicit memory system associated with consciously recalled images or symbols is available [52,53]. In the view developed here, these implicit relational representations encode the "deep structure" of the early parent-infant affective dialog, including the deletions and distortions in the dialog that will eventually constitute internalized mental processes. The authors argue that such intrapsychic mental processes originate in characteristics of the two-person dialog from very early in life.

The dimensions of the parent-infant dialog most relevant to the later development of dissociation appear to be the contradictory communications, failures to respond, withdrawing behaviors, disoriented behaviors, and role-confused behaviors that override the infant's attachment cues but are not, in and of themselves, explicitly hostile or intrusive. In such instances, the caregiver behaves in ways that have the effect of "shutting out" the child from the process of dialog. This shutting out of the child's contribution to the regulatory process eventually leaves the child without an internalized form of relational dialog, or internal working model, that can provide a sense of safety and reliable comfort in times of distress.

In the case of an abusive parent, it is clear how the child's attempts to participate in the parent-child dialog may be shut out; however, this invalidation of the child's input can also occur without the degree of deviation represented by abusive parenting. Whitmer [54] described dissociation from a psychodynamic perspective as a process of simultaneously knowing and not knowing and related this process to the difficulty dissociative individuals experience when engaging in verbalization or meaning-making of their sensations and perceptions. He postulated that one cannot truly "know" his own experience until he is seen, recognized, and reflected on by the other. In essence, then, dissociated experiences around fearful affects are not necessarily experienced and then lost or defended against, but may instead be "unthinkable" in that they have gone unrecognized by central attachment figures. This model suggests that the etiology of dissociation does not lie in an individual, intrapsychic process but represents a dynamic, interactive dialogic process that originates in the interchange between the self and the other. That which occurs in this dialogic process may then become intrapsychic by way of internalization. In the case of primary failure of the parent-infant dialog, the child is faced with a lack of integrated affective, symbolic, and interactive dialog with the parent so that this lack of integration, in the form of dissociation, is eventually internalized by the child. Thus, this model postulates that for an individual to be able to experience more fully integrated mental states, a collaborative dialog between the parent and child must be created. This dialog must be elaborated with the collaboration of the child, such that the parent elicits the child's contributions and actively considers his experience, and an expression of this consideration on the part of the parent is demonstrated back to the child in developmentally appropriate ways that will be understood by the child. Conversely, the parent's inability to acknowledge the child's experiences or needs while in dialog (in other words, shutting out the child) may result in the child's failure to understand or integrate these same self-experiences, eventually leading to the development of dissociative symptomatology.

A final clinical example, in which there was a frightening childhood experience in the context of a nonabusive family, provides a vivid illustration of how the pivotal absence of a regulating parent-child dialog may be related to dissociative phenomena. A young man, whom the authors call Nate, presented for treatment with a severe generalized anxiety disorder and intense fears of abandonment in his short and unstable romantic relationships. As the treatment relationship progressed over a 3-year period, he began to comment on the therapist's reliability and to have increasingly frightening nightmares of being killed, tortured, or mutilated. These increasingly fearful images finally culminated in a fugue state one evening that lasted several hours and was accompanied by chills, nausea, and diarrhea. In this state, which he said was like "dreaming while he was awake," he became increasingly frantic as he experienced himself being in a refugee camp desperately trying to match up young children with their mothers, only to find that they kept getting separated again.

He called the therapist and she scheduled an extra session to meet the next day. When he arrived at the session, he sat down and said that he had had trouble taking off his coat as he came into the office. It was difficult, he said, because there were two of him in the coat. One persona was a young boy named Buddy, who was the one who loved people and had feelings. Buddy's name was the same as the name of the boy in the movie *Fried Green Tomatoes* who was killed by a train when his foot became stuck in the railroad tracks. The other person in his coat was a hostile and distrustful boy named Max, whose job it was to protect Buddy and drive away anyone who tried to get close to him. As he left the session, he said to his therapist of 3 years, "I just want you to know that if I left treatment now, I wouldn't remember who you are."

In subsequent sessions, Nate alternated between being enraged at the therapist and beginning to recall images of being hospitalized unexpectedly for several weeks at age 4.5 years for a serious infection. As he recalled this experience, which he only remembered in a fragmentary way, several pivotal scenes emerged. He remembered that he was told by his family that they were going for a drive and then he found himself in the hospital. After he had been admitted, his parents told him they were going to park the car and would be back in a minute, but they did not return. His mother did not drive, so his parents only visited him once a week on Sundays. In one particularly poignant session, he remembered his parents coming to visit and seeing his mother looking at him very upset and frightened. He said, "I knew that she needed someone to help her and a part of me slipped out through a crack in the floor." Later in the same session he said, "I think I forgot my mother when I was in the hospital." His tendency to dissociate at moments of neediness continued into his adult life.

At the time that these images of his hospitalization were being explored in treatment, the extended separation from his parents while he was hospitalized was viewed as traumatic by definition and as fully accounting for the severity of his symptoms. It was not until much later in the treatment that he and his therapist more fully appreciated how deeply he felt his mother's sense of helplessness and anxiety throughout his childhood and how role-reversed his relationship with his mother had been and continued to be.

Accordingly, the research results previously reviewed and Nate's account of his early hospitalization point to the relational context of this event as critical to whether or not a dissociative solution occurred. If his parents had been able to tolerate his sadness and rage and remain in a collaborative and psychologically containing dialog with him throughout that experience, would there have been a dissociative outcome? Nate seemed to have internalized a way of being in which his extreme distress, his affective aliveness, was subordinated to the needs of his parent and excluded from the dialog. This internalization was theoretically the only available route to maintain some form of involvement with his mother, by reducing her stress and colluding in not knowing his feelings.

Summary

The first clinical implication of the theory and research reviewed in this article is that the capacity of attachment figures for modulating fearful arousal in a responsive dialog with the child has a major impact on the development of dissociative symptoms over time. A second clinical implication is that traumatic events are often discrete occurrences, whereas disturbed parental affective communications are often an enduring, day-in-day-out feature of the childhood years. In contrast to a more discrete traumatic event, the parent's responses to the child's foundational needs for comfort and soothing are worked into the fabric of identity from a very early age. They are also worked into the fabric of the child's biologic stress regulation. Therefore, the resolution of discrete traumatic events in treatment may come about more quickly than the resolution of long-standing patterns of role-reversal, disorientation, and disrupted forms of affective communication in the transference. Among dissociative young adults, current research results indicate that disrupted communication patterns with attachment figures tend to be a subtle and implicit part of dyadic interaction from a very early age and, therefore, may be extremely difficult for the patient to articulate until forms of a healthier and more genuine implicit and explicit dialog around heightened affective experiences are worked out in the therapeutic relationship.

This hypothesis regarding the importance of the quality of the parent-child dialog in the genesis of dissociative tendencies has important implications for treatment that are compatible with trauma theory. It highlights the importance of trauma survivors being "heard" in their journey to recovery. Herman [55] described dissociation as the "internal mechanism by which terrorized people are silenced." This internal mechanism may parallel the manner in which infants vulnerable to developing dissociation are silenced or shut out of collaborative dialog with their parent, setting the stage for the later lack of affectively alive collaborative dialog often seen in adults who have dissociative processes.

What is important about this model of the parent-child dialog is that it may help to address the current gaps in the dissociation literature that emphasize traumatic experience rather than ongoing parent-child processes in the generation of adult dissociative disorders. It offers a framework for understanding why individuals vary so greatly in the development of dissociation in response to trauma. This model may provide a better understanding of nontraumatized individuals who dissociate and of individuals traumatized by war or other nonfamilial experiences who do not develop dissociation. This model may also provide a more nuanced understanding of Liotti's [9] work regarding the relationship between infant disorganization and dissociation by adding to the model a finer description of the particular relational transactions that underlie disorganization in infancy and dissociation in early adulthood.

Although the studies reviewed in this article provide empiric evidence regarding the long-term predictive power of infant disorganization and the parent-infant dialog, these factors are not necessarily the only or even the most important factors in this development. Clearly, such development occurs within a complex web of environmental, societal, familial, and genetic factors that are all likely to interact in ways that we have only begun to understand. Accordingly, more research is needed that includes strong measures of family relational process to expand our understanding of how these relational factors may interact with genetic, biologic, and trauma-related processes to influence the development of dissociation over the life span. Collaborative efforts between trauma clinicians and attachment researchers to document diagnosable adult dissociative disorders in longitudinal cohorts will also shed light on the clinical impact in adulthood of processes related to childhood attachment disorganization.

References

[1] Putnam FW. Dissociation in children and adolescents. New York: Guilford Press; 1997.
[2] Kluft RP. Multiple personality in childhood. Psychiatr Clin North Am 1984;7(1): 121–34.
[3] Braun BG, Sachs RG. The development of multiple personality disorder: predisposing, precipitating and perpetuating factors. In: Kluft RP, editor. Childhood antecedents of multiple personality. Washington, DC: American Psychiatric Press; 1985. p. 37–74.
[4] Mann BJ, Sanders S. Child dissociation and the family context. J Abnorm Child Psychol 1994;22:373–88.
[5] Malinosky-Rummell RR, Hoier TS. Validating measures of dissociation in sexually abused and non-abused children. Behav Assess 1991;13:341–57.
[6] Egeland B, Susman-Stillman A. Dissociation as a mediator of child abuse across generations. Child Abuse Negl 1996;20(11):1123–32.
[7] Barach PM. Multiple personality disorder as an attachment disorder. Dissociation 1991; 4(3):117–23.
[8] Bowlby J. Attachment and loss, vol. 2. Separation. New York: Basic; 1973.
[9] Liotti G. Disorganized/disoriented attachment in the etiology of the dissociative disorders. Dissociation 1992;5(4):196–204.
[10] Main M, Hesse E. Parents' unresolved traumatic experiences are related to infant disorganized attachment status: is frightened and/or frightening parental behavior the linking mechanism? In: Greenberg M, Cicchetti D, Cummings EM, editors. Attachment in the preschool

years: theory, research and intervention. Chicago: University of Chicago Press; 1990. p. 161–84.

[11] Lyons-Ruth K, Bronfman E, Parsons E. Maternal disrupted affective communication, maternal frightened or frightening behavior, and disorganized infant attachment strategies. In: Vondra J, Barnett D, editors. Atypical patterns of infant attachment: theory, research and current directions. Monogr Soc Res Child Dev 1990;64:67–96.

[12] Lyons-Ruth K, Bronfman E, Atwood G. A relational diathesis model of hostile-helpless states of mind. Expressions in mother-infant interactions. In: Solomon J, George C, editors. Attachment disorganization. New York: Guilford Press; 1999. p. 33–70.

[13] Ogawa J, Sroufe LA, Weinfield NS, et al. Development and the fragmented self: a longitudinal study of dissociative symptomatology in a non-clinical sample. Dev Psychopathol 1997; 4:855–79.

[14] Bernstein E, Putnam FW. Development reliability and validity of a dissociation scale. J Nerv Ment Dis 1986;174:727–35.

[15] Egeland B, Sroufe LA. Developmental sequelae of maltreatment in infancy. New Dir Child Dev 1981;11:77–92.

[16] Dutra L, Lyons-Ruth K. Maltreatment, maternal and child psychopathology, and quality of early care as predictors of adolescent dissociation. Presented at the Biennial Meeting of the Society for Research in Child Development. Atlanta, GA; 2005.

[17] Schuder M, Lyons-Ruth K. "Hidden trauma" in infancy: attachment, fearful arousal, and early dysfunction of the stress response system. In: Osofsky J, editor. Trauma in infancy and early childhood. New York: Guilford Press; 2004. p. 69–104.

[18] American Psychiatric Association. Diagnostic and statistical manual of mental disorders. 4th edition. Washington, DC: American Psychiatric Association; 1994.

[19] Bowlby J. Attachment and loss, vol. 1 Attachment. London: Hogarth Press, Institute of Psychoanalysis; 1969.

[20] Lyons-Ruth K, Jacobvitz D. Attachment disorganization: unresolved loss, relational violence, and lapses in behavioral and attentional strategies. In: Cassidy J, Shaver P, editors. Handbook of attachment: theory, research, and clinical implications. New York: Guilford Press; 1999. p. 520–54.

[21] Spangler G, Grossmann KE. Biobehavioral organization in securely and insecurely attached infants. Child Dev 1993;64:1439–50.

[22] Seligman MED. Helplessness: on depression, development and death. San Francisco (CA): Freeman; 1975.

[23] Taylor SE, Klein LC, Lewis BP, et al. Biobehavioral responses to stress in females: tend-and-befriend, not fight-or-flight. Psychol Rev 2000;107:411–29.

[24] O'Connor TG, Rutter M, the English and Romanian Adoptees Study Team. Attachment disorder behavior following early severe deprivation: extension and longitudinal follow-up. J Am Acad Child Adolesc Psychiatry 2000;39(6):703–12.

[25] Atlas-Corbett A. Indiscriminate attachment behavior in infancy and maternal psychosocial problems [honors thesis]. Waltham (MA): Brandeis University; 2005.

[26] Riley C. Indiscriminate attachment behavior in infancy as risk factor for preschool behavior problems [honors thesis]. Cambridge (MA): Harvard University; 2005.

[27] Spangler G, Schieche M. Emotional and adrenocortical responses of infants to the strange situation: the differential function of emotional expression. Int J Behav Dev 1998;22: 681–706.

[28] Ashman SB, Dawson G, Panagiotides H, et al. Stress hormone levels of children of depressed mothers. Dev Psychopathol 2002;14:333–49.

[29] Gunnar M, Mangelsdorf S, Larson M, et al. Attachment, temperament and adrenocortical activity in infancy: a study of psychoendocrine regulation. Dev Psychopathol 1989;25:355–63.

[30] Spangler G, Grossmann K. Individual and physiological correlates of attachment disorganization in infancy. In: Solomon J, George C, editors. Attachment disorganization. New York: Guilford Press; 1999. p. 95–124.

[31] Hertsgaard L, Gunnar M, Erickson MF, et al. Adrenocortical responses to the strange situation in infants with disorganized/disoriented attachment relationships. Child Dev 1995; 66(4):1100–6.

[32] Essex M, Klein M, Eunsuk C, et al. Maternal stress beginning in infancy may sensitize children to later stress exposure: effects on cortisol and behavior. Biol Psychiatry 2002;52:776–84.

[33] Coplan JD, Andrews MW, Owens MJ, et al. Persistent elevations of cerebrospinal fluid concentrations of corticotropin-releasing factor in adult nonhuman primates exposed to early-life stressors: implications for the pathophysiology of mood and anxiety disorders. Proc Natl Acad Sci U S A 1996;93:1619–23.

[34] Francis D, Diorio J, Liu D, et al. Nongenomic transmission across generations of maternal behavior and stress responses in the rat. Science 1999;286:1155–8.

[35] Ames EW. Spitz revisited: a trip to Romanian "orphanages" [C.P.A. section]. Dev Psychol Newslett 1990;9(2):3–4.

[36] Carlson M, Dragomir C, Earls F, et al. Cortisol regulation in home-reared and institutionalized Romanian children. Soc Neurosci Abstracts 1995;698:1.

[37] Carlson M, Earls F. Psychological and neuroendocrinological sequelae of early social deprivation in institutionalized children in Romania. Ann N Y Acad Sci 1997;807:419–28.

[38] Kroupina M, Gunnar MR, Johnson DE. Report on salivary cortisol levels in a Russian baby home. Minneapolis (MN): Institute of Child Development, University of Minnesota; 1997.

[39] Fisher P, Gunnar M, Chamberlain P, et al. Preventive intervention for maltreated preschool children: impact on children's behavior, neuroendocrine activity, and foster parent functioning. J Am Acad Child Adolesc Psychiatry 2000;39:1356–64.

[40] Gilles EE, Berntson GG, Zipf WB, et al. Neglect is associated with a blunting of behavioral and biological stress responses in human infants. Presented at the International Conference of Infant Studies. Brighton, England, 2000.

[41] van IJzendoorn MH, Schuengel C, Bakermans-Kranenburg MJ. Disorganized attachment in early childhood: meta-analysis of precursors, concomitants, and sequelae. Dev Psychopathol 1999;11:225–49.

[42] Carlson V, Cicchetti D, Barnett D, et al. Disorganized/disoriented attachment relationships in maltreated infants. Dev Psychopathol 1989;25:525–31.

[43] Goldberg S, Benoit D, Blokland K, et al. Atypical maternal behavior, maternal representations and infant disorganized attachment. Dev Psychopathol 2003;15:239–57.

[44] Grienenberger J, Kelly K. Maternal reflective functioning and caregiving: links between mental states and observed behavior in the intergenerational transmission. Presented at the biennial meeting of the Society for Research in Child Development. Minneapolis, MN; 2001.

[45] Madigan S, Pederson D, Moran G. Unresolved states of mind, disorganized attachment relationships, and anomalous mother-infant interactions. Dev Psychol, in press.

[46] Sroufe LA, Jacobvitz D, Mangelsdorf S, et al. Generational boundary dissolution between mothers and their preschool children: a relational systems approach. Child Dev 1985;56: 317–25.

[47] Main M, Solomon J. Procedures for identifying infants as disorganized/disoriented during the Ainsworth strange situation. In: Greenberg M, Cicchetti D, Cummings EM, editors. Attachment in the preschool years: theory, research and intervention. Chicago: University of Chicago Press; 1990. p. 121–60.

[48] NICHD Early Child Care Research Network. Child-care and family predictors of preschool attachment and stability from infancy. Dev Psychopathol 2001;37(6):847–62.

[49] Lyons-Ruth K, Holmes B, Hennighausen K. Prospective longitudinal predictors of borderline and conduct symptoms in late adolescence: the early caregiving context. Presented at the Biennial Meeting of the Society for Research in Child Development. Atlanta: Georgia; 2005.

[50] Lyons-Ruth K, Block D. The disturbed caregiving system: relations among childhood trauma, maternal caregiving, and infant affect and attachment. Infant Ment Health J 1996;17:257–75.

[51] Ainsworth MDS, Blehar M, Waters E, et al. Patterns of attachment: a psychological study of the strange situation. Hillsdale (NJ): Erlbaum; 1978.

[52] Lyons-Ruth K. The two-person unconscious: intersubjective dialogue, enactive relational representation, and the emergence of new forms of relational organization. In: Aron L, Harris A, editors. Relational psychoanalysis, vol. II. Hillsdale (NJ): Analytic Press; 2005. p. 311–49.

[53] Stern D. The interpersonal world of the infant. New York: Basic Books; 1985.

[54] Whitmer G. On the nature of dissociation. Psychoanal Q 2001;70:807–37.

[55] Herman JL. Complex PTSD: a syndrome in survivors of prolonged and repeated trauma. J Trauma Stress 1992;5:377–91.

ELSEVIER
SAUNDERS

PSYCHIATRIC
CLINICS
OF NORTH AMERICA

Psychiatr Clin N Am 29 (2006) 87–112

Posttraumatic Personality Disorder: A Reformulation of Complex Posttraumatic Stress Disorder and Borderline Personality Disorder

Catherine C. Classen, PhD[a,b,c,*],
Clare Pain, MD, FRCPC[a,d], Nigel P. Field, PhD[e],
Patricia Woods, RN, CPMHN(C)[b]

[a]Department of Psychiatry, University of Toronto, Toronto, ON, Canada
[b]Trauma Therapy Program, Department of Psychiatry, Sunnybrook & Women's College
Health Sciences Centre, Toronto, ON, Canada
[c]Women's Mental Health Research Program, Centre for Research in Women's Health,
Toronto, ON, Canada
[d]Department of Psychiatry, University of Western Ontario, London, ON, Canada
[e]Pacific Graduate School of Psychology, Palo Alto, CA, USA

There is a growing recognition among clinicians who treat individuals who are chronically traumatized that the *Diagnostic and Statistical Manual, 4th Edition* (*DSM-IV*) [1] does not provide an adequate diagnostic category to capture the full range of symptomatology with which these individuals frequently present. Borderline personality disorder (BPD) and posttraumatic stress disorder (PTSD) often are considered the best diagnostic options. Alone or together, however, these categories do not describe the full range of symptomatology for individuals suffering as a result of chronic traumatization. Furthermore, they do not provide an adequate framework for understanding etiology or how to treat these individuals. New diagnostic categories are needed to better account for the range of symptom constellations that can result from chronic traumatization.

This article draws on the work of leaders in the field of chronic traumatization and attachment and offers an idea for conceptualizing BPD and two new diagnostic categories, called posttraumatic personality disorder–disorganized (PTPD-D) and posttraumatic personality disorder–organized

* Corresponding author. Sunnybrook and Women's College Health Sciences Centre, 76 Grenville Street, Room 956, Toronto, ON M5S 1B2, Canada.
  E-mail address: catherine.classen@sw.ca (C.C. Classen).

0193-953X/06/$ - see front matter © 2005 Elsevier Inc. All rights reserved.
doi:10.1016/j.psc.2005.11.001
psych.theclinics.com

(PTPD-O). These three disorders are categorized according to the presence or absence of disorganized attachment and more or less of a history of chronic child abuse (Fig. 1). This article proposes that PTPD requires a history of extensive chronic traumatization beginning in childhood. When children who have disorganized attachment also experience chronic traumatization, this can lead to PTPD-D. Chronic child abuse of individuals who have organized attachment can lead to PTPD-O. This article proposes that a diagnosis of BPD occurs with individuals who have a disorganized attachment and who have a less severe history of child abuse.

This article presents a reformulation of complex PTSD [2], otherwise known as disorders of extreme stress not otherwise specified (DESNOS) [3], and of BPD. In the interest of encouraging a new way of thinking about these disorders and their relation to one another and wanting to use language that describes these conditions more accurately, the term, PTPD, is used to capture PTSD plus complex PTSD (or DESNOS). This article argues that complex PTSD/DESNOS is a chronic adaptation to PTSD and that severe, unresolved chronic traumatization in childhood leads to more than a collection of symptoms—it actually shapes the personality, meeting the definition of a personality disorder according to the *DSM-IV*. In addition, this article contends that disorganized attachment underlies BPD and, thus, the symptoms characteristic of BPD are viewed as adaptations to living with a disorganized attachment pattern. Someone diagnosed with PTPD-D is living with the consequences of severe chronic childhood traumatization and disorganized attachment. Thus, PTPD-D is a melding of complex PTSD/DESNOS and BPD. A person diagnosed with PTPD-O has an organized attachment pattern and also lives with the consequences of severe chronic childhood traumatization. Such a person's coping strategies, however, include symptoms related only to complex PTSD/DESNOS and not symptoms characteristic of BPD. The authors choose to leave the BPD label untouched because of its long history and consequent familiarity.

Two fictional case examples are presented to support the argument for the creation of two new diagnostic categories, PTPD-O and PTPD-D. This is followed by a discussion of the limitations of PTSD as a classification

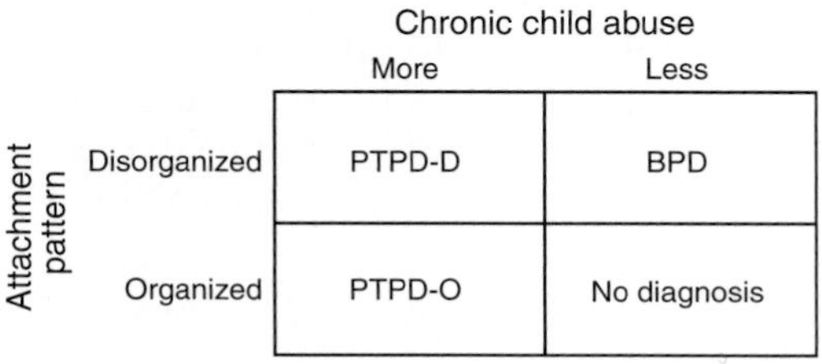

		Chronic child abuse	
		More	Less
Attachment pattern	Disorganized	PTPD-D	BPD
	Organized	PTPD-O	No diagnosis

Fig. 1. Three diagnostic classifications based on attachment pattern and the presence or absence of chronic child abuse.

for survivors of chronic abuse in childhood and a brief discussion of problems with the diagnostic category of BPD. Research comparing PTSD and BPD is presented and discussed in the context of the proposed conceptualization of BPD and the organized and disorganized classifications of PTPD. Discussion continues of the conditions that lead to the development of disorganized attachment and the relationship of disorganized attachment to BPD. The effect of severe, chronic traumatization in childhood is discussed, including the response of the child when directly experiencing the abuse as well as the child's response to living in the abusive environment. The personality adaptations to severe chronic traumatization, which are suggested as resulting in PTPD, are described. PTPD is discussed in the context of attachment. Individuals are described who have an organized attachment pattern that exhibits PTPD (PTPD-O) or a disorganized attachment pattern that exhibits PTPD (PTPD-D). This article concludes with discussion of treatment implications.

Case examples

The two fictional cases in this article are composites of the types of cases the authors have seen that fit their criteria for PTPD. The first fictional case describes someone who has an organized attachment pattern, has been traumatized extensively and chronically, and who meets criteria for PTPD-O. The second fictional case describes someone who has a disorganized attachment pattern, experienced extensive chronic traumatization, and meets criteria for PTPD-D. In attempting to categorize these survivors, their complex experiences are simplified. Although it is not possible to flesh out all the ways in which these individuals were traumatized and neglected or the ways in which they experienced loss and deprivation, there are important subtle but distinct differences between these two types of patients and these differences determine treatment and outcome. Rationale for the categorization of these two fictional cases is provided with presentation of the argument for creating these two new diagnostic categories.

Posttraumatic personality disorder–organized

Gay is a slight, young-looking, 50-year-old divorced mother of two adult children. She has not worked for some years and is on a disability pension for depression. As a child, Gay was one of seven siblings growing up in eastern Canada. Even though her parents were poor and busy, she felt loved by them and believed she could ensure a place in their hearts by never causing them any trouble. She saw how tired her parents were, worn down by poverty and hard work, and how little energy and resources they had to go around. Being good, never making a fuss, and not having needs were ways she could ensure her acceptability. She never thought to tell her parents about the sexual and physical abuse she suffered from their neighbor.

Gay's abuse began when she was 6 years old. Her recollection of what happened is sketchy. She has memories of the neighbor giving her candy, but when she tries to think of what happened when he took her into his bedroom, she becomes afraid and dissociates into a numb amnestic state. The abuse stopped when she was 12 and sent to live with her single aunt. Her aunt needed a companion and Gay went to school and "paid her way" as her aunt's housekeeper. She was frightened and helpless when her aunt died suddenly, in front of her, of a cardiac event, 2 years after Gay moved in with her. She felt guilty and responsible for her aunt's death because, in her shock, she had found it difficult to dial for the ambulance. She returned home but interrupted her education to marry early so that she could relieve her parents of the burden of her care. Her husband was frightening and physically and sexually abusive toward her. He became increasingly dependent on drugs and theft to pay for his addiction and eventually was jailed for armed robbery. Before this, Gay was stalked by him and feared he would kill her. Gay's daughter also reports her father sexually abused her.

Before coming into the trauma program, Gay had received minimal treatment with antidepressants and supportive counseling by her family doctor. In the trauma program, for the past 3 years, she has been in an outpatient group and an individual treatment program. She now is well enough psychologically to be able to reflect on her progress in therapy and on her past. Superficially, she seems shy and quiet. Although liked by everyone in the program, she never seems to recognize the warmth and acceptance of others. She feels soiled and unacceptable and shrinks from any voluntary social contact; nevertheless, she is unable to prevent herself from being chronically taken advantage of by others. She complains of an ongoing state of general malaise and low energy. She suffers from insomnia, headaches, and occasional panic attacks during which she cannot speak and believes she is going to have a heart attack. She reports that she has felt suicidal for as long as she can remember. She has no history of self-harm or substance use.

Although Gay attended group therapy regularly, for the first year or more she was mostly "zoned out" and occasionally cried silently without being able to identify why. When she joined the program she rarely was conscious of hunger, found no pleasure from food, and needed to remind herself to eat because she knew she "should." Encouraged by the group to become more assertive, she expressed fear of being seen as "selfish" and stated she did not deserve to stand up for herself. Gay says she had not realized how afraid and unsafe she felt all the time until she learned to ground herself more reliably in the present. With this capacity, her voice grew stronger and became consistently audible, and she became more comfortable with eye contact. Somewhat to the surprise of the staff and with minimal encouragement, she divorced her abusive husband, who was in jail, contacted her estranged son, and tentatively began to call him regularly. Still in treatment, she remains socially isolated, although less so than before, perhaps because she can consider how and when to say no, which, for example, frees her from long telephone calls from people who take advantage of her time. With a growing confidence in her ability to recognize what she feels and why, she has joined a back-to-work retraining program and hopes to work part time in a local charity shop.

Posttraumatic personality disorder–disorganized

Dee is 25 years old, unemployed, single, and supported on welfare. Her 8-year-old son has lived with his paternal grandparents from infancy. The court is determining whether or not to award Dee supervised visits. Three suicide attempts since the legal battle began have led to a psychiatric referral by the crisis unit.

Dee reports a childhood history of unresolved loss, inconsistent parenting, an absence of clear boundaries or structure, and emotional, sexual, and physical abuse and neglect. A brother, almost two years older, was a toddler when he drowned in the bathtub. When she was growing up, her mother kept his room as a "shrine" and used alcohol to deal with her grief. Dee's alcoholic father left home when she was 3 years old. Dee was abused sexually for 4 years beginning at age 10 by a maternal uncle, who gave her money and bought her clothes. She reported the abuse by her uncle but was beaten violently by her mother and forced to apologize to her uncle for lying. After this, she decided, "What's the point?" and has not spoken of the abuse since then. Her mother's boyfriend touched her inappropriately and abused her physically throughout her early teens. When she talks about the abuse, she appears emotionally detached and her thoughts become disorganized.

Dee has self-injured since age 13 and states that it "helps me feel real, it takes the deadness away for a while." She also began using drugs at age 14 and minimizes her current marijuana use, as "it's only weed—it makes me calm." In grade 11, Dee left school after becoming pregnant by her boyfriend, Paul, who is 5 years her senior, an alcoholic, and became increasingly abusive during Dee's pregnancy. She left him only to return again and repeated this pattern several times until she learned he was seeing someone else. Dee made her first suicide attempt after this discovery. She worked at odd jobs occasionally, leaving because of conflict or an inability to tolerate the structure. She has difficulty keeping friends and her involvements tend to be brief and intense. Her living situation became increasingly unstable; with no reliable accommodation, she moved between friends, hostels, and her mother's home. After the baby's birth, custody was awarded to Paul's parents. Dee made several suicide attempts when she lost custody of her baby and began using drugs again.

In the clinician's office, Dee complained angrily that she had "no supports" and rejected recommendations to see a therapist. She stated that she planned to report her family doctor for neglecting to respond to her many crisis calls. During the evaluation, it became increasingly clear that her treatment providers likely were frustrated by her frequent crises and her angry inability to accept help. She complained that she was always thinking of others but "no one is there when I need them." As the interview was ending, she told the clinician that she had faith in her skills because "you are a specialist" and that "no one else can help me." When she was reminded that the meeting was for an assessment, not ongoing treatment, her expression then shifted to one of shock and angry entitlement. She left the office and was found by the receptionist in the washroom, making cuts on her arm.

These fictional cases illustrate the two PTPD categories, one with an organized attachment (Gay) and one with disorganized attachment (Dee). Although both fictional cases share the experience of extensive chronic traumatization, they differ in their early attachment history, quality of their relationships, and their views of self.

The differences in their early attachment experiences are significant. The first 6 years of Gay's life were relatively stable. Although family resources were limited and her parents often preoccupied with making ends meet, she believed they loved her. Gay's ability to adapt to her early environment and become "invisible" or "need nothing" enabled her to feel a sense of control over ensuring their love. Despite the underlying insecurity that living in poverty instilled in her, the quality of her attachment to her parents was predictable and benign. Dee, alternatively, had a mother who was distracted and unavailable to her emotionally because of alcohol and grief. Dee's description of her mother suggests that she was unresolved in relation to the death of her son, which, along with her alcoholism, may have led to the mother behaving in a frightening or frightened manner toward Dee, promoting a disorganized attachment in Dee. Furthermore, her father also was an alcoholic and left when she was 3 years old, again providing an unlikely source of secure attachment and a significant early loss.

It is not surprising that Gay and Dee differ in their relational patterns. Given Gay's strong attachment to her parents and the difficult financial conditions in which her family was living, Gay learned her security was contingent on her parents' needs being met. At an early age, she took on the burdens of her overworked mother, learning that a child so useful and with so few stated needs was valued and corresponding behaviors reinforced. Dee, alternatively, had a much less reliable background than Gay. Dee's parents were unavailable, unpredictable, and, at times, abusive. Dee's home life was chaotic, and she learned not to rely on adults for emotional or practical support. Neglect alternated with punishment, and both seemed random and capricious.

These early relational patterns are reflected in the interpersonal relationships of both adult women. Dee felt chronically angry and let down by people around her and was unable to have stable or long-term relationships. Gay felt defective and had difficulties standing up for herself and let others needs take precedence over her own. Dee's relational life was chaotic, whereas Gay's consistently was constrained.

Gay and Dee had significant, chronic traumatization during childhood. Gay experienced protracted abuse by a neighbor, which was secret and aversive. It seems to have been frightening and humiliating, resulting in her use of amnestic and numbing dissociative defenses. Gay's vulnerability to the abuse and silence about it also may have been connected to a feeling that she needed to protect her parents from further difficulties and was congruent with her paradoxic sense of worth because she never complained or expressed her needs. Despite her hard work, Gay's inability to protect her aunt and the suddenness of her aunt's death left Gay with the certainty that, although responsible for the needs of the adults in her life, she was inadequate to the task. This, followed by a frightening, coercive, and abusive marriage, virtually ensured that all of her beliefs and experiences of herself as inadequate, too visible and needy, guilty, and shameful remained entrenched. Gay's coping strategies included isolation, dissociation, making herself "small," and denying her own needs and boundaries.

In early adolescence, Dee was abused for several years by her uncle and her mother's boyfriend. Her attempt to seek protection by her mother was met with disbelief and anger and resulted in violent punishment and blame. The physically abusive relationship with the father of her child reinforced her profound ambivalence about relationships and her anger with not getting from them what she needed. Her suicide attempts, cutting, and use of drugs were strategies that she used to manage overwhelming feelings of rage and fear. Dee lives in a state of crisis, which replicates her experience in her home. Dee does not trust what she is told and moves quickly to negative assumptions and outbursts of anger, which keeps people at a safe distance. She feels misunderstood and victimized by the health care system, which results in a push-pull relationship with her health providers. In turn, they are frustrated by Dee's relational style of dismissing her pain, trauma, and losses and her preference for substances and chaos while she also insists on help and then rejects the help that is offered.

Gay and Dee were abused and neglected significantly. They experienced overwhelming affect states, which they dealt with in somewhat different ways: Gay by dissociating, withdrawing, and having somatic complaints and Dee by dissociating, self-harm, drugs, and demanding and engaging in further interpersonal disputes. Neither is able to integrate the complicated traumatic and neglectful experiences they have had or make sense of them and understand their behavior in light of them. Consequently, their sense of self has been organized by this failure and the failure of their attachment figures to help them understand themselves and others. Despite their similarities, there are significant differences in these two fictional case presentations.

Recommendations for working with each of these types of patients are provided at the end of this article. First is a discussion of the definition of trauma and the classifications of PTSD and BPD; then, a model of PTPD is presented.

What is a trauma?

According to the *DSM-IV*, a traumatic event has occurred if "the person experienced, witnessed, or was confronted with an event or events that involved actual or threatened death or serious injury, or a threat to the physical integrity of self or others" and "the person's response involved intense fear, helplessness, or horror." In the case of children, the response "may be expressed instead by disorganized or agitated behavior" [1]. Although the *DSM* provides a definition of a traumatic event, the concept of trauma tends to be used differently in the PTSD/trauma and attachment literature. For the purpose of this article, a distinction is made between traumatization that occurs during infancy as a result of misattunements in the attachment relationship because of a frightened or frightening caregiver [4] and traumatization that occurs as a result of physical, emotional, or sexual abuse or extreme neglect, beginning either at infancy or later in childhood. The latter type of traumatization objectively is much more extreme and is the type of traumatization that leads to accusations of child abuse. In the attachment context, traumatization can occur because of far more subtle behaviors on the part of a caregiver. Specifically, it is the degree of responsive attunement of a protective caregiver that largely determines the extent to which infants or very young children register an event as a major threat to psychologic integrity and not its more "objective" threat value as understood from the vantage point of adults [5]. Thus, the notion of trauma in the attachment literature (see the article by Lyons-Ruth et al elsewhere in this issue) is in sharp contrast to trauma as it is defined in the *DSM* and the trauma literature. In this article, chronic traumatization refers to experiences of physical, emotional, or sexual abuse or extreme neglect occurring at anytime during childhood.

Limitations of posttraumatic stress disorder as a classification for those who are chronically traumatized

The *DSM-IV* diagnosis of PTSD is intended to capture the pathologic consequences of experiencing one or more traumatic events. The diagnosis of PTSD originally was designed to account for the stress responses of combat veterans to the trauma of war. Over time, however, this diagnosis has been shown as failing to capture the full range of consequences for all types of traumas, including combat trauma [6,7].

The limitations of PTSD are recognized in the literature on chronic traumatization [2,3,8,9] and are reflected in the concept of complex PTSD [2] and DESNOS [3]. The DESNOS classification originally was proposed as a new diagnostic category for inclusion in the *DSM-IV*, but, instead, the constellation of symptoms was noted as "associated features of PTSD" in the *DSM-IV* and included "impaired affect modulation; self-destructive and impulsive behavior; dissociative symptoms; somatic complaints; feelings of ineffectiveness, shame, despair, or hopelessness; feeling permanently damaged; a loss of previously sustained beliefs; hostility; social withdrawal; feeling constantly threatened; impaired relationship with other; or a change from the individual's previous personality characteristics." This syndrome often is associated with sustained or repeated interpersonal trauma during childhood or adolescence but also it may be associated with sustained trauma in later life or as a late consequence of chronic PTSD. (The authors believe that it is possible to develop PTPD as a result of extreme or chronic traumatization that occurs during adulthood, such as might occur when someone is held hostage under brutal conditions for a period of time or experiences significant torture. These types of conditions are excluded from this analysis, because they are beyond the scope of this article.) DESNOS attempts to link the persistent difficulties and symptoms in several domains as one disorder. These domains extend beyond the three PTSD clusters of re-experiencing, avoidance and numbing, and hyperarousal to include affect dysregulation, alterations of consciousness, alterations in self-perception, difficulty with interpersonal relationships and profound identity disturbances, somatization, and alterations in systems of meaning [10].

The *DSM-IV* field trial for PTSD finds that PTSD, somatization, dissociation, and affect dysregulation are all highly interrelated and the authors conclude that the PTSD diagnosis does not adequately cover the extent of the difficulties experienced by many who are diagnosed with PTSD [11]. A national comorbidity study finds that PTSD is highly comorbid, with 79% having at least one other axis 1 diagnosis [12]. The limitation of PTSD as a diagnosis also is reflected in the *International Statistical Classification of Diseases, 10th Revision*, which, along with PTSD, includes the diagnosis, "enduring personality change after catastrophic experience" [13]. The term, "complex PTSD," as opposed to "simple PTSD," is used in the literature to highlight when PTSD is accompanied by a host of other symptoms. It has become clear that responses to chronic interpersonal trauma extend well beyond intrusion, avoidance, and hyperarousal.

Although DESNOS is not included in the *DSM-IV* as a separate disorder, it has generated a great deal of interest. Many who treat individuals who are chronically traumatized view DESNOS as doing a better job of delineating the symptoms associated with chronic traumatization [2,8,14–16]. In addition, BPD also has come to be seen as a consequence of chronic traumatization [8,17]. BPD is shown to be distinct from but also overlapping with DESNOS [11]. An important difference is that BPD has been viewed as an attachment disorder [18–20] and DESNOS a disorder of self-regulation [14,15,21].

Reconceptualizing borderline personality disorder

From the moment that Stern first coined the term, borderline, in 1938 [22], this diagnosis has been problematic, reflected in the fact that it took until 1980 before it was introduced into the *DSM*. The broad symptom categories of BPD include affective disturbance, disturbed cognition, impulsivity, and intense unstable relationships. In the *DSM-IV*, five of nine criteria are required to diagnose BPD. The validity of this diagnosis long has been questioned [23] and over time, this diagnosis has come to be viewed as vague, stigmatizing, and pejorative [8,14,24]. BPD's stigmatization is critiqued as gender specific and, although the cause of BPD remains an open question, BPD has come to be viewed as a female disorder [8,25].

In line with Judith Herman's position, the authors posit that it is for sociopolitical reasons that environmental factors only recently have been given serious consideration as an etiologic explanation [14]. The collision of two historical developments in psychiatry has made the identification of important etiologic factors possible: (1) the collection of data on the high rates of child abuse (especially among females) and its deleterious effects and (2) the growing appreciation of attachment theory and the importance of attachment patterns to mental health. In addition, the influence of the women's movement [14] and feminist models of treatment [26] on the field of trauma and the impact they have had on understanding BPD must be acknowledged.

Practitioners are now in a better position to appreciate the role of environment, in particular the familial environment, in the development of BPD. BPD is a disorder profoundly affected by the early attachment environment and the broader relational environment. The meaning of broader relational environment extends beyond the mother or primary caregiver to include the potential effect of fathers, sons, uncles, daughters, grandparents, neighbors, and so forth. Theoreticians recognize the "remarkable resistance to acknowledging the appalling early experience of most borderline patients" [27] and resistance to acknowledging the connection between relational trauma and disorganized attachment in the development of the disorder [28]. The authors agree and contend that the extent and effect of childhood abuse and grossly impaired patterns of parent-child communication need to be recognized and understood in the context of the specific attachment environment to have a full appreciation of this disorder.

What is the relationship between borderline personality disorder and posttraumatic stress disorder?

The empiric literature suggests that there is a strong relationship between BPD and PTSD but that these disorders also are distinct. In recent years, there have been several studies that examine their relationship. It seems that rates of comorbid BPD and PTSD are high. One study finds 56% of patients who have BPD have PTSD and 68% of patients who have PTSD are diagnosed with BPD [29]. Research also suggests a diagnosis of BPD increases vulnerability to developing PTSD [30–32] and that PTSD can exacerbate borderline symptoms [32].

Research suggests that a diagnosis of comorbid BPD and PTSD leads to greater pathology and dysfunction than either diagnosis alone. Women who have comorbid PTSD and BPD compared with PTSD only are found to score higher in dissociation, anger expression, anxiety, interpersonal problems, and general symptomatology [33]. Another study finds that borderline patients who have PTSD have greater general dysfunction and more hospitalizations compared with BPD only or other patients who are personality disordered and who have comorbid PTSD [34]. Women who have a diagnosis of BPD only or BPD plus PTSD also are more prone to suicide and impulsivity compared with other women who are personality disordered and have PTSD [34]. Overall, research suggests that individuals who have comorbid BPD and PTSD are worse off than those who have either BPD or PTSD only, although this is not supported in all studies [35].

There also is research on the relationship of child abuse with BPD and PTSD. Zlotnick and colleagues examine the rates of sexual, physical, verbal, and emotional abuse and neglect in women who have PTSD plus BPD, BPD only, and those who have PTSD plus some other personality disorder [34]. They find that although all groups have histories of child abuse, both the personality-disordered PTSD group and the PTSD plus BPD group had higher rates in each type of child abuse compared with the BPD only group. There was no difference in rates of neglect across the three groups. This suggests that more extreme abuse in childhood is associated with PTSD.

Heffernan and Cloitre focus on women survivors of child sexual abuse and compare PTSD groups who did and did not have BPD [33]. They find no differences in severity and frequency of abuse, number of perpetrators, whether or not the perpetrator was a family member, or revictimization during childhood when comparing women who had PTSD only with women who had PTSD and BPD. Women who had PTSD plus BPD compared with women who had PTSD only were found to have more severe histories of physical and verbal abuse by their mothers and an earlier onset of abuse. These findings show some consistency with the Zlotnick study in that both groups had PTSD and there were no differences in many of the indicators of severity of childhood abuse. However, the differences they did find are consistent with the view the BPD is an attachment disorder.

These studies comparing PTSD and BPD provide preliminary evidence for the proposed conceptualization of PTPD-D, PTPD-O, and BPD. In Zlotnick's study, both PTSD groups had extensive chronic traumatization in childhood and significantly more child abuse than the pure BPD group [34]. The two PTSD groups likely meet this article's definition of PTPD-D and PTPD-O. If so, this study supports the suggestion that severe chronic traumatization in childhood leads to PTPD, whereas less severe traumatization in childhood is associated with BPD. Heffernan and Cloitre focus on women survivors of child sexual abuse and compare PTSD groups who did and did not have BPD [33]. This article's definitions suggest that they were comparing PTPD-D with PTPD-O, given the severity and chronicity of the childhood abuse reported. If so, then a difference is not expected in severity of abuse between these two groups. Thus, finding no differences in severity and frequency of abuse, number of perpetrators, or revictimization during childhood agrees with the model in this article. At the same time, they also find earlier onset of sexual abuse and greater physical and verbal abuse by a mother or stepmother among women who had PTSD and BPD (or PTPD-D, in this article's terms) compared with women who had PTSD (or PTPD-O). This suggests a profound failure to protect by an attachment figure, and, again, is in line with this article's model. The only finding in this study that is not in line with this article's model is that there is no difference in whether or not the perpetrator was a family member. This variable includes attachment figures, and a greater number of attachment figures as perpetrators in the PTSD plus BPD group was expected. In general, however, the findings from these two studies are consistent with this article's conceptualization of PTPD and BPD.

Disorganized attachment and borderline personality disorder

Attachment theorists propose that disorganized attachment lies at the core of BPD and is characterized by unintegrated schemas of self-with-other involving an attachment figure [5,18,19,36–38]. This literature on disorganized attachment provides a framework for explaining important commonalities between BPD and PTPD-D and for distinguishing these disorders from PTPD-O. The authors consider PTPD-O to be more advantageous than either BPD or PTPD-D, because it involves an organized attachment pattern. In distinguishing types of PTPD according to organized versus disorganized attachment, the authors acknowledge that organized attachment includes securely and insecurely attached individuals [19]. The authors use the classification of organized versus disorganized, because research suggests that it is the disorganization of the attachment relationship that accounts for the disturbances associated with maltreatment [39].

Attachment theorists demonstrate that the primary caregiver plays a pivotal role in assisting the infant and young child in modulating and managing their affective states. The caregivers' capacity to accurately track the child's ongoing affective experiences accurately in the service of assisting the child in regulating unmanageable affects and levels of physiologic arousal provides the underpinnings for later effective autoregulation of affect. The child gradually internalizes these functions, initially supplied by the caregiver in the course of normal development [37,38]. Thus, a sensitively attuned attachment figure enables the child to achieve a secure attachment style, resulting in an integrated sense of self, which is evident in a stable self-concept and the child's capacity to reflect on and modulate his or her affects [19,37]. (The attachment literature identifies attachment security versus insecurity as a distinct dimension from organized versus disorganized. Attachment security is viewed as an outcome of effective parenting. Insecure forms of attachment involve some degree of compromise in caregiving effectiveness, resulting in suboptimal attachment patterns. Nevertheless, as long as the attachment pattern is organized, securely and insecurely attached infants have a more or less integrated sense of self.)

It is the significant failure of the caregiver to protect the child from overwhelming distress and, in particular, failure to provide reassurance and reparation under conditions in which the caregiver may have contributed inadvertently or intentionally to the child's distress, that place the child at risk of not achieving a reliably integrated self. The child's experience of the caregiver as the source of fear and reassurance produces strong conflicting motivations. Such failure in the caregiving reparative function is believed to play a central role in the development of disorganized attachment [40]. Disorganized attachment in infancy and early childhood is considered to be the developmental precursor to the dissociated self-with-other schemas found in BPD [19,36]. The manifestation of dissociated self-with-other schemas often is referred to as "splitting."

There is a growing consensus that disorganized attachment underlies BPD [5,18,19,36–38]. The profound failure of the caregiver to be attuned to the child's needs leads to an inability to integrate representations of self-with-other [41] and deficits in self-reflective and metacognitive capacities [41,42] and in self-regulation [41]. In the authors' model, these difficulties are evident in BPD and PTPD-D. Unfortunately, individuals who have PTPD-D have the added burden of having to deal with the psychologic impact of more extensive, chronic traumatization, which implies a greater burden of fear and the difficulties associated with having a frightened and frightening primary caregiver.

The hypothesized development of posttraumatic personality disorder

Stage 1: the child's response

Lenore Terr divides childhood trauma into broad categories, type I and type II traumas [43]. Type I traumas are single events, whereas type II traumas are long-standing, multiple, or repeated experiences that, as Judith Herman points out [14], occur only in the context of circumstances in which the trauma is predictable and there is no escape. This is the experience of children abused by family members or by other familiar adults. Typically, the child will have either a trusting or dependent relationship with an adult or both. When the adult repeatedly betrays that trust by physically or sexually abusing the child, the child is usually powerless to stop it and must resort to whatever means she can to protect herself. In the moment, this often takes the form of dissociation. The child "escapes" by using her mind to go somewhere else. She might separate herself from her body (depersonalization) and watch what is happening from, for instance, a crack in the ceiling. She will remain psychologically distanced or detached until it is safe to return. When she returns, she returns to a different state where the fear and confusion have remitted, a state of being bereft of emotional contextualizing cues. This makes it easier to ignore what happened. Ignoring what happened is necessary because to remember directly is too threatening. Furthermore, whether the caregiver was available to provide support and protection or was a perpetrator or accessory to the abuse has direct bearing on the extent to which the child is capable of integrating trauma (combining affective and cognitive elements with a coherent narrative of the event) [44].

The child who is chronically traumatized inevitably swings between states of dissociative numbing and detachment and a constant state of alertness to environmental cues that predicts a repetition of their trauma. This leads to such hyperarousal symptoms as hypervigilance, difficulty concentrating, or being startled easily. Long after the traumatic experience is over, reminders of the trauma trigger these hypo- and hyperaroused states; the adult once again lives the experience of the abused child. The repeated abuse and the child's adaptation to it eventually shapes and distorts the child's sense of self and of the world. Sometimes, this can lead to a dissociative disorder, such as dissociative identity disorder. In other cases, it can lead to PTPD or comorbid dissociative and PTPDs.

Stage 2: posttraumatic personality disorder is a secondary adaptation to posttraumatic stress disorder symptoms

Krystal [45] suggests that failure of initial PTSD symptoms to resolve provokes a secondary adaptation to them. The authors propose that it is this secondary adaptation to PTSD symptoms that Herman, van der Kolk, and others call complex PTSD or DESNOS and that forms the basis of PTPD. (This theoretic stance is consistent with work that has looked at emotional tone in a family as a "bias" in development, much as it is a bias in chaos and complexity theory [46]). This is especially so if the traumatic experience remains ongoing, as in the case of chronic child abuse. If PTSD is characterized by the failure to process traumatic experience as truly having ended, or as part of the past, adaptation to a chronically aroused fear system requires extreme defensive measures that influence every aspect of a patient's psychic life. For example, severe avoidance, chronic numbing states, and an over-reliance on dissociation may help manage overwhelming affect states associated with the unresolved traumatic experiences [15], but it also seriously impedes a person's day-to-day functioning, having an impact on a person's sense of self, significant personal relationships, and navigation of interpersonal groups and communities. In support of the proposal that PTPD is a secondary adaptation to PTSD symptoms, Luxenburg and colleagues [15] note how the symptoms of PTSD re-emerge as successful treatment for DESNOS is under way. The implication is that as the secondary defenses diminish, the original disorder re-emerges.

In arguing that there is a personality adaptation to unresolved symptoms of PTSD, the authors suggest that the chronic activation of the fear system is at the heart of PTPD (either with or without disorganized attachment). This accounts for the affect dysregulation considered by some to be the core dysfunction resulting from unresolved trauma [11,15,47,48]. The chronic invocation of the fear system induces physiologic hyperarousal accompanying the expectation of danger, flashbacks of the original trauma, and impulses to flee or fight. Chronically traumatized individuals inevitably cycle from hyper- to hypoarousal states, the latter described more classically as dissociative.

Although dissociation is described variously as a process, skill, number of different symptoms, mental structure, psychologic defense, and deficit in integrative capacity [49], usually clinicians refer to dissociation as the subjective experience of detachment or separation from the sense of self and that frequently it is provoked by reminders of severe inescapable trauma. These hypo- and hyperarousal states, with their attendant affects and behavior, prevent the processing of experience in the here and now. So, too, the capacity to learn, explore, and adapt is impaired significantly by the need of a mind to manage unstable, shifting affects and their psychologic consequences. The impairment in the capacity to adapt and grow, especially during the formative years of childhood, leads to the development of a personality disorder, because individuals are forced, in a sense, to accommodate or grow around these defensive strategies and unprocessed experiences. To use developmental psychologist, Kurt Fischer's particularly apt phrase, this leads to children "growing up strangely" [50], resulting in a PTPD.

The authors submit that PTPD meets the *DSM-IV* definition of a personality disorder, which is defined as "an enduring pattern of inner experience and behavior that deviates markedly from the expectations of the individual's culture, is pervasive and inflexible, has an onset in adolescence or early adulthood, is stable over time, and leads to distress or impairment" [1]. Growing up in the context of chronic child traumatization has a relentless effect on a child's sense of self and the world. Ayoub and Fischer describe maltreated children as being on a "different" developmental pathway [51]. The developing self-system somehow must accommodate the experience of chronic traumatization, including the defensive strategies learned along the way. The authors argue in this article that this different developmental pathway shapes the inner experience and behaviors of an abuse survivor, leading to persistent distress and impairment.

Posttraumatic personality disorder and the attachment context

The necessity and type of secondary defensive attempts to keep some measure of biopsychosocial stability in individuals who are chronically traumatized vary depending on the quality of their early attachments and leads to either PTPD-O or PTPD-D.

Posttraumatic personality disorder–organized

PTPD-O includes individuals who are chronically traumatized and who have a consistently organized attachment pattern that can be either secure or insecure. Secure children have the capacity for the most adaptive connection with an important other because their earliest attachments are with a responsive attuned other who considers and relates to them as separate (and separately motivated) individuals and whose response as caregivers is to allay fear and protect from danger. For children who have an insecure attachment pattern, it also is organized insofar as it is an adaptive response to a less adequate caregiver. They have a capacity for connection with others even though it is somewhat compromised. Thus, secure and insecure children have had the experience of being able to maintain some connection to their early attachment figures.

Given these early nontraumatizing relational experiences, these children have developed more or less a capacity to recognize the malevolence of the perpetrator. Adults who have PTPD-O are less likely to show type D attachment patterns on the Adult Attachment Interview and more likely show secure, avoidant, or anxious-ambivalent patterns. As discussed previously, dissociative defenses are common in children who cannot escape sexual and physical abuse by a caretaker. In these children, a layer of dissociative defenses is added because of their need to avoid knowing what they know. They need to veil the cause of their fear states from self-reflective awareness. Without help from another, these traumatic events cannot be known and contained within the mind of a child. If the trauma never was recognized by significant others in a child's life, such as with Gay's sexual abuse, Stern [52] states, "such experience is screened out prior to its articulation; it remains undeveloped...and is excluded from the self system, along with whatever implications it might have had." Stern and others take this idea one step further: that the undeveloped experience remains a part of the self-system, but in an unformulated manner, and results in the child growing along an abnormal developmental pathway [53,54]. For example, it becomes increasingly important for the integrity of the self to not know there is something terrifying that is not known. With no safe caregiver to stop the abuse and help understand and reflect on it, the child cannot allow herself to "know" what happened and, as a result, the events cannot be integrated fully. Instead, the events go unmarked and unknown and the affects of terror, shame and anger are kept at bay by the detachment and ultimate compartmentalization of inner experience [55].

This complex inhibition leaves large parts of the child's past unintegrated and individuals who have PTPD-O in chronically aroused states of fear. The fight, flight, and dissociative defenses are triggered easily. This results in an inability to attend adequately to the experience of the present. The experience of fear and its invalidation or invisibility to a caregiver becomes fodder for the child's self-blaming and shaming explanations for unspoken traumatic experiences. The child comes to believe that the abuse must be deserved, that the perpetrator recognized her dirty, disposable core nature, confirmed by the fact no one intervened. The sense of a secretly damaged self leads to the interpretation of internal cues through this belief in badness; wanting or need, for instance, is derided by individuals as shameful or embarrassing. Relationships with other people may seem superficially on track but to a traumatized person they provide little warmth and intimacy. They are filtered through the lens of a self that believes it is deeply unworthy.

Although some of these adaptations can seem analogous to borderline phenomena, despite similarities and overlap between PTPD-O and BPD, there are some important differences. Building on the clinical observations of Luxenburg and colleagues [15], individuals who have PTPD-O, as opposed to those who have BPD, have less ability to experience or sustain access to positive emotions. Although individuals who have BPD can oscillate from intense positive feelings associated with idealization of others to intense negative feelings associated with the denigration of others, individuals who have PTPD-O tend to feel far more negative affect in general because of their self-negation, formed by the more pressing need to manage and placate others. They are more avoidant of others, whereas individuals who have BPD are more approach focused. In patients who have PTPD-O, the use of avoidance in their response to fear of the trauma becoming reactivated also explains the more phobic response toward others, in contrast to the complex, contentious engagements of individuals who have BPD. Individuals who have PTPD-O attempt to regulate their affect states alone and not with the help of others, although, paradoxically, they learn to direct their attention outwards to monitor their environment, including other people. They learn to please, placate, and manage others to avoid conflict. Thus, on the surface, they may seem pleasant. They tend to feel extremely anxious in the presence of others, chronically tracking for the signs of danger. Dissociation is not brief and transient as it is in BPD but a chronic and frequent state in PTPD. Finally, although their sense of self is less confused than in BPD, the self-abnegation, fear, and chronic dissociative defenses reinforce permanent feelings of damage and alienation from others.

Posttraumatic personality disorder–disorganized

Individuals who have PTPD-D struggle with the consequences of disorganized attachment and chronic childhood traumatization. Unlike individuals who are chronically traumatized and have an organized attachment pattern (PTPD-O) and, thus, a relatively stable sense of self, persons who are chronically traumatized and have disorganized attachment lack a stable sense of self and have little experience of primary attachments that are not fear based. In addition, persons who have PTPD-D are chronically adapted to overwhelming fear states as a result of significant chronic childhood abuse. Individuals who have PTPD-D have the full spectrum of DESNOS symptoms, PTSD symptoms, and the symptoms of BPD.

Individuals who have PTPD-D have a longing for and fear of interpersonal connection. Thus, unlike individuals who have PTPD-O, who prefer to self-regulate alone, these individuals use an approach-avoidance strategy in relationships. As with those who have BPD, these individuals fear and chronically predict their abandonment. In addition, chronic traumatization involving the use of power, intimidation, or violence by an abuser instills fear and anger and reinforces disorganization. Persons who have PTPD-D use either dissociative adaptations to escape or engage in angry and violent acting out, often in ways similar to how adults communicated in their chaotic childhood. As disorganized individuals become dependent on and fearful of their perpetrator, their behavioral manifestations as adults may be either helpless or hostile interpersonal stances or the two in alternation [56]. Thus, unlike persons who have PTPD-O, who are actively avoidant, the PTPD-D person is likely to take an alternating passive-dependent or aggressive stance in relationships. Terrified of abandonment and bored without intense ambivalent interactions, they quickly burn out friends, family, and caregivers. Furthermore, these individuals constantly monitor their environment for danger and usually misattribute motivations to the other. In combination with their difficulty recognizing danger in their environment, this renders these individuals highly prone to revictimization, which only reinforces behaviors, feelings, and beliefs associated with PTPD-D.

An important difference in the childhood experiences of those who develop PTPD-D from those who develop BPD is in the degree to which the fear system is activated. Given the intensity of fear evoked by exposure to more extreme chronic abuse, those who have a history of early childhood abuse likely show significant deficits in their ability to regulate their affect. In cases where a primary caregiver has perpetrated the abuse, the disjunctiveness of the parent's behavior during the abuse episode from how the parent is likely to behave during other times is likely to result in more pronounced dissociation of such experiences than in the case of less overt maltreatment. This helps explain the greater prominence of dissociative symptoms in individuals who have PTPD-D relative to BPD. In BPD, dissociative symptoms are not pervasive and typically are transient responses to stress [15,57]. In patients who have PTPD-D, alternatively, dissociation is more prevalent as they must manage the overwhelming fear that easily is triggered by reminders of the abuse that occur in everyday experience.

Affect-regulating behaviors in individuals who have PTPD-O and those who have PTPD-D can involve several behaviors aimed at subduing internal tension and often involve self-harm. For instance, both types of individuals may use drugs or alcohol to "feel better." Other behaviors include self-injury, such as cutting, which has the paradoxic effect of improving how they feel. In individuals who have PTPD-O, these behaviors may be hidden and private, because their purpose strictly is affect regulation. With PTPD-D, however, such behaviors more likely involve affect management and communicating relational needs. Recognizing these differences is helpful for treating clinicians.

Implications of this typology for treatment

This section on treatment constitutes a brief series of comments to facilitate more comprehensive treatment strategies. These strategies can be combined easily with existing clinical guidelines for the treatment of individuals who are chronically traumatized and those who have BPD. This proposed typology hopes to add another lens through which the phenomenology and suffering of clients who have chronic trauma disorders is illuminated and also hopes to validate and reinforce experienced clinicians' continuing observations, thoughtful evaluations, and refinement of treatment strategies and techniques for clients who are chronically frightened and whose coping involves significant personality adaptations. Treatment implications for patients who have PTPD-O and the PTPD-D are approached within a phase-orientated treatment orientation and treatment of BPD is discussed only as it helps elucidate this. The fictional cases of Gay and Dee, as examples of one patient who has PTPD-O and one who has PTPD-D, are used to illustrate the clinical examples.

There are three phases of treatment commonly used to guide the treatment of individuals who are traumatized [14,24]. Phase one refers to the stabilization of patients. Phase two involves the specific focus on past traumatic experiences that remain unintegrated. Techniques aimed at helping patients to assimilate whatever is unprocessed or unreflected on in their past usually are used at this point in treatment. Phase three involves the re-entry of individuals into their lives after their understanding and coming to terms with their traumatic pasts. There is a reorganizing of defenses and coping abilities after treatment of chronic fear states. Consequently, life choices, plans, and relationships take on a different quality and emphasis, as if a whole life is reclaimed and reworked.

Phase one

Focusing on the stabilization phase for patients who have PTPD-O or PTPD-D requires early attention to their dissociative phenomena. Although these patients have multiple symptoms and difficulties, little useful work can occur until they are less afraid of staying engaged in their present experience. Therapy for these two types of patients has a greater focus on grounding and a present felt sense of safety than for patients who have BPD, who are locked less chronically into fear states. For patients, such as Gay and Dee, developing the capacity to stay present and grounded and attend to their somatic, emotional, and cognitive reactions is the essential component to beginning therapeutic work. Stabilization for Dee includes helping her to become free of substance use, usually done in conjunction with a specialized drug and addiction team and program.

Gay (PTPD-O) is an example of a woman whose chronic fear is "invisible," although superficially she does not look beside herself with fear, this is her subjective experience most of the time, especially in the company of another person. She remains detached or outside her subjective sense of self most of the time because she is frightened most of the time. Everyone liked Gay in the trauma program; she was compliant and agreeable. She seemed to listen, nodded and smiled faintly, and was composed and kindly. Gay was not able to muster any reflective sense of self to be able to consider whether or not she actually agreed with what was said to her. She could not take in the good will and fondness others had of her. It is easy for inexperienced therapists to miss how successfully patients who have PTPD-O "hide in plain sight," meaning that their chronic fear states go unseen and unremarked on by others. Their profoundly negative sense of self also precludes almost any familiarity with tolerance for positive affect. Experience in this case teaches that often clinicians do not know how well their patients camouflage their fear. Asking directly how distressed they are on a Subjective Units of Distress Scale of 0 to 10 (0 meaning no distress and 10 the maximum imaginable) often is the only way to find out, early in a treatment.

There often is more chaos in the life of patients who have PTPD-D, such as Dee. They may have a wider range of affective tone in their engagement with others compared with individuals who have PTPD-O. There is a greater capacity for experiencing positive and negative affects compared with those who have PTPD-O. Relational idealization and disappointments are more pronounced in patients who have BPD or PTPD-D.

As discussed previously, patients who have PTPD are characterized by significant affect dysregulation. They have a combination of dissociative numbing and distancing from their emotions that may alternate with emotional flooding. Paradoxically, this seems to enhance their tendency to interpret their emotions as calls to action or avoidance, to be more fearfully reactive to intense affect. Once patients are able to stay more fully present, mindfully naming and recognizing their emotions and their immediate causes, they are less obliged to take action and can initiate a more regulated internal experience and a less chaotic social environment.

The use of psychoeducation is remarkably therapeutic for both types of PTPD early in treatment. Recognizing how abuse and fear have led to the seven domains or symptom clusters of DESNOS can be validating and reassuring and helps build a therapeutic alliance. Developing this common understanding also serves as a secure base of shared perspective, from which nonadaptive behavior and other relational difficulties may be recognized as etiologically related to the past and their adaptation to it. Because this shared frame considers all behavior, suffering and difficulties as adaptive responses to an abusive and disconfirming past, the groundwork for undercutting negative sense of self is laid. The shift toward an empathic appreciation of their own strength, courage, and fortitude in the face of unrelenting hardship is slow to evolve, making early self-care a frequent topic of therapeutic challenge.

Of particular importance is that Gay (PTPD-O) was chronically suicidal and Dee (PTPD-D) made several suicide attempts. Therapists need to differentiate between self-abuse, which generally is aimed at trying to regulate affect and stay alive, from the wish, plan, or behaviors aimed at ending one's life. Recognizing behaviors that create high risk for self-harm, especially for Dee, is a vital part of developing stability. The use of contracts in therapy, clarifying mutually agreed-upon rules about suicidal thoughts and impulses, can be helpful, in particular for patients who have PTPD-D. Therapists need to ensure, however, that they not only are loophole-free but also sealed with eye contact and often a handshake. Being helped in this concrete way to keep their word can be highly supportive for patients. They may feel more securely "held" by the bonds of such a contract. The mortar of the contract is in the feeling of the relationship between patient and therapist. Contracts, in and of themselves, are no guarantee of safety. For patients who have PTPD-D or PTPD-O, the role of brief voluntary hospitalizations is discussed as a way to short-circuit suicide attempts. For patients who have PTPD-O, often this takes the place of a more formally agreed-upon antisuicide contract, because they are more relationally resourced.

As Gay and Dee each attain a measure of biopsychosocial stability, which may involve the judicious use of psychotropics, their differences start to become more evident. Whereas once Gay achieved even a modest degree of stability (discussed previously), she surprised her therapists by being able to divorce her abusive husband and search out her estranged son—actions Gay had wanted to do for years. Once Dee's dissociative numbness began to remit, she needed considerably more focus on the frame and boundaries of therapy and on her relationship with her therapist. The presence of felt affect was frightening and destabilizing. She needed to learn to identify felt feelings and how to tolerate and resolve them. Dee's failure to settle and work in therapy annoyed her therapist, who also realized that with less dissociation Dee's chronic relational pattern was emerging. Dee behaved with her therapist just as she had learned to behave with her mother, stepfather, and boyfriends. Her approach-avoidance strategy was played out as feeling positive one minute with her therapist and angrily berating her the next, as though a calm consistent relationship was less predictable or even frightening. This should be pointed out gently and often to Dee, with the therapist suggesting that her devaluing words were perhaps a preemptive strike, a protection against being left.

Failure to recognize and explore these relational repetitions of early empathic failures can lead patients to drop out of therapy or become increasingly angry and upset within it, but never really staying and working or leaving physically. For patients who have PTPD-D, the challenge is to develop a positive dependency or a healthy reliance on a therapist. It can be easy for therapists either to fall into the trap of seeing a patient like Dee as having BPD only or as having PTDP-O only. With one type of misunderstanding of a patient's need to modulate affects and relational distance, a patient's adaptation to the presence of chronic fear is underacknowledged; with the other type, her need for more relationally attuned work is overlooked.

Phase two

In phase two, working through recollections of traumatic experience can start with both types of patients who have PTPD as long as they have a relatively more stable sense of self-in-therapy and an ongoing prepared-ness to prioritize stability over trauma work at any time. This is acquired somewhat more reliably in the group that has PTPD-O. Stability within phase two requires that any attempt to explore the past be titrated to ensure that swings between hyperarousal and hypoarousal states connected with dissociation are kept to a minimum. This may be retraumatizing when it oc-curs. Appropriate positive reinforcement goes a long way toward assisting these patients in remembering their grounding techniques when difficult ma-terial from the past threatens to destabilize them. Patients who have PTPD-D usually need help slowing down their wish to access past traumatic states, which can destabilize them dramatically. They often put too much emphasis on the urgency and centrality that desensitizing themselves to past trauma plays, failing to appreciate that relevant aspects of their past are played out minute by minute within the therapeutic dyad and often are addressed more safely and more successfully in the here-and-now relational context.

Recalling traumatic experience with patients who have BPD is not a ma-jor focus of work, although it might be easy to be persuaded that it is by such patients. Their memories of bad times are less screened off from their awareness, the abuse is less pervasive and severe than for patients who have PTPD, and they are less amnestic for their past. Whatever traumatic expe-riences they may have had is less the issue than the lack of their relational skills. It is likely, however, that the affect concerning their memories is not integrated adequately—it may be incongruent or somehow exaggerated and inauthentic as it is with Dee. This work is undertaken best as their mem-ories disturb or interfere with a therapeutic relationship.

Phase three

Phase three for patients who have PTPD-O or PTPD-D requires clear on-going work on investing in relationships outside of therapy. Patients who are chronically traumatized often are phobic of any type of relationship, in particular intimate ones. The therapeutic relationship is central to therapy in all three groups of patients in this discussion. For the patients who have PTPD-O or PTPD-D, therapists constantly need to find ways to challenge their reliance on therapy as a relational substitute for social bonds outside the consulting room. Problem-solving the details of new relationships and interpersonal relational competance are useful with patients who have PTPD. Phase three for PTPD-D, however, requires additional focus on de-velopment of a cohesive sense of self and tolerance for being alone. Having relied so heavily on chaotic relational re-enactments for a sense of familiar-ity, therapeutic encouragement is required to help patients develop a sense of self that can exist stably without the need for intense ambivalent relation-ships. Focus on work or school is helpful at this stage. With PTPD-O and PTPD-D, there is a period in phase three when the clear gains patients make become obvious to patients and therapists alike. Paradoxically, it is this experience that can be anxiety provoking, a type of latter day rapprochement, when returning to previous (mal-)adaptation no longer is possible and the experience of relative gains in psychologic health is too fragile to count on securely. This passes, however, as patients, with therapist assistance, develop experience and confidence in building a life worth living and move toward the termination of therapy.

Summary

This article proposes two new diagnostic categories intended to capture the full range of consequences that can arise as a result of chronic childhood traumatization. Although complex PTSD (or DESNOS) is intended to reflect the consequences of chronic traumatization, the domains that DESNOS describes are characterized more accurately as a personality disorder, more specifically, a PTPD. Furthermore, there are two types of PTPD, one involving organized attachment and the other involving disorganized attachment, both determined by early attachment experiences. Both are associated with PTSD. PTPD-D is the category that represents the comorbid condition of BPD and DESNOS. PTPD-O, alternatively, represents DESNOS without BPD. Understanding the effect of chronic traumatization in the context of either organized or disorganized attachment has specific treatment implications.

This model is offered as a vehicle for furthering the authors' collective thinking and understanding of the consequences of chronic traumatization. It also is their hope that this model stimulates research in an effort to test its validity and, ultimately, that it helps inform clinical practice.

References

[1] American Psychiatric Association. Diagnostic and statistical manual of mental disorders. 4th edition. Washington, DC: American Psychiatric Association; 1994.

[2] Herman JL. Complex PTSD: a syndrome in survivors of prolonged and repeated trauma. J Trauma Stress 1992;5:377–91.

[3] van der Kolk BA, Roth S, Pelcovitz D, et al. Complex PTSD: results of the PTSD field trial for DSM-IV. Washington, DC: American Psychiatric Association; 1993.

[4] Hesse E, Main M, Abrams K, et al. Unresolved states regarding loss or abuse can have "second-generation" effects: disorganization, role inversion, and frightening ideation in the offspring of traumatized, non-maltreating parents. In: Solomon M, Siegel D, editors. Healing trauma: attachment, mind, body, and brain. New York: W.W. Norton; 2003; p. 57–106.

[5] Lyons-Ruth K, Yellin C, Melnick S, et al. Expanding the concept of unresolved mental states: hostile/helpless states of mind on the Adult Attachment Interview are associated with disrupted mother-infant communication and infant disorganization. Dev Psychopathol 2005;17:1–23.

[6] Yehuda R, McFarlane AC. Conflict between current knowledge about posttraumatic stress disorder and its original conceptual basis. Am J Psychiatry 1995;152:1705–13.

[7] Ford JD. Disorders of extreme stress following war-zone military trauma: associated features of posttraumatic stress disorder or comorbid but distinct syndromes? J Consult Clin Psychol 1999;67:3–12.

[8] Courtois CA. Complex trauma, complex reactions: assessment and treatment. Psychoth Theory Res Practice Training 2004;41(4):412–25.
[9] Roth S, Newman E, Pelcovitz D, et al. Complex PTSD in victims exposed to sexual and physical abuse. J Trauma Stress 1997;10:539–55.
[10] Pelcovitz D, van der Kolk B, Roth S, et al. Development of a criteria set and a structured interview for disorders of extreme stress (SIDES). J Trauma Stress 1997;10:3–16.
[11] van der Kolk BA, Pelcovitz D, Roth S, et al. Dissociation, somatization, and affect dysregulation: the complexity of adaptation to trauma. Am J Psychiatry 1996;153:83–93.
[12] Kessler RC, Sonnega A, Bromet E, et al. Posttraumatic stress disorder in the National Comorbidity Survey. Arch Gen Psychiatry 1995;52:1048–60.
[13] World Health Organization. The ICD-10 classification of mental and behavioural disorders: clinical descriptions and diagnostic guidelines. Geneva: World Health Organization; 1992.
[14] Herman JL. Trauma and recovery. New York: Basic Books; 1992.
[15] Luxenberg T, Spinazzola J, van der Kolk BA. Complex trauma and disorders of extreme stress (DESNOS) diagnosis, part one: assessment. Directions Psychiatry 2001;21: 363–92.
[16] Luxenberg T, Spinazzola J, Hidalgo J, et al. Complex trauma and disorders of extreme stress (DESNOS) part two: treatment. Directions Psychiatry 2001;21:395–414.
[17] Briere J. Therapy for adults molested as children. 2nd edition. New York: Springer Publishing Company; 1996.
[18] Holmes J. Borderline personality disorder and the search for meaning: an attachment perspective. Aust N Z J Med 2003;37:524–31.
[19] Liotti G. Trauma, dissocation, and disorganized attachment: three strands of a single braid. Psychother Theory Res Practice Training 2004;41:472–86.
[20] Gunderson JG. The borderline patient's intolerance of aloneness: insecure attachments and therapist availability. Am J Psychiatry 1996;153:752–8.
[21] Harvey M. An ecological view of psychological trauma and trauma recovery. J Trauma Stress 1996;9:3–23.
[22] Stern A. Psychoanalytic investigation of therapy in the borderline group of neuroses. Psychoanal Q 1938;7:467–89.
[23] Paris J. Borderline personality disorder: a multidimensional approach. Washington, DC: American Psychiatric Press; 1994.
[24] Chu JA. Rebuilding shattered lives: the responsible treatment of complex post-traumatic and dissociative disorders. New York: John Wiley & Sons; 1998.
[25] Zanarini MC, Williams AA, Lewis RE, et al. Reported pathological childhood experiences associated with the development of borderline personality disorder. Am J Psychiatry 1997; 154:1101–6.
[26] Brown LS. Feminist paradigms of trauma treatment. Psychother Theory Res Practice Training 2004;41:464–71.
[27] Golynkina K, Ryle A. The identification and characteristics of the partially dissociated states of patients with borderline personality disorder. Br J Med Psychol 1999;72:429–45.
[28] Blizard R. Chronic relational trauma disorder: a new paradigm for borderline personality and the spectrum of dissociative disorders. Presented at The International Society for the Study of Dissociation 21st International Fall Conference. New Orleans, 2004.
[29] Shea MT, Zlotnick C, Weisberg RB. Commonality and specificity of personality disorder profiles in subjects with trauma histories. J Pers Disord 1999;13:199–210.
[30] Yen S, Shea MT, Battle CL, et al. Traumatic exposure and posttraumatic stress disorder in borderline, schizotypal, avoidant and obsessive-compulsive personality disorders: findings from the Collaborative Longitudinal Personality Disorders Study. J Nerv Ment Dis 2002; 190:510–8.
[31] Golier J, Yehuda R, Bierer LM, et al. The relationship of borderline personality disorder to posttraumatic stress disorder and traumatic events. Am J Psychiatry 2003;160: 2018–24.

[32] Axelrod SR, Morgan CA, Southwick SM. Symptoms of posttraumatic stress disorder and borderline personality disorder in veterans of Operation Desert Storm. Am J Psychiatry 2005;162:270–5.

[33] Heffernan K, Cloitre M. A comparison of posttraumatic stress disorder with and without borderline personality disorder among women with a history of childhood sexual abuse: etiological and clinical characteristics. J Nerv Ment Dis 2000;188:589–95.

[34] Zlotnick C, Johnson DM, Yen S, et al. Clinical features and impairment in women with borderline personality disorder (BPD) with posttraumatic stress disorder (PTSD), BPD without PTSD, and other personality disorders with PTSD. J Nerv Ment Dis 2003;191:706–13.

[35] Zlotnick C, Franklin CL, Zimmerman M. Is comorbidity of posttraumatic stress disorder and borderline personality disorder related to greater pathology and impairment? Am J Psychiatry 2002;159:1940–3.

[36] Blizard RA. Disorganized attachment, development of dissociated self states, and a relational approach to treatment. J Trauma Dissociation 2003;4:27–50.

[37] Fonagy P, Gergely G, Jurist EL, et al. Affect regulation, mentalization, and the development of the self. New York: Other Press; 2002.

[38] Schore A. The effects of early relational trauma on right brain development, affect regulation, and infant mental health. Infant Ment Health J 2001;22:201–69.

[39] Lyons-Ruth K, Jacobvitz D. Attachment disorganization: unresolved loss, relational violence, and lapses in behavioral and attentional strategies. In: Cassidy J, Shaver PR, editors. Handbook of attachment: theory, research, and clinical applications. New York: Guilford Press; 1999.

[40] Solomon J, George C. The place of disorganization in attachment theory: linking classic observations with contemporary findings. In: Solomon J, George C, editors. Attachment disorganization. New York: Guilford Press; 1999. p. 3–32.

[41] Liotti G. Il nucleo del Disturbo Borderline di Personalità: un'ipotesi integrativa [The nucleus of the Borderline Personality Disorder: an integrative hypothesis]. Psicoterapia 1999; 5(16/17):53–65 [in Italian].

[42] Fonagy P, Steele M, Steele H, et al. Attachment, the reflective self, and borderline states: the predictive specificity of the adult attachment interview and pathological emotional development. In: Goldberg S, Muir R, Kerr J, editors. Attachment theory: social, developmental, and clinical perspectives. Hillsdale (NJ): Analytic Press; 2000.

[43] Terr LC. Childhood traumas: an outline and overview. Am J Psychiatry 1991;148:10–20.

[44] Lieberman AF. Traumatic stress and quality of attachment: reality and internalization in disorders of infant mental health. Infant Ment Health J 2004;25:336–51.

[45] Krystal H. Integration and self-healing: affect, trauma, alexithymia. Hillsdale (NJ): Analytic Press; 1988.

[46] Stechler G, Kaplan S. The development of the self—a psychoanalytic perspective. Psychoanal Study Child 1980;35:85–105.

[47] Ford J, Kidd T. Early childhood trauma and disorders of extreme stress as predictors of treatment outcome wiht chronic posttraumatic stress disorder. J Trauma Stress 1998;11: 743–61.

[48] Lang PJ. The emotion probe: studies of motivation and attention. Am Psychol 1995;50: 372–85.

[49] van der Hart O, Nijenhuis E, Steele K, et al. Trauma-related dissociation: conceptual clarity lost and found. Aust N Z J Psychiatry 2004;38:906–14.

[50] Fischer KW, Pipp SL. Development of the structures of unconscious thought. In: Meichenbaum KBD, editor. The unconscious reconsidered. New York: Wiley; 1984. p. 88–148.

[51] Ayoub CC, Fischer KW. Developmental pathways and intersections among domains of development. In: McCartney K, Phillips D, editors. Blackwell handbook on early childhood development. Malden (MA): Blackwell, in press.

[52] Stern DB. Unformulated experience: from dissociation to imagination in psychoanalysis. Hillsdale (NJ): Analytic Press; 1997.

[53] Fischer KW, Ayoub C, Singh I, et al. Psychopathology as adaptive development along distinctive pathways. Dev Psychopathol 1997;9:749–79.

[54] Chefetz RA. The paradox of "detachment disorders": binding-disruptions of dissociative process. Psychiatry 2004;67:246–55.

[55] Allen JG. Traumatic relationships and serious mental disorders. New York: John Wiley & Sons; 2001.

[56] Fonagy P. Attachment theory and psychoanalysis. New York: Other Press; 2001.

[57] Darves-Bornoz JM, Lemperiere T, Degiovanni A, et al. Sexual victimization in women with schizophrenia and bipolar disorder. Soc Psychiatry Psychiatr Epidemiol 1995;30:78–84.

PSYCHIATRIC
CLINICS
OF NORTH AMERICA

Psychiatr Clin N Am 29 (2006) 113–128

Neurobiology of Dissociation: Unity and Disunity in Mind–Body–Brain

Paul A. Frewen, MA[a], Ruth A. Lanius, MD, PhD[b],*

[a]*Department of Psychology, The University of Western Ontario,*
339 Windermere Road, P.O. Box 5339, London, Ontario N6A 5A5, Canada
[b]*Department of Psychiatry, The University of Western Ontario, 339 Windermere Road,*
P.O. Box 5339, London, Ontario N6A 5A5, Canada

This article reviews studies of the neural correlates of dissociative experiences as assessed by functional neuroimaging (positron emission tomography [PET] and functional magnetic resonance imaging [fMRI]). Current PET and fMRI studies are reviewed in reference to van der Kolk and colleagues' [1] organizing psychologic constructs: primary, secondary, and tertiary dissociation. We believe the distinctive neural correlates of primary and secondary dissociative experiences, observed in response to reminders of previous psychologic trauma in individuals who have posttraumatic stress disorder (PTSD), support state-phase models of animal defensive reaction to external threat [2,3]. Furthermore, disconnection of neural pathways normally linking self-awareness with emotional body-state perception could occasion the development of dissociative identities in traumatized children.

Primary dissociation

As defined by van der Kolk and colleagues [1], primary dissociation refers to the intrusion into conscious awareness of fragmented traumatic memories, primarily in sensory rather than verbal form: "Memories of the trauma are initially experienced as fragments of the sensory components of the event—as visual images; olfactory, auditory, or kinesthetic sensations; or

---

This work is supported by grants #MOP 49543 from the Canadian Institutes of Health Research; #M931D5 from the Ontario Mental Health Foundation; #MA9477 from the Canadian Psychiatric Research Foundation; and a Canada Graduate Scholarship from the Social Sciences & Humanities Research Council of Canada.
* Corresponding author.
E-mail address: ruth.lanius@lhsc.on.ca (R.A. Lanius).

doi:10.1016/j.psc.2005.10.016   *psych.theclinics.com*

intense waves of feelings." These phenomenologic responses, cued by reminders of past traumatic events, represent a defining diagnostic feature of PTSD and are often associated with psychophysiologic arousal, as indexed by increased heart-rate and electrical skin conductance [4]. In our own studies, approximately 70% of individuals diagnosed with PTSD display this prototypical symptom profile in response to verbal reminders of their traumatic events.

Several functional neuroimaging studies have examined the neural correlates of this response using a script-driven imagery paradigm [5–19]. This paradigm involves exposing an individual to an audio script that briefly recounts a personally traumatic experience in their life. The individual is instructed to recall sensory aspects of the event while listening to the script. Through subtraction analysis, areas of neural response to traumatic script-driven imagery are demarcated from areas involved in processing nontraumatic memories, or compared with neural processing involved in some other nonaffective baseline task (eg, while monitoring one's breathing). In turn, areas of neural activation are identified that differentiate PTSD symptom-responses from those of trauma-exposed nonpsychiatric controls, the latter typically reporting no to very limited subjective emotional impact of the experimental paradigm.

We review the results of such comparisons at length in a separate recent article [20], and therefore this article only summarizes the principal findings. The most replicated findings include less response of the anterior cingulate cortex (ACC) (Brodmann areas [BAs] 24 & 32) and medial prefrontal cortex (mPFC) (BAs 9 & 10) in individuals who have PTSD compared with nonpsychiatric controls (Fig. 1) [8,10,17,18,21]. Based on the results of other studies in cognitive and affective neuroscience, these structures are known to serve several key emotion-processing functions. The ACC is involved in the executive (effortful, intentional) control of attention in terms of regulating emotional [22,23], cognitive [24,25], and autonomic [26–28] responses. In patients who have PTSD, the relative inactivity of the ACC during trauma script-imagery is therefore in accord with clinical observations that these patients are unable to modulate their automatic affective response to cues of their traumatic experiences. This response may be partly mediated by an overactive amygdala [16,29,30], which is known to be involved in fear conditioning and selective attention to threat [31,32]. Studies have found pronounced amygdala response to external fearful stimuli (eg, emotional facial expressions) in PTSD [33–35].

In contrast, the mPFC is normally active during self-reflective thought [36–39] and when individuals are in a state of quiet ease (ie, "free-floating" mental awareness), and often deactivates during tasks requiring concentrated mental effort [40]. Therefore, less activation of mPFC during trauma script-driven imagery in PTSD is consistent with a hyperarousal response marshaled to cope with perceived current threat. Studies have found an inverse correlation between mPFC and amygdala activation to fearful stimuli in PTSD [7,35].

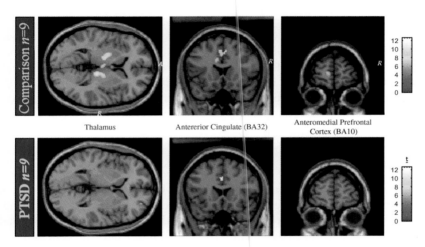

Fig. 1. Primary dissociative response to script-driven imagery of traumatic events. Areas of significant Blood-Oxygen-Level-Dependent fMRI response to script-driven imagery of traumatic events in individuals who have PTSD (primary dissociative response) and comparison (nonpsychiatric control) subjects ($P = .001$, $k = 10$).

In addition to replicating the robust ACC and mPFC effects, Lanius and colleagues [8,10] identified reduced thalamic activation during symptom-provocation in patients who had PTSD, as have others (see Fig. 1) [21,41]. Llinás [42] describes intrinsic thalamocortical oscillatory activation as characterizing normal waking consciousness and dream states. According to this theory, temporal integration of thalamic-modulated sensory input with high-order cortical representations constitutes the platform on which felt perceptions of being a unitary self existing in an external world (ie, of temporal consciousness and reality) are synthesized. Relative lack of thalamic activation during primary-dissociative "reliving" in PTSD may exemplify dysregulation in the normal dynamic communication between thalamus and cortex, during which thalamic inputs representing the objective sensed state of the external world fail to influence cortical representations. In turn, our observations of distributed right-hemispheric cortical activation in PTSD during symptom provocation, in the relative absence of thalamic input, might mediate memory-derived altered conscious perceptions (ie, primary dissociation and the reliving sense) [12,43].

In summary, extant findings are generally in concordance with clinical observations that suggest that, rather than processing traumatic memories reflectively (ie, with no more than moderate arousal and while maintaining consciousness of the current self, environmental, and temporal context), primary dissociative responses in PTSD involve the emotional and phenomenologic reliving of traumatic memories as if they are occurring at the moment of recall. These experiences may correspond with initial amygdala hyperresponsivity to trauma fear cues, temporarily increasing the salience of sensory associations recorded in occipital and parietal somatosensory regions, and superseding the influence on consciousness of less immediately affect-inducing language-mediated symbolic associations (eg, those stored in the left hippocampus; [44]). Coupled with a relative lack of response modulation through the ACC and mPFC, the increased salience of traumatic sensory-memory representations may exceed the influence of sensory-thalamic inputs on cortex, resulting in traumatic memory-derived perceptual distortions invading consciousness.

Secondary dissociation

In comparison with primary dissociation, which emphasizes sensations of reliving traumatic memories, van der Kolk and colleagues [1] define secondary dissociation as the mental "leaving" of the body and observing what happens from a distance during moments of trauma. van der Kolk and colleagues [1] emphasize that such psychologic distancing of one's conscious awareness from one's body limits pain and distress, and "puts people out of touch with the feelings and emotions related to the trauma; it anesthetizes them." Although secondary dissociation is acknowledged as a commonly associated feature of PTSD as it is defined by the *Diagnostic and Statistical Manual of Mental Disorders, Fourth Edition* (DSM-IV), and is often referred to as *peritraumatic dissociation* in the contemporary literature, these symptoms are not a central diagnostic mark of PTSD, but are prominent in the diagnosis of depersonalization disorder. In a PET study during which subjects performed a verbal learning and memory task, Simeon and colleagues [45] observed reduced metabolism in BA 22 of the right superior temporal gyrus and in area 21 of the middle temporal gyrus, and increased metabolism in areas 7B and 39 of the parietal lobe and area 19 of the left occipital lobe in patients who had depersonalization disorder compared with nonpsychiatric controls. These findings are consistent with visual and somatosensory abnormalities reported by patients who have depersonalization disorder, who commonly feel that their psychological self or mind is somehow detached from their physical self or body. Simeon and colleagues speculate that such distortions in body schema represent functional lesions that have similar (if less dramatic) psychologic symptoms to structural lesions of the parietal lobe, the latter often resulting in well-recognized neurologic syndromes, such as neglect.

Three neuroimaging investigations of dissociative responses to trauma-script–driven imagery have been published to date [9,11,13]. In a case study [11], autonomic (heart rate change) and neural responses were compared in a husband and wife who developed PTSD after being exposed to the same traumatic event but who exhibited differing psychologic reactions. (The couple was trapped in their car after a multivehicle accident where they witnessed a child from another vehicle burn to death, and feared for their own lives.) In this instance, the husband displayed a primary dissociative reliving response to the script-driven imagery paradigm, which included elevated subjective fear and increased heart rate, and was associated with increased activation relative to baseline in several neural areas distributed across the limbic, frontal, and temporal lobes. In comparison, the wife displayed a secondary dissociative response, reporting afterward that she felt "extremely numb" and "frozen." Her heart rate did not change significantly from baseline in response to imagery of her traumatic experience, and she exhibited increased neural activity confined to areas around the parietal-occipital juncture (right precuneus, bilateral cuneus, and bilateral lingual gyrus; BAs 18 & 19). Although generalizations regarding the neurobiology of primary versus secondary dissociative responses are appropriately reserved in this instance given the uniqueness of the sample, the study does illustrate that the same traumatic event can be experienced differently by individuals, and that these differences can be observed at psychologic and neural levels of analysis.

In a larger script-imagery fMRI study [9], brain activation was compared between seven individuals who exhibited a secondary dissociative response and 10 nonpsychiatric controls who reacted nonaffectively. Secondary dissociative responses did not exhibit the significant increase in heart rate typically associated with primary dissociative reliving responses [4]. In contrast to findings of decreased ACC and mPFC function typically observed during primary dissociative reliving, individuals who had PTSD who demonstrated a secondary-type dissociative response showed increased right ACC and mPFC activity compared with nonpsychiatric controls. This response suggests a possible enhanced suppression of limbic emotion circuits in secondary dissociation.

In addition, individuals who had secondary-type dissociative PTSD showed more significant activation of the superior and middle temporal gyri (BA 38, 39), the right precuneus (parietal lobe, BA 7), and the left cuneus (occipital lobe, BA 19). Increased temporal lobe activation in secondary dissociation is consistent with hypotheses that draw parallels between psychologic trauma-induced depersonalization and experiences provoked by temporal lobe epilepsy [46,47]. In addition, our fMRI results were broadly consistent with Sierra and Berrios' [48] corticolimbic model of dissociation. This model posits that limbic emotional response (eg, amygdala) is suppressed through increased mPFC activation and increased right dorsolateral PFC activation and ACC inhibition, resulting in hypervigilance for external threat or self-perception. Although we did not observe differential activation in the amygdala, this structure is known to respond more robustly to external threat stimuli (eg, aversive or threatening pictures or sound) relative to emotion generated through episodic recall or imagination [49]. In addition, the amygdala appears to respond automatically and rapidly mainly to the onset of threat (including unconscious stimuli [32,50]) rather than over a long duration. This temporal profile is thus unlikely to be captured with the script-driven imagery paradigm. Increased ACC activation observed in our study differs, however, from the decreased activation predicted by Sierra and Berrios [48], and therefore these findings await clarification by additional research.

We believe these results, as exemplified at a neurobiologic level of analysis, support the validity of van der Kolk and colleagues' [1] categorical distinctions between primary and secondary dissociation. We also believe these differences support state-phase models of animal defensive reaction to external threat. Nijenhuis and colleagues [3] reported that animals display different characteristic behavioral patterns in response to predators, depending on their physical and temporal proximity to the source of threat. These phases can be categorized as pre-encounter, postencounter, and circa-strike defense. The pre-encounter period is defined by behavioral patterns characteristic of nonthreat (eg, eating, foraging). The postencounter period is when the animal may flee, freeze, or attack when it becomes aware that a predator is present. Researchers believe postencounter response selection is determined by an estimation of the degree of safety each behavioral option would predictably engender. Freezing behavior is not simply thought of as a lack of protective behavior (ie, a lack of fight or flight) or an inactive form of protection, but rather an active and organized behavioral and neurobiologic defensive state in its own right. For one, the freezing state is regarded as best selected when movement might transmit the animal's specific location to its predator. In its postencounter form, freezing is regarded as a hypervigilant and hyperaroused state of readiness, wherein the animal is prepared for subsequent action (eg, fight or flight). When an animal is about to be attacked, which is the circa-strike defense phase, freezing behavior may nevertheless continue and be combined with analgesia. Such immobility is believed to potentially reduce the likelihood of continued attack in cases when aggressive defensive behavior is unlikely to be successful.

Parallels between the postencounter flight and freezing behavior on the one hand and circa-strike freezing on the other might be drawn between primary dissociation and secondary dissociation, respectively. During primary dissociative reliving, the fragmented memories experienced in patients who have PTSD are typically infused with a strong sense of trepidation. Dissociative reliving episodes are often elicited following a startle response, may include a marked sense of fear, and tend to prompt an action tendency (flight or freezing). In contrast, secondary dissociative responses are not associated with intense fear, and no action tendency seems to be provoked. Freezing or immobility in the latter instance is typically experienced as an automatically generated process, rather than the result of a judgment (at least semiconscious) about the effectiveness of survival-promoting behavior.

Accordingly, although freezing behavior is associated with hypervigilance, arousal, and readiness for action during the postencounter phase, freezing during circa-strike is associated with a relative blinding of awareness; decreased arousal; numbing and analgesia; and inactivity. Therefore, during secondary dissociation it seems as though, at least for a transitory period, the mind has given up on the body and the capacity to alter the situation (helplessness). For these moments, the individual has seemingly concluded that escape is extremely unlikely, and thus has made no efforts toward that end. In this state, the mind reflexively relinquishes executive control to a lower-order survival mechanism principally based on increased pain tolerance. Researchers have hypothesized that the parasympathetic nervous system may play a role in such secondary dissociative responses. For example, Schore [51] has speculated that activity of the dorsal vagal complex in the medulla may increase dramatically in the dissociative state, thus leading to decreases in blood pressure, metabolic activity, and heart rate despite increases in circulating adrenaline.

The extant literature is not currently developed enough to validate many of the above inferences, or to study their neural correlates. Initial steps have been taken toward this goal, however. For example, in a recently published study (Fig. 2) [13], the functional connectivity of the left thalamus in individuals who had PTSD who displayed secondary dissociative reactions (n = 10) was compared with the connectivity found in nonpsychiatric controls (n = 10). Our original study of secondary dissociative responses in PTSD [9] did not show statistically-significant group differences in thalamic activation, which discriminated between primary dissociative PTSD and nonpsychiatric controls [8]. Specifically, patients who had secondary dissociative PTSD and nonpsychiatric controls exhibited increased thalamic activation in response to trauma script-driven imagery relative to baseline. However, although subtraction analyses can identify brain areas whose activation significantly co-varies with a given task, functional connectivity analyses identify correlations between different brain areas that coactivate during the task, thereby potentially revealing functional neural networks or systems mediating psychologic processes. The functional connectivity of a region may

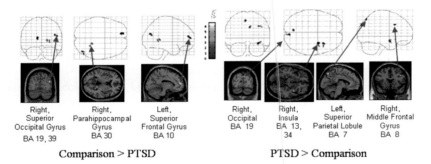

| Right, Superior Occipital Gyrus BA 19, 39 | Right, Parahippocampal Gyrus BA 30 | Left, Superior Frontal Gyrus BA 10 | Right, Occipital BA 19 | Right, Insula BA 13, 34 | Left, Superior Parietal Lobule BA 7 | Right, Middle Frontal Gyrus BA 8 |

Comparison > PTSD   PTSD > Comparison

Fig. 2. Functional connectivity analyses of left thalamus [-14 -164] in comparison subjects and individuals who have PTSD (secondary dissociative). Blood-Oxygen-Level-Dependent (BOLD) fMRI response in cortex where correlations with BOLD response in left thalamus during script-driven imagery of traumatic events were significantly different in individuals who had PTSD (secondary dissociative response, n = 10) and comparison (nonpsychiatric control, n = 10) subjects.

differ between individuals and groups, despite similar levels of overall activation in the region.

Although the sensory thalamus may remain online during secondary dissociation, its transmissions with cortex appeared to be disturbed in our functional connectivity study [13]. Nonpsychiatric controls exhibited more significant coactivation with left thalamus in left superior frontal gyrus (BA 10), right parahippocampal gyrus (BA 30), and the right superior occipital gyrus (BA 19, 39) when compared with the patients who had secondary dissociative PTSD. In comparison, patients who had secondary dissociative PTSD showed more significant coactivation with left thalamus in right insula (BA 13, 34), left parietal lobe (BA 7), right middle frontal gyrus (BA 8), superior temporal gyrus (BA 38, 34), and right cuneus (BA 19) relative to nonpsychiatric controls. In interpreting these results, we focused on the generally verbal (left-lateralized) compared with nonverbal (right-lateralized) pattern of activation in nonpsychiatric controls and secondary dissociative PTSD, respectively, and specifically the altered activity of the right insula in patients who have PTSD. The right insula is a region known to be involved in conveying bodily states (eg, of the viscera, of pain) to the brain [52,53].

At least two recent lines of inquiry suggest the idea that altered body perception plays a key role in secondary dissociative PTSD. The first is that of Nijenhuis and colleagues [54], who have associated depersonalization disorder and dissociative disorders with a psychologic construct labeled *somatoform dissociation* [54]. These researchers have shown that psychologic dissociation, which refers to disruptions in memory, consciousness, and identity, commonly accompanies somatoform dissociation, involving disturbances in sensation (including pain), movement, and bodily function. As a self-report measure of this phenomenon, this group has developed the Somatoform Dissociation Questionnaire [55], which includes test items such as, "My body, or a part of it, feels numb" or is "insensitive to pain," and, "It is as if my body, or a part of it, has disappeared." Following this line of evidence, we are currently examining the neural correlates of thermal pain perception using fMRI during the script-imagery paradigm in individuals who have PTSD, and expect to find differences in response to pain between individuals who display primary and secondary dissociative responses to trauma cues.

A second line of inquiry suggesting disturbed body perception in secondary dissociative PTSD comes from our recent study relating the psychologic construct of alexithymia to dissociative experiences in PTSD [56]. *Alexithymia* refers to difficulties identifying and labeling emotional states, and is most commonly assessed with a self-report measure named the Toronto Alexithymia Scale. The 20-item version (TAS-20) includes test items such as, "I am often confused about what emotion I am feeling," and, "It is difficult for me to find the right words for my feelings" [57]. We believe deficits in the conscious awareness of bodily states are integral to the alexithymia construct because the substance that is felt during an emotional feeling seems inherently to be a particular bodily state [58]. Associations between trait alexithymia and secondary dissociative states may develop over the course of chronic childhood physical and sexual abuse [56]. Specifically, with increased repetition and automatization of secondary dissociative processes during situations of long-standing abuse, the priming of the dissociative state may become sensitized and increasingly automatic and unconscious. In addition, repetitious entry into secondary dissociative states may produce progressively more marked departures from external reality and consciousness for self. As dissociative individuals become increasingly less aware of and connected with their identity, feelings, body, and surroundings, they may become alexithymic and thereby deficient in how much they are able to cognitively understand their emotional experiences. In addition, with little cognitive insight about their emotional feelings, dissociative-alexithymic individuals are correspondingly unable to regulate their affective responses (eg, through ACC) in an adaptive coping manner.

In a currently unpublished study [59], baseline TAS-20 scores were predictive of patterns of primary dissociative responses to script-imagery in PTSD (Fig. 3). Specifically, greater alexithymia in patients who had PTSD was associated with increased activity bilaterally in thalamus, insula (BA 13, 47), and posterior cingulate cortex (PCC) (BA 23, 29, 31). Increased insular activation may relate to representations of current bodily state in patients who have PTSD and alexithymia, although the bodily representations that are encoded are likely to be dysregulated from other verbal and frontal systems. The association between increased PCC activation during traumatic imagery and increased levels of alexithymia may be related to increased activation of valenced memory retrieval processes or altered pain perception [60].

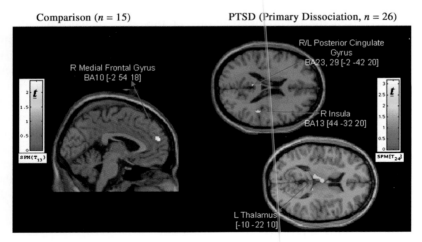

Fig. 3. Positive correlations between Toronto Alexithymia Scale (TAS-20) scores and Blood-Oxygen-Level-Dependent fMRI signal in response to script-driven imagery of traumatic events in individuals who had PTSD (primary dissociative response) and comparison (nonpsychiatric control) subjects ($P = .05$, $k > 5$). L, left; R, right.

A study by Phillips and colleagues [61] further supports the notion that emotional response to threatening stimuli is altered in depersonalization disorder (DD). Consistent with findings that electrical skin conductance response to affective stimuli is blunted in patients who have DD [62], Phillips and colleagues found that these patients failed to differentiate between objectively aversive and neutral scenes in their emotional response ratings to threatening and aversive pictures: "Many depersonalized patients said that they saw and understood the content of the pictures but did not experience an emotional response" [61]. Neural correlates of this experience included a relative absence of activation in left insula, bilateral cingulate gyrus (BA 24, 32), lingual (BA 19) and superior temporal gyri (BA 22, 42), and left inferior parietal lobule (BA 40). They also found greater global cerebral blood flow to neutral compared with aversive stimuli in patients who have DD, with the opposite result (to be expected) from nonpsychiatric controls [61]. The comparative absence of insular, temporal, and parietal response to aversive relative to neutral stimuli in patients who have DD is consistent with a general dampening of affect and arousal during emotion-challenge, and altered body-state mapping. During depersonalization episodes, it would thus appear that the individuals' senses of mind (through left-brain–mediated conscious internal language and reasoning functions) versus body (through right-hemisphere and limbic lobe functions) are divided.

Most of Phillips and colleagues' [61] results for aversive pictures, however, differ from our results for secondary dissociative PTSD responses to script-driven imagery. The reasons for these discrepancies are likely manifold, including the degree to which subjects experienced depersonalization symptoms during scanning, and the degree to which subjects responded emotionally and with self-relevance to the paradigm. These measures may have been higher in our study given the personalized nature of the script-imagery paradigm. Moreover, differences in results may be partly because of differences in symptom origin. Symptom origin may have been heterogeneous (eg, caused by past drug abuse, undiagnosed neurologic conditions) in Phillips and colleagues' sample, but was always associated with a traumatic event (peritraumatic dissociation) in our sample. What is clear and compelling from the study by Phillips and colleagues is that patients who are depersonalized reveal a relative absence of neural and emotional response to normally highly aversive visual stimulation, despite understanding that they should feel an emotion in response to the pictures (ie, they generally know that their response to aversive stimuli deviates from the norm). These findings are consistent with the notion that secondary dissociation represents a psychologic distancing of mind from body, and of self from external environment.

Tertiary dissociation

van der Kolk and colleagues [1] define tertiary dissociation as the development of "ego states that contain a traumatic experience, or complex identities with distinctive cognitive, affective, and behavioural patterns." They also assert that states or identities may represent different emotions (eg, pain, fear, anger) or different components of one or more traumatic experiences, and are central to the diagnostic profile of dissociative identity disorder (DID) [1].

Although significant progress has been made in understanding tertiary dissociation at psychologic and phenomenologic levels of analysis, little is known about the neurobiology underlying tertiary dissociation. Recent key findings observe that attachment disorganization and relational trauma that occur in early childhood are robust predictors of dissociative experiences subsequently reported during adolescence and adulthood [63,64]. These findings likely parallel the plastic and susceptible nature of brain microarchitecture at this formative period of development (see article by Lyons-Ruth elsewhere in this issue). An inaugural study published by Reinders and colleagues [65], studied 11 women who had DID in a PET script-imagery paradigm under different identity-state conditions. The authors report that, as a result of treatment, the patients in their sample had developed the ability to perform self-initiated and self-controlled switches between one of their neutral and one of their traumatic personality states at the time of scanning. In an ingenious experimental design, neural activity was recorded under four conditions: when they listened to a neutral memory while experiencing the neutral personality state (NPS) and while experiencing the trauma personality state (TPS), and when they listened to a trauma memory while experiencing the NPS and while experiencing the TPS. Although the neutral memory script was regarded as a personal experience by each of these personality states, the trauma memory was experienced as self-relevant and involved episodic retrieval for the TPS only.

Brain activation to the neutral scripts did not differ between NPS and TPS. In contrast, activation in left parietal operculum and left insula during the traumatic script was greater in the TPS than the NPS. In comparison, NPS was associated with greater activation than TPS in right mPFC (BA 10), bilateral middle frontal gyrus (BA 6), bilateral intraparietal sulcus (BA 7/40), and bilateral parietal-occipital sulcus (BA 18, precuneus). Finally, no differences in brain activation were found during the NPS when processing the neutral and traumatic scripts. Reinders and colleagues [65] relate their results to studies of differences between autobiographic and nonautobiographic episodic memory retrieval, which generally show increased mPFC involvement in the former [37–39]. In addition, Reinders and colleagues interpret increased parietal-occipital blood flow during NPS processing of traumatic memories as reflective of a low level of somatosensory awareness and integration in DID NPS.

Future neuroimaging studies of tertiary dissociation are needed. The generalizability of Reinders and colleagues' [65] study is limited because their DID sample had already developed the capacity to switch between NPS and TPS. Neuroimaging studies of a more natural automatic and subtle shift between identity-states are needed, which might take the form of repeated test scans during which patients are asked about their current identity-states while processing state/identity-relevant and -irrelevant stimuli, and asked to make judgments about the stimuli. Stimuli appropriate for such a study might include self-referential or affective judgments concerning trauma cues, and personality-trait adjectives and demographic descriptors (eg, "child" versus "adult"). Another methodology might entail having patients who have DID view pictures of themselves while experiencing distinct identity-state conditions.

A significant impediment to programmatic research concerning the neurobiology of tertiary dissociation, however, is the current lack of broad-spectrum theories through which empiric hypotheses can be derived and tested. Specification of such a theory is beyond the scope of this article, although future neuropsychiatric theories of DID will need to address a few issues. One issue is where neuropsychiatrists should 'look' in their attempts to locate different dissociative identities in the brain. To the extent that differing identity-states are complex, it is unlikely that encoded neural representations of the different states will be found simply in discrete areas of the brain (eg, adjacent columns in a structure). Rather, it is far more likely that identity-states will be encoded within distributed representations across shared neuron groups. For example, whereas Broca's and Wernicke's areas encode representations mediating language processing for all dialects, significant differences between languages (eg, between English and Chinese) are associated with only subtle differences in neural structure [42]. The same can be expected of the neural representations that encode distinct identity-states in DID (eg, in mPFC). In addition, complex identity-states involving particular stereotyped but nevertheless elaborate individualized sets of thoughts, feelings, and actions will presumably occupy distributed representations essentially across the whole brain, rather than in only a few key structures. An important step toward differentiating between these distributed cortical representations will involve mining bottom-up associations. For example, disturbances in neural activity at lower levels of the nervous system (eg, brain-stem, thalamus, cerebellum) appear to exert greater influence on the topography of somatosensory cortex than do intraregional processes [66].

However, to the extent that less complex identity-states might be organized in terms of context-dependent behavioral functions or goals, use of neuroimaging to study these states becomes more tractable. Specifically, different identity-states might be probed as characteristic information-processing modes and, like different emotions, such states might be distinguished by their response to external input (eg, extent of approach behavior versus withdrawal, external versus self-focused attention). In other words, distinctive identity-states not only differ in the contents of consciousness but also might be associated with differences in the way external information is processed across neural subsystems. Such patterns of response can be studied through functional connectivity analysis [67].

Summary

This article reviews the results of PET and fMRI studies of primary, secondary, and tertiary dissociation. Primary versus secondary dissociative experiences appear to have distinctive neural correlates, which are consistent with the proposed functional role these behaviors have in defensive engagement with sources of external threat. Amygdalar and insular hyperactivity in combination with ACC, mPFC, and thalamic hypoactivity in PTSD during primary dissociative reliving is consistent with the idea that brain centers that facilitate conscious, volitional, and controlled contact with the external world are temporarily overridden by affective-sensory associations that come to consciousness in the form of thoughts, images, and bodily sensations. In contrast, increased mPFC and ACC activity in secondary dissociative experiences, in combination with distributed temporal-parietal activity, is consistent with a suppression of bodily affect when individuals are reminded of trauma combined with abnormalities in self and the somatosensory awareness such hypersuppression might create. Finally, advances in clinical and neuropsychiatric theory will improve understanding of the neurobiology of tertiary dissociation and DID. The multiple senses of mind that emerge from the single brain of the patient who has DID will likely be best understood as representations distributed within and across neural regions rather than occupying distinctive territories.

References

[1] van der Kolk BA, Van der Hart O, Marmar CR. Dissociation and information processing in posttraumatic stress disorder. In: van der Kolk BA, McFarlane AC, Weisaeth L, editors. Traumatic stress: the effects of overwhelming experience on mind, body, and society. New York: Guilford Press; 1996. p. 303–27.

[2] Foa EB, Zinbarg R, Rothbaum BO. Uncontrollability and unpredictability in post-traumatic stress disorder: an animal model. Psychol Bull 1992;112:218–38.

[3] Nijenhuis ERS, Vanderlinden J, Spinhoven P. Animal defensive reactions as a model for trauma-induced dissociative reactions. J Trauma Stress 1998;11:243–60.

[4] Orr SP, McNally RJ, Rosen GM, et al. Psychophysiologic reactivity: implications for conceptualizing PTSD. In: Rosen GM, editor. Posttraumatic stress disorder: Issues and controversies. New York: John Wiley & Sons; 2004. p. 101–26.

[5] Bremner JD, Narayan M, Staib LH, et al. Neural correlates of memories of childhood sexual abuse in women with and without posttraumatic stress disorder. Am J Psychiatry 1999a;156: 1787–95.

[6] Driessen M, Beblo T, Mertens M, et al. Posttraumatic stress disorder and fMRI activation patterns of traumatic memory in patients with borderline personality disorder. Biol Psychiatry 2004;55(6):603–11.

[7] Gilboa A, Shalev AY, Laor L, et al. Functional connectivity of the prefrontal cortex and the amygdala in posttraumatic stress disorder. Biol Psychiatry 2004;55(3):263–72.

[8] Lanius RA, Williamson PC, Densmore M, et al. Neural correlates of traumatic memories in posttraumatic stress disorder: a functional MRI investigation. Am J Psychiatry 2001;158:1920–2.

[9] Lanius RA, Williamson PC, Boksman K, et al. Brain activation during script-driven imagery induced dissociative responses in PTSD: a functional MRI investigation. Biol Psychiatry 2002;52:305–11.

[10] Lanius RA, Williamson PC, Hopper J, et al. Recall of emotional states in posttraumatic stress disorder: an fMRI investigation. Biol Psychiatry 2003;53:204–10.

[11] Lanius RA, Hopper JW, Menon RS. Individual differences in a husband and wife who developed PTSD after a motor vehicle accident: a functional MRI case studyAm J Psychiatry 2003b;160(4):667–9.

[12] Lanius RA, Williamson PC, Densmore M, et al. The nature of traumatic memories: a 4-T fMRI functional connectivity analysis. Am J Psychiatry 2004;161(1):36–44.

[13] Lanius RA, Williamson PC, Bluhm RL, et al. Functional connectivity of dissociative responses in posttraumatic stress disorder: a functional magnetic resonance imaging investigation. Biol Psychiatry 2005;57:873–84.

[14] Britton JC, Phan KL, Taylor SF, et al. Corticolimbic blood flow in posttraumatic stress disorder during script-driven imagery. Biol Psychiatry 2005;57:832–40.

[15] Osuch EA, Benson B, Geraci M, et al. Regional cerebral blood flow correlated with flashback intensity in patients with posttraumatic stress disorder. Biol Psychiatry 2001;50:246–53.

[16] Rauch SL, van der Kolk BA, Fisler RE, et al. A symptom provocation study of posttraumatic stress disorder using positron emission tomography and script driven imagery. Arch Gen Psychiatry 1996;53:380–7.

[17] Shin LM, McNally RJ, Kosslyn SM, et al. Regional cerebral blood flow during script-driven imagery in childhood sexual abuse-related PTSD: a PET investigation. Am J Psychiatry 1999;156(4):575–84.

[18] Shin LM, Whalen PJ, Pitman RK, et al. An fMRI study of anterior cingulate function in posttraumatic stress disorder. Biol Psychiatry 2001;50:932–42.

[19] Shin LM, Orr SP, Carson MA, et al. Regional cerebral blood flow in the amygdala and medial prefrontal cortex during traumatic imagery in male and female Vietnam veterans with PTSD. Arch Gen Psychiatry 2004;61(2):168–76.

[20] Lanius RA, Bluhm R, Lanius U, et al. A review of neuroimaging studies of hyperarousal and dissociation in PTSD: heterogeneity of response to symptom provocation. J Psychiatr Res, in press.

[21] Bremner JD, Staib L, Kaloupek D, et al. Neural correlates of exposure to traumatic pictures and sound in Vietnam combat veterans with and without posttraumatic stress disorder: a positron emission tomography study. Biol Psychiatry 1999b;45:806–16.

[22] Ochsner KN, Bunge SA, Gross JJ, et al. Rethinking feelings: an fMRI study of the cognitive regulation of emotion. J Cogn Neurosci 2002;14:1215–29.

[23] Phan KL, Fitzgerald DA, Pradeep JN, et al. Neural substrates for voluntary suppression of negative affect: a functional magnetic resonance imaging study. Biol Psychiatry 2005;57: 210–9.

[24] Botvinick MM, Braver TS, Barch DM, et al. Conflict monitoring and cognitive control. Psychol Rev 2001;108:624–52.

[25] Bush G, Luu P, Posner MI. Cognitive and emotional influences in the anterior cingulate cortex. Trends Cogn Sci 2000;4:215–22.

[26] Critchley HD, Corfield DR, Chandler MP, et al. Cerebral correlates of autonomic cardiovascular arousal: a functional neuroimaging investigation in humans. J Physiol 2000;523: 259–70.

[27] Critchley HD, Melmed RN, Featherstone E, et al. Volitional control of autonomic arousal: a functional magnetic resonance study. Neuroimage 2002;16:909–19.

[28] Critchley HD, Mathias CJ, Josephs O, et al. Human cingulate cortex and autonomic control: converging neuroimaging and clinical evidence. Brain 2003;126:2139–52.

[29] Liberzon I, Taylor SF, Amdur R, et al. Brain activation in PTSD in response to trauma-related stimuli. Biol Psychiatry 1999;45:817–26.

[30] Pissiota A, Frans O, Fernandez M, et al. Neurofunctional correlates of posttraumatic stress disorder: a PET symptom provocation study. Eur Arch Psychiatry Clin Neurosci 2002;252: 68–75.

[31] LeDoux JE. Emotion circuits in the brain. Annu Rev Neurosci 2000;23:155–84.

[32] Whalen PJ. Fear, vigilance, and ambiguity: initial neuroimaging studies of the human amygdala. Current Directions in Psychological Science 1998;7:177–88.

[33] Protopopescu X, Pan H, Tuescher O, et al. Differential time courses and specificity of amygdala activity in posttraumatic stress disorder subjects and normal control subjects. Biol Psychiatry 2005;57:464–73.

[34] Rauch SL, Whalen PJ, Shin LM, et al. Exaggerated amygdala response to masked facial stimuli in posttraumatic stress disorder: a functional MRI study. Biol Psychiatry 2000; 47(9):769–76.

[35] Shin LM, Wright CI, Cannistraro PA, et al. A functional magnetic resonance imaging study of amygdala and medial prefrontal cortex responses to overtly presented fearful faces in posttraumatic stress disorder. Arch Gen Psychiatry 2005;62:273–81.

[36] Gallagher HL, Frith CD. Functional imaging of 'theory of mind'. Trends Cogn Sci 2003;7: 77–83.

[37] Johnson SC, Baxter LC, Wilder LS, et al. Neural correlates of self-reflection. Brain 2002;125: 1808–14.

[38] Kelley WM, Macrae CN, Wyland CL, et al. Finding the self? An event-related fMRI study. J Cogn Neurosci 2002;14:785–94.

[39] Ochsner KN, Knierim K, Ludlow DH, et al. Reflecting upon feelings: an fMRI study of neural systems supporting the attribution of emotion to self and other. J Cogn Neurosci 2004;16: 1746–72.

[40] Gusnard DA, Akbudak E, Shulman GL, et al. Medial prefrontal cortex and self-referential mental activity: relation to a default mode of brain function. Proc Natl Acad Sci U S A 2001; 98:4529–64.

[41] Liberzon I, Taylor SF, Fig LM, et al. Alteration of corticothalamic perfusion ratios during a PTSD flashback. Depress Anxiety 1996–97;4:146–50.

[42] Llinás RR. I of the vortex: from neurons to self. Boston: Massachusetts Institute of Technology: MIT press; 2002. p. 126.

[43] Krystal JH, Bremner JD, Southwick SM, et al. The emerging neurobiology of dissociation: implications for the treatment of posttraumatic stress disorder. In: Bremner JD, Marmer CR, editors. Trauma, memory, and dissociation. Washington (DC): American Psychiatric Press; 1998. p. 321–63.

[44] Brewin CR. A cognitive neuroscience account of posttraumatic stress disorder and its treatment. Behav Res Ther 2001;39(4):373–93.

[45] Simeon D, Guralnik O, Hazlett EA, et al. Feeling unreal: a PET study of depersonalization disorder. Am J Psychiatry 2000;157:1782–8.

[46] Teicher MH, Glod CA, Surrey J, et al. Early childhood abuse and limbic system rating in adult psychiatric outpatients. J Neuropsychiatry Clin Neurosci 1993;5:301–6.

[47] Teicher MH, Ito Y, Glod CA, et al. Preliminary evidence for abnormal cortical development in physically and sexually abused children using EEG coherence and MRI. In: Yehuda R, McFarlane AC, editors. Psychobiology of posttraumatic stress disorder, vol. 821. New York: The New York Academy of Sciences; 1997. p. 160–75.

[48] Sierra M, Berrios GE. Depersonalization: neurobiological perspectives. Biol Psychiatry 1998;44:898–908.

[49] Phan KL, Wager T, Taylor SF, et al. Functional neuroanatomy of emotion: a meta-analysis of emotion activation studies in PET and fMRI. Neuroimage 2002;16:331–48.

[50] Morris JS, Ohman A, Dolan RJ. Conscious and unconscious emotional learning in the human amygdala. Nature 1998;393:467–70.

[51] Schore AN. The effects of relational trauma on right brain development, affect regulation, and infant mental health. Infant Mental Health J 2001;22:201–69.

[52] Craig AD. How do you feel? Interoception: the sense of the physiological condition of the body. Nat Rev Neurosci 2002;3:655–66.

[53] Critchley HD, Wiens S, Rotchtein P, et al. Neural systems supporting interoceptive awareness. Nat Neurosci 2004;7:189–95.

[54] Nijenhuis ERS. Somatoform dissociation. phenomena, measurement and theoretical issues. Assen (Netherlands): Van Gorcum & Company; 1999.

[55] Nijenhuis ERS, Spinhoven P, Van Dyck R, et al. The development and psychometric characteristics of the Somatoform Dissociation Questionnaire (SDQ-20). J Nerv Ment Dis 1996; 184:688–94.

[56] Frewen PA, Lane R, Lanius RA. Alexithymia and emotional awareness in posttraumatic stress disorder I: a psychometric study. Manuscript in preparation, 2005.

[57] Bagby RM, Parker JDA, Taylor GJ. The twenty-item Toronto Alexithymia Scale-I: Item selection and cross-validation of the factor structure. J Psychosom Res 1994;38:23–32.

[58] Damasio A. The feeling of what happens: body and emotion in the making of consciousness. Fort Worth (TX): Harcourt College Publishers; 1999.

[59] Frewen PA, Lane R, Lanius RA. Alexithymia and emotional awareness in posttraumatic stress disorder II: a fMRI study. Manuscript in preparation, 2005.

[60] Nielsen FA, Balslev D, Hansen LK. Mining the posterior cingulate: Segregation between memory and pain components. Neuroimage, in press.

[61] Phillips ML, Medford N, Senoir C, et al. Depersonalization disorder: Thinking without feeling. Psychiatry Res 2001;108:145–60.

[62] Sierra M, Senior C, Dalton J, et al. Autonomic response in depersonalization disorder. Arch Gen Psychiatry 2002;59:833–8.

[63] Ogawa JR, Sroufe LA, Weinfield NS, et al. Development and the fragmented self: longitudinal study of dissociative symptomatology in a nonclinical sample. Dev Psychopathol 1997; 9:855–79.

[64] Lyons-Ruth K. Dissociation and the parent-infant dialogue: a longitudinal perspective from attachment research. J Am Psychoanal Assoc 2003;51(3):883–911.

[65] Reinders AA, Nijenhuis ER, Paans AM, et al. One brain, two selves. Neuroimage 2003;20: 2219–25.

[66] Jones EG. Cortical and subcortical contributions to activity-dependent plasticity in primate somatosensory cortex. Annu Rev Neurosci 2000;23:1–37.

[67] Ramnani N, Behrens TEJ, Penny W, et al. New approaches for exploring anatomical and functional connectivity in the human brain. Biol Psychiatry 2004;56:613–9.

ELSEVIER
SAUNDERS

Psychiatr Clin N Am 29 (2006) 129–144

PSYCHIATRIC
CLINICS
OF NORTH AMERICA

Dissociative Disorders as a Confounding Factor in Psychiatric Research

Vedat Sar, MD[a],*, Colin Ross, MD[b]

[a]Clinical Psychotherapy Unit and Dissociative Disorders Program,
Medical Faculty of Istanbul, Istanbul University, 34390 Capa, Istanbul, Turkey
[b]Colin A. Ross Institute for Psychological Trauma, 1701 Gateway, Suite 349,
Richardson, TX 75080, USA

Dissociation is a confounding factor in the entire spectrum of psychiatric disorders. The lack of dissociative disorder sections in widely used general psychiatric assessment instruments has led to neglect of this phenomenon for many decades. Recent studies have benefited, however, from standardized diagnostic interviews and rating scales that make the specific assessment of dissociative disorders and dissociation reliable and valid. From the perspectives of both diagnosis and treatment, studies concerning childhood trauma need to include dissociation as a variable. This article focuses on the evidence-based literature available to date. Besides examining empirical studies, also suggested are how measures of dissociation can be incorporated in research including treatment outcome studies for a variety of disorders in psychiatry.

Trauma, dissociation, and psychiatric comorbidity

As phenomenologic classification systems, the Diagnostic and Statistical Manuals (DSM) of the American Psychiatric Association have increasingly allowed concurrent diagnoses [1]. As a result, comorbidity has become one of the central issues in clinical psychiatry. High levels of comorbidity for many DSM disorders, however, cannot be simply an artifact of overinclusive or imprecise diagnostic criteria; they must reflect a multifactorial etiology for psychiatric disturbances and a need for multimodal treatment strategies in daily clinical practice. In this sense, psychiatric research has lagged behind clinical practice and experience; studies conducted on "pure" diagnostic populations hardly reflect the "real" clinical situation [2,3].

* Corresponding author.
 E-mail address: vsar@istanbul.edu.tr (V. Sar).

0193-953X/06/$ - see front matter © 2005 Elsevier Inc. All rights reserved.
doi:10.1016/j.psc.2005.10.008

Nevertheless, comorbidity in psychiatry is related to certain risk factors rather than being common to all patients. Apparently, developmental traumas are one of these risk factors. A 12-month follow-up study covering mood, anxiety, and substance use disorders in the general population demonstrated that the odds ratios for parental psychiatric history and childhood trauma were higher for individuals with comorbid conditions than for those with pure disorders [4].

In epidemiologic studies of posttraumatic stress disorder (PTSD) in the general population, three risk factors were identified: (1) pre-existing psychiatric disorders, (2) a family history of psychiatric disorders, and (3) childhood trauma [5]. Several studies documented the existence of a relationship between childhood trauma and dissociation, including one prospective study [6,7]. Patients with dissociative disorders report the highest frequency of childhood trauma among all psychiatric categories [8] and have extensive psychiatric comorbidity in both DSM axes [9].

A number of psychiatric disorders, including personality disorders, either have dissociative disorder comorbidity or contain dissociative symptoms in their diagnostic criteria [10–15]. Childhood sexual abuse and dissociation are independently associated with several other indicators of mental health disturbance including suicidality, self-mutilation, and sexual aggression [16]. Overall, besides the main diagnosis, in many but not all cases, childhood trauma, dissociation, self-mutilation, suicidality, and excessive psychiatric comorbidity together form a significant additional cluster [2]. This pattern is not only significant for nosologic reasons, but it is also a clinical problem well known to professionals who work with difficult patients.

Mood disorders and schizophrenia

Overall, childhood trauma increases the risk for positive psychotic symptoms in the general population [17]. Among patients with psychotic disorders involving auditory hallucinations, 38.5% reported childhood sexual abuse [18]. Childhood trauma is associated with higher levels of depression and dissociation, and is linked to a tendency to regard the voices of auditory hallucinations as more malevolent.

The same three features (depression, dissociation, and auditory hallucinations) were all associated with the age at first reported abuse, with a younger age of first experience being related to higher levels of psychopathology in all instances. Schizophrenic patients with a comorbid dissociative disorder have more severe childhood trauma histories, more comorbidity, and higher scores for both positive and negative symptoms [19]. Among patients with schizophrenia, higher levels of borderline traits are uniquely related to the report of childhood sexual abuse [20], whereas dissociation correlates with both emotional and physical abuse [10].

Once thought to be pathognomonic for schizophrenia, schneiderian first-rank symptoms also have been recognized among patients with bipolar disorder [21,22]. Additionally, first-rank symptoms are more common in dissociative identity disorder than in schizophrenia [23]. Schneiderian symptoms are highly related to other dissociative symptom clusters and to childhood trauma even in the general population [24].

Data about childhood trauma among patients with bipolar disorder also present interesting findings. In a group of bipolar disorder patients, a significant association was found between reported childhood trauma (sexual abuse) and auditory hallucinations [25]. Rapid-cycling bipolar disorder patients differ from non–rapid-cycling ones with respect to a history of childhood physical or sexual abuse, history of drug abuse, bipolar I disorder subtype, and number of lifetime depressive and manic episodes [26]. The prevalence of these features increases progressively with episode frequency. In this study, subjects with rapid cycling versus non–rapid cycling demonstrated rates of PTSD of 8.5% versus 3.6%, drug abuse or dependence of 27.3% versus 17.2%, any anxiety disorder at the rate of 50.2% versus 30.7%, and history of physical or sexual abuse as a child of 40.1% versus 24.1% or only during adolescence at rates of 10.8% versus 6.3%. These were some of the most salient of characteristics distinguishing these groups. Rapid-cycling subjects were associated with much higher rates of trauma-related symptoms than non–rapid-cycling subjects.

In another study, early stress (self-report of early physical or sexual abuse was used as the primary index) was associated with earlier onset of bipolar disorder; a more adverse course of illness; more axis I, II, and III comorbidities; lack or loss of ongoing social and medical supports; and an increased incidence of serious suicide attempts [27]. These relationships suggest that a link also may exist between childhood trauma and dissociation among patients with bipolar disorder.

The impact of childhood trauma history within the mood disorders spectrum is not limited to bipolar disorder. Depressed women with a childhood sexual abuse history reported more childhood physical abuse, childhood emotional abuse, and parental conflict in the home, compared with depressed women without a childhood sexual abuse history [9]. The two groups (with and without childhood sexual abuse) were similar in the severity of depression, but the women with a childhood sexual abuse history were more likely to have attempted suicide, or to have engaged in deliberate self-harm. The women with childhood sexual abuse also became depressed earlier in life, were more likely to have panic disorder, and were more likely to have reported a recent assault.

In a controlled study on patients with chronic forms of major depression, among those with a history of early childhood trauma (loss of parents at an early age, physical or sexual abuse, or neglect), psychotherapy alone was superior to antidepressant monotherapy. Moreover, the combination of psychotherapy and pharmacotherapy was only marginally superior to psychotherapy alone among the childhood abuse cohort [28]. In clinical practice, dissociative patients' chronic (double) depression and suicidality are usually resistant to standard biologic treatment modalities suitable for depressive disorders but respond positively to successful treatment of the dissociative disorder. Surveys demonstrate that unrecognized comorbid conditions are primary factors causing and maintaining a patient's depression [29]. The single disease model fails to account for the extensive comorbidity of most or all difficult patients.

Further complicating the understanding of schizophrenia and mood disorders, a dissociative disorder itself may take the form of a psychosis [30,31]. Although it has never been part of official classification systems, dissociative psychosis (formerly hysterical psychosis) has been recognized by clinicians without official sanction [32,33]. Dissociative psychosis is an acute condition that does not last longer than a few weeks. Although dissociative psychosis may mimic an acute schizophrenic, manic, or delirious condition, the disorder ceases abruptly and without any sequelae (ie, no schizotypal symptoms remain as is usual for a schizophrenic psychosis) [32]. Occasionally, amnesia may remain for the period of acute psychosis. This is further evidence of the dissociative nature of the episode. Dissociative psychosis may also occur in patients with dissociative identity disorder as a result of decompensation after an acute stressful life event [34,35].

As a trauma-induced psychosis, dissociative psychosis can be linked to the psychogenic or reactive psychosis concepts of European psychiatry [36–39]. There is clinical evidence that among special populations, such as immigrants and communities under war conditions, severe stress and extremely traumatic experiences may take the form of a brief reactive psychosis and not the form of the classical PTSD [40–42]. Many of these patients may have had dissociative psychosis. Familiarity with dissociative phenomena is important to give the correct diagnosis and treatment and to avoid unnecessary hospitalization or neuroleptic treatment.

Although these observations underline the impact of childhood trauma and dissociation in the phenomenology of psychotic disorders, a possible direct relation may exist between dissociative phenomena and schizotypy, although it remains to be illuminated. In one study, both pathologic and nonpathologic dissociation were predicted by the dimension of schizotypy, even after the contribution of childhood trauma had been removed [43]. In contradiction to this finding, in another study, although the depersonalization disorder group had higher schizotypy scores than the healthy control group, when depersonalization disorder participants with axis II disorders were excluded, within the remaining pure depersonalization disorder group, dissociation and schizotypy scores were not significantly correlated [44].

Borderline personality disorder and posttraumatic stress disorder

The relation of dissociation to PTSD and acute stress disorder is a widely disputed area that requires further study. The findings available to date are, however, thought-provoking. For instance, among road traffic accident survivors, all measures of dissociation, particularly persistent dissociation 4 weeks after the accident, predicted chronic PTSD severity at 6 months [45]. Dissociative symptoms predicted subsequent PTSD over and above the other PTSD symptom clusters.

In a study of acutely burned children there were two pathways to PTSD. Frequency of PTSD was proportional to the size of the child's burn. The pathways were distinguished by either a mediator of the level of separation anxiety or the level of acute dissociation [46]. In another study, persistent dissociation was more strongly associated with acute stress disorder severity and intrusive symptoms than was peritraumatic dissociation [47]. In this study, persistent rather than peritraumatic dissociation was the best predictor of posttraumatic psychopathology.

Patients with borderline personality disorder (BPD) and a dissociative disorder have high levels of reported childhood trauma [15,48]. Childhood trauma was one of six significant predictors of multiple prior hospitalizations for BPD patients: age 26 or older, a history of quasipsychotic thought, lifetime number of self-mutilative efforts and suicide attempts, a childhood history of reported sexual abuse, and a history of being physically or sexually assaulted in adulthood [49].

In a comparison of BPD patients with healthy controls, familial neurotic spectrum disorders, childhood sexual abuse, separation from parents, and unfavorable parental rearing styles predicted a BPD diagnosis [50]. In an unselected sample of women attending clinical psychology services, sexual abuse was associated with the extent of depression, somatization, compulsive behavior, phobic symptoms, and BPD characteristics [51]. In this study, dissociation served as a mediator in that link.

In another study, Hudziak and coworkers [52] found no cases of pure BPD (ie, BPD without comorbidity). It is possible, but remains to be investigated, that these other comorbid disorders define patients more appropriately with regard to choice of treatment, natural history, outcome, and family illness patterns than does BPD itself. Dissociative disorders are one of these comorbid conditions.

BPD, which affected 8.5% of college students in one study (Sar and coworkers, unpublished data), may be a type of posttraumatic syndrome involving the mechanism of dissociation [6]. Dissociation in response to childhood traumata may be at the core of the pathogenic process that results in symptomatology embodied in the diagnoses of both BPD and dissociative disorders.

BPD and dissociation could be related to each other in several different ways. For instance, it could be that borderline features develop in response to living with the core symptoms of dissociation. In one study, higher thought suppression (a dissociation between cognitions) mediated the relationship between negative affective intensity or reactivity and BPD symptoms, after controlling for a history of childhood sexual abuse [53].

Chronic efforts to suppress (dissociate) unpleasant thoughts may in some cases be a regulatory strategy underlying the relationship between intense negative emotions and BPD symptoms.

Dissociative disorders have also been reported as one of the most common comorbid conditions in gender identity disorders [54]. Identity disturbance, which is a characteristic of BPD, is partly related to a history of sexual abuse [55]. The association with early trauma and PTSD, however, does not seem to be unique to BPD among others [56].

A recent survey of a random national sample of experienced clinicians in North America yielded the finding that a significant proportion (53.3%) of their patients with BPD had a dissociative disorder diagnosis on axis I [57]. Empirical studies support this observation: in one study, 64% of the outpatients with DSM-III-R BPD had a DSM-IV dissociative disorder [15]. The percentage of DSM-IV BPD patients with a dissociative disorder is 72.5% for college students and 69.2% for women with DSM-III-R BPD in the general population (Sar and coworkers, unpublished data) [58]. There are other conceptually significant findings: for instance, 30% of patients with BPD have persistent hallucinations, which may be dissociative in nature [59]. High levels of dissociative experiences have been shown in a substantial subgroup of BPD patients [60]. Inversely, patients with dissociative disorder have high rates of BPD comorbidity [9]. This evidence further supports the relationship between dissociation and BPD .

There is a large phenomenologic overlap between BPD and dissociative disorders. This overlap is not adequately accounted for by the ninth diagnostic criterion for BPD introduced in the DSM-IV, which consists of "transient dissociative phenomena and paranoid ideation." This criterion mentions stress-related transient dissociative phenomena as a feature of BPD only, confounds it with a qualitatively different feature, such as paranoid ideation, and the possibility of a dissociative disorder comorbidity as a separate diagnosis remains hidden. Unfortunately, many otherwise high-quality studies on BPD [61,62] and discussions on suspected cases [63] simply omit dissociative disorders as a possible axis I comorbidity.

Impulsive-compulsive spectrum

Disorders and behavior that are usually considered to belong to the impulsive-compulsive spectrum (eg, obsessive-compulsive disorder, eating disorders, substance use disorders, suicidality, self-mutilation) have various relations to childhood trauma and dissociation. Among these, suicidality and self-mutilation, in particular, are two issues of special importance for clinicians working in general psychiatric settings [64]. Self-harm leads to repeated hospitalizations, is difficult to treat successfully, and has forensic implications. Violent behavior may also have relations to childhood trauma and dissociation [65,66].

Childhood physical and sexual abuse is correlated independently with repeated suicidal behavior and self-mutilation [67]. Patients with dissociative disorders are usually preoccupied with suicidal ideas, which seem to be related to dissociative psychopathology rather than being merely a component of a concurrent depressive disorder. In accordance with this notion, a study on patients with BPD found that affective instability was the criterion most strongly associated with suicidal behavior [68]. Patients with profound affect instability ought to be screened for the presence of a dissociative disorder.

Because major depressive disorder did not significantly predict suicidal behavior in this study, the reactivity associated with affective instability (more so than negative mood states) seemed to be a critical element in predicting suicidal behavior. It is an unanswered question, and a topic for future research, whether this reactivity is an element of the mood disorder or better understood as dissociative in nature. Another study demonstrated that greater lability, in terms of anger and anxiety, and oscillation between depression and anxiety [69] was related to BPD. There was no relationship, however, between BPD and oscillation between depression and elation. This finding further suggests that some of the reactivity and instability in borderline personality may be dissociative, rather than being caused by other comorbid mood disorders.

Patients with eating disorders are also at risk for self-injurious behavior and this is related to comorbid dissociative phenomenology and traumatic experiences [13]. A total of 15.8% of patients with obsessive-compulsive disorder and 18.8% of patients with trichotillomania had Dissociative Experiences Scale (DES) [70] scores of 30 or above in one study [12]. Significant positive correlations were found between DES scores and emotional, sexual, and physical abuse, and physical neglect scores in both diagnostic groups. In the dissociative subgroup of obsessive-compulsive patients, the study documented an increased incidence of a lifetime history of tics, Tourette's syndrome, bulimia nervosa, and BPD. Among patients with trichotillomania, significantly more high dissociators than low dissociators reported lifetime kleptomania and depersonalization disorder. The authors consider this comorbidity pattern to be an increased incidence of impulse dyscontrol disorders among high dissociators in both disorders.

In a large group of treatment-seeking inpatients with drug or alcohol abuse, the prevalence of dissociative disorders was 17.2% [11]. A total of 64.9% of the dissociative group reported that their dissociative experiences started before the onset of substance use; the interval between onset of dissociation and onset of substance abuse averaged 3.6 years with a range of 1 to 11 years. The dissociative patients in this study were younger, had shorter remission durations, and tended to use drugs rather than alcohol; the number of substances used was correlated with the severity of the current dissociative disorder. Female gender, childhood emotional abuse, and suicide attempts predicted a dissociative disorder diagnosis in this sample. In another study, the prevalence of dissociative disorders increased to 26% among inpatients with drug abuse (Tamar-Gurol and coworkers, unpublished data). It is noteworthy that significantly more chemically dependent inpatients with a dissociative disorder cease participation in their treatment program prematurely, compared with patients with no comorbid dissociative disorder [11].

Somatoform dissociation and general medicine

A high proportion of women primary care patients report abusive experiences in childhood and adulthood and mental health problems [71]. Somatoform presentations and the need to formulate inclusive differential diagnoses means that conversion and somatization disorders are of particular interest for general medicine. For example, pseudoseizures have become a major study area in neurology. Among outpatients who were admitted to a primary health care institution in Turkey, the prevalence of conversion symptoms in the preceding month was 27.2%. The lifetime rate of a conversion disorder in this sample was 48.2% [72].

High sexual abuse rates have been found for pseudoseizures [73], somatization disorder [74], and conversion disorder patients in general [14,16]. The prevalence of dissociation was significantly higher among fibromyalgia patients compared with other rheumatic disorder patients in another study [75]. A total of 30.5% to 47.4% of patients with conversion disorder have a DSM-IV dissociative disorder on axis I [14,76]. Consistent with these data, a new concept of somatoform dissociation has been proposed recently that could elucidate the basic mechanism in this spectrum of disorders [77].

Allegedly an acute and monosymptomatic condition, conversion disorder is frequently part of a more chronic and complex disorder [14]. Patients with conversion disorder have overall psychiatric symptom scores close to those of general psychiatric patients, suggesting high general psychiatric comorbidity [78]. A total of 89.5% of patients with conversion disorder had at least one psychiatric diagnosis in a 2-year follow-up [14]. It is noteworthy, that among patients with conversion disorder, a concurrent dissociative disorder is a significant predictor of higher general psychiatric comorbidity including somatization disorder, dysthymic disorder, major depression, BPD, self-destructive behavior, suicide attempts, and childhood trauma [14]. As such, conversion disorder and somatization disorder provide a diagnostic and therapeutic challenge not only for psychiatrists, but also for clinicians working in general medicine. Clearly, patients in these diagnostic groups need screening for the presence of a dissociative disorder.

How measures of dissociation could be incorporated in studies of other disorders

Measures of dissociation could be incorporated into studies of etiology, phenomenology, biology, natural history, genetics, family dynamics, or any other aspect of mental health and addictions. This tends not to occur because dissociation is not part of the mind set of many researchers, because researchers in other areas are not familiar with the scientific literature on dissociation, and because the dissociative disorders are not included in widely used measures like the Structured Clinical Interview for DSM-III-R [79].

The trauma model of schizophrenia [3,19,22] predicts specific relationships between trauma, dissociation, comorbidity, and psychotic symptoms that cannot be tested without valid and reliable measures of dissociation. The model proposes the existence of a dissociative subtype of schizophrenia characterized by severe childhood trauma, dissociative symptoms, auditory hallucinations, and extensive comorbidity. Statistically, all these elements would correlate positively with each other if the model is correct. Consider as an example the main multicenter clinical trial of quetiapine that resulted in its receiving approval from the Food and Drug Administration [80].

In this trial, 361 participants with acute exacerbations of schizophrenia were randomized to several different doses of quetiapine, haloperidol, or placebo. The most effective dose of quetiapine was 150 mg. Only 29% of participants were classified as responders to this dosage, however, where responder status was defined as a 40% or greater drop in baseline psychosis scores.

The trauma model predicts that in this trial, the response rate to quetiapine would be higher among participants scoring under 10 on the DES [70] than among participants scoring over 30. Within schizophrenia, DES scores should be powerful predictors of psychosis scores, treatment resistance, comorbidity, reported childhood trauma, and a range of phenomenologic and biologic variables not addressed in the quetiapine trial. These relationships were not evident in the quetiapine trial because there were no measures of dissociation or psychologic trauma, and because comorbidity on axis I was an exclusion criterion, as it is throughout the psychopharmacology literature. According to the trauma model, psychosis and dissociation scores should covary (the higher the DES score, the more positive symptoms of schizophrenia are present); however, in the high-DES individual, the psychotic symptoms should be less responsive to medication and more responsive to psychotherapy. From the perspective of conventional psychiatry, this prediction is paradoxical, but it is consistent with the replicated finding that positive symptoms of schizophrenia are more frequent in dissociative identity disorder than in schizophrenia [3]. The idea is that within the dissociative subtype of schizophrenia, positive symptoms are more frequent, and also more trauma-driven and responsive to psychotherapy.

In studies of bipolar mood disorder, measures of dissociation might correlate with childhood trauma, comorbidity, symptom severity, and response to mood-stabilizing medication. In high DES scorers, more of the affective and behavioral instability might be caused by trauma and dissociation. Response to agents effective for mood disorders might be poorer. High DES scores, then, would predict treatment resistance to mood stabilizers and could be used to triage participants into a cognitive therapy arm of a treatment study.

In such a design, participants would be randomized to one of four groups: (1) medication-cognitive therapy, (2) placebo-cognitive therapy, (3) medication-no cognitive therapy, and (4) placebo-no cognitive therapy. The trauma model predicts that participants with high DES scores respond better to placebo-cognitive therapy than to medication-no cognitive therapy. By identifying a subgroup with high levels of trauma, dissociation, and comorbidity, such a methodology would also, potentially, separate out a subgroup with a more pure, endogenous biologic etiology.

The relationship between trauma, dissociation, and comorbidity is especially important in BPD. Dissociation should be a powerful predictor of phenomenology, history, and response to medication and psychotherapy in BPD. The design of a possible psychotherapy treatment study of borderline personality that incorporates dissociation as a key variable is described elsewhere [81].

One benefit of including measures of trauma, dissociation, and comorbidity in psychiatric research is that such measures could identify and separate out the environmental noise that confounds much biologic research to date, thereby making it easier to identify subgroups within any diagnostic category with a predominantly endogenous, genetic, or biologic etiology. This benefit could accrue all across axis I and II, no matter what other variables were the focus of research.

How omission of dissociative disorders in differential diagnosis confounds and weakens studies on other disorders

Among patients with bipolar disorder adult comorbid PTSD was significantly associated with childhood sexual abuse, among other variables [82]. Severe childhood abuse was reported by about half of bipolar patients, but only one third of abused patients developed PTSD. Risk for PTSD rose in a linear fashion with the number of childhood abuse subtypes present. Adult sexual abuse was significantly more likely to be associated with PTSD if childhood sexual abuse was present rather than absent.

The authors of this study [82] propose that childhood sexual abuse may sensitize individuals who are predisposed to bipolar disorder also to develop eventual PTSD; however, possible mechanisms of this phenomenon remain obscure. The question arises whether assessment of comorbid dissociative disorders contributes to illumination of this link. The psychiatric outcome of traumatic experiences (particularly childhood trauma) is not limited to PTSD; although dissociation is closely related to development of PTSD [43–45], in response to trauma some individuals develop PTSD without a dissociative disorder, some develop a dissociative disorder without PTSD, and many develop both.

In general, identifying an additional group among individuals without PTSD by screening for dissociative disorders increases the overall rate of discovery of patients who developed a psychiatric disorder in the aftermath of traumatic experiences, no matter what primary diagnosis was being examined in a given study.

Schneiderian symptoms during a first manic episode identify a subgroup of patients with poorer short-term outcome [21]. First-rank symptoms are common in dissociative disorders [23], and they are highly related to other dissociative symptom clusters and to childhood trauma even in the general population [24]. The link between early stress (childhood trauma) and poor outcome in bipolar disorder should be explored in future studies [27]; study of comorbid trauma-related dissociative disorders might lead to interesting observations about the mechanism of schneiderian symptoms and treatment resistance in bipolar disorder.

In a 6-year follow-up study on BPD, Zanarini and coworkers [83] reported that substance-use disorders were most closely associated with the failure to achieve remission from BPD. Because comorbid dissociative disorders were not screened for in that study, despite prior evidence that they are common in BPD [15,57], a possible contribution of dissociation to negative outcome in the study could not be identified. In other samples of substance users, patients with comorbid dissociative disorders are over-represented among drop-outs from treatment programs [11,84]. The lack of screening for dissociative disorders among these psychiatric disorders may lead to misleading study results, confounding of data, and lost opportunities to understand better how to direct more disturbed patients to proper treatments.

Testing for and identifying dissociative disorders in research protocols

Assessment tools developed for evaluation and screening of dissociative disorders range from easy-to-administer short and structured instruments to comprehensive inventories that try to document dissociative psychopathology in all its aspects. As in anxiety research, state and trait dissociation can be assessed separately; self-rating or clinician administered scales exist for both purposes [70,85]. The differentiation of trait and state dissociation may be especially important in future neurobiologic research. Assessment measures for somatoform [86] and peritraumatic dissociation [87] also have been developed.

Structured interviews like the Dissociative Disorders Interview Schedule [88] and semistructured clinical interviews like the Structured Clinical Interview for DSM-IV Dissociative Disorders [89] are crucial for obtaining a dissociative disorder diagnosis in research studies. Until general psychiatric interview schedules, such as the Structured Clinical Interview for DSM-III-R [79], include sections for dissociative disorders, to identify comorbid dissociative disorders, a selected combination of these assessment tools should be adopted as additional measures. For a more comprehensive evaluation of dissociative phenomena, a Multidimensional Inventory of Dissociation has been developed recently [90]. In addition to clinical evaluation and standardized measuring tools, use of projective assessments, such as Rorschach test, is also possible (see the article by Brand and coworkers elsewhere in this issue); however, more data are needed to uncover the potentials of this valuable instrument for assessment of dissociative disorders [91].

Summary

Overall, this article suggests from several aspects that long-lasting omission of dissociative disorders in general psychiatric research has led to significant information loss and to misdirection of both financial and human resources. It is proposed that measures of dissociation should be incorporated in a wide range of research into mental health and addictions. Given the findings from research on dissociative disorders in the last two decades, this area of psychopathology has the potential to transform today's psychiatry.

References

[1] American Psychiatric Association. Diagnostic and statistical manual of mental disorders. 4th edition. Washington: American Psychiatric Association; 1994.
[2] Ross CA. The trauma model: a solution to the problem of comorbidity in psychiatry. Richardson (TX): Manitou Communications; 2000.
[3] Ross CA. Schizophrenia: innovations in diagnosis and treatment. New York: The Haworth Press; 2004.
[4] De Graaf R, Bijl RV, Simit F, et al. Risk factors for 12-month comorbidity of mood, anxiety, and substance use disorders: findings from the Netherlands Mental Health Survey and Incidence Study. Am J Psychiatry 2002;159:620–9.
[5] Breslau N. Epidemiologic studies of trauma, posttraumatic stress disorder, and other psychiatric disorders. Can J Psychiatry 2002;47:923–9.
[6] Chu JA, Dill DL. Dissociative symptoms in relation to childhood physical and sexual abuse. Am J Psychiatry 1990;147:887–92.
[7] Ogawa JR, Sroufe LA, Weinfield NS, et al. Development and the fragmented self: longitudinal study of dissociative symptomatology in a nonclinical sample. Dev Psychopathol 1997; 4:855–79.
[8] Gladstone GL, Parker GB, Mitchell PB, et al. Implications of childhood trauma for depressed women: an analysis of pathways from childhood sexual abuse to deliberate self-harm and revictimization. Am J Psychiatry 2004;161:1417–25.
[9] Ellason JW, Ross CA, Fuchs DL. Lifetime axis I and II comorbidity and childhood trauma history in dissociative identity disorder. Psychiatry 1996;59:255–66.
[10] Holowka DV, King S, Sahep D, et al. Childhood abuse and dissociative symptoms in adult schizophrenia. Schizophr Res 2003;60:87–90.
[11] Karadag F, Sar V, Tamar-Gürol D, et al. Dissociative disorders among inpatients with drug or alcohol dependency. J Clin Psychiatry 2005;66:1247–53.
[12] Lochner C, Seedat S, Hemmings SMJ, et al. Dissociative experiences in obsessive-compulsive disorder and trichotillomania: clinical and genetic findings. Compr Psychiatry 2004;45: 384–91.

[13] Paul T, Schroeter K, Dahme B, et al. Self-injurious behavior in women with eating disorders. Am J Psychiatry 2002;159:408–11.

[14] Sar V, Akyüz G, Kundakci T, et al. Childhood trauma, dissociation and psychiatric comorbidity in patients with conversion disorder. Am J Psychiatry 2004;161:2271–6.

[15] Sar V, Kundakci T, Kiziltan E, et al. Axis I dissociative disorder comorbidity of borderline personality disorder among psychiatric outpatients. J Trauma Dissociation 2003;4:119–36.

[16] Simeon D, Guralnik O, Schmeidler J, et al. The role of childhood interpersonal trauma in depersonalization disorder. Am J Psychiatry 2001;158:1027–33.

[17] Janssen I, Krabbendam L, Bak M, et al. Childhood abuse as a risk factor for psychotic experiences. Acta Psychiatr Scand 2004;109:38–45.

[18] Offen L, Waller G, Thomas G. Is reported childhood sexual abuse associated with the psychopathological characteristics of patients who experience auditory hallucinations? Child Abuse Negl 2003;27:919–27.

[19] Ross CA, Keyes B. Dissociation and schizophrenia. J Trauma Dissociation 2004;5:69–83.

[20] Lysaker PH, Wickett AM, Lancaster RS, et al. Neurocognitive deficits and history of childhood abuse in schizophrenia spectrum disorders: associations with cluster B personality traits. Schizophr Res 2004;68:87–94.

[21] Conus P, Abdel-Baki A, Harrigan S, et al. Schneiderian first rank symptoms predict poor outcome within first episode manic psychosis. J Affect Dis 2004;81:259–68.

[22] Gonzales-Pinto A, Van Os J, Perez De Heredia JL, et al. Age-dependence of schneiderian psychotic symptoms in bipolar patients. Schizophr Res 2003;61:157–62.

[23] Kluft RP. First rank symptoms as a diagnostic clue to multiple personality disorder. Am J Psychiatry 1987;144:293–8.

[24] Ross CA, Joshi S. Schneiderian symptoms and childhood trauma in the general population. Compr Psychiatry 1992;33:269–73.

[25] Hammersley P, Dias A, Todd G, et al. Childhood trauma and hallucinations in bipolar affective disorder: preliminary investigation. Br J Psychiatry 2003;182:543–7.

[26] Kupka RW, Luckenbaugh DA, Post RM, et al. Comparison of rapid-cycling and non-rapid-cycling bipolar disorder based on prospective mood ratings in 539 outpatients. Am J Psychiatry 2005;162:1273–80.

[27] Leverich GS, Perez S, Luckenbaugh DA, et al. Early psychosocial stressors: relationship to suicidality and course of bipolar illness. Clin Neurosci Res 2002;2:161–70.

[28] Nemeroff CB, Heim CM, Thase ME, et al. Differential responses to psychotherapy versus pharmacotherapy in patients with chronic forms of major depression and childhood trauma. Proc Natl Acad Sci U S A 2003;100:14293–6.

[29] Parker GB, Malhi GS, Crawford JG, et al. Identifying paradigm failures contributing to treatment-resistant depression. J Affect Dis 2005;87:185–91.

[30] Hollender MH, Hirsch SJ. Hysterical psychosis. Am J Psychiatry 1964;120:1066–74.

[31] Hirsch SJ, Hollender MH. Hysterical psychosis: clarification of the concept. Am J Psychiatry 1969;125:909–15.

[32] Öztürk OM, Gögüs A. Agir regressif belirtiler gösteren histerik psikozlar [Hysterical psychoses presenting with severe regressive symptoms]. In: Proceedings of the 9th National Congress of Psychiatry and Neurology. Ankara, Turkey: Meteksan; 1973. p. 155–64.

[33] Van der Hart O, Witztum E, Friedman B. From hysterical psychosis to reactive dissociative psychosis. J Trauma Stress 1992;6:43–64.

[34] Tutkun H, Yargic LI, Sar V. Dissociative identity disorder presenting as hysterical psychosis. Dissociation 1996;9:241–9.

[35] Sar V, Ozturk E. Psychotic presentations of dissociative identity disorder. In: Dell P, O'Neil J, editors. Dissociation and dissociative disorders: DSM-V and beyond. In press.

[36] Strömgren E. Psychogenic psychoses. In: Hirsch SR, Shepherd M, editors. Themes and variations in European psychiatry. Bristol: Wright; 1974. p. 97–120.

[37] Strömgren E. The development of the concept of reactive psychoses. Psychopathology 1986; 20:62–7.

[38] Ungvari GS, Leung HCM, Tang WK. Reactive psychosis: a classical category nearing extinction? Psychiatry Clin Neurosci 2000;54:621–4.
[39] Ungvari GS, Mullen PE. Reactive psychoses revisited. Aust N Z J Psychiatry 2000;34: 458–67.
[40] Grisaru N, Irwin M, Kaplan Z. Acute psychotic episodes as a reaction to severe trauma in a population of Ethiopian immigrants to Israel. Stress Health 2003;19:241–7.
[41] Kozaric-Kovacic D, Borovecki A. Prevalence of psychotic comorbidity in combat-related post-traumatic stress disorder. Mil Med 2005;170:223–6.
[42] Ozek M. Soziale umstrukturierung als provokationsfaktor depressiver psychosen [Social restructuralization as provoking factor for depressive psychoses]. In: Problems of provocation of depressive psychoses. Graz, Austria; 1971. p. 109–15.
[43] Irwin HJ. The relationship between dissociative tendencies and schizotypy: an artifact of childhood trauma? J Clin Psychol 2001;57:331–42.
[44] Simeon D, Guralnik O, Knutelska M, et al. Dissection of schizotypy and dissociation in depersonalization disorder. J Trauma Dissociation 2004;5:111–9.
[45] Murray J, Ehlers A, Mayou RA. Dissociation and post-traumatic stress disorder: two prospective studies of road traffic accident survivors. Br J Psychiatry 2002;180:363–8.
[46] Saxe G, Stoddard F, Hall E, et al. Pathways to PTSD, Part I: Children with burns. Am J Psychiatry 2005;162:1299–304.
[47] Panasetis P, Bryant RA. Peritraumatic versus persistent dissociation in acute stress disorder. J Trauma Stress 2003;16:563–6.
[48] Zanarini MC, Williams AA, Lewis RE, et al. Reported pathological childhood experiences associated with the development of borderline personality disorder. Am J Psychiatry 1997; 154:1101–6.
[49] Zanarini MC, Frankenburg FR, Khera GS, et al. Treatment histories of borderline inpatients. Compr Psychiatry 2001;42:144–50.
[50] Bandelow B, Krause J, Wedekind D, et al. Early traumatic life events, parental attitudes, family history, and birth risk factors in patients with borderline personality disorder and healthy controls. Psychiatry Res 2005;134:169–79.
[51] Ross-Gover J, Waller G, Tyson M, et al. Reported sexual abuse and subsequent psychopathology among women attending psychology clinics: the mediating role of dissociation. Br J Clin Psychol 1998;37:313–26.
[52] Hudziak JJ, Boffeli TJ, Kriesman JJ, et al. Clinical study of the relation of borderline personality disorder to Briquet's syndrome (hysteria), somatization disorder, antisocial personality disorder, and substance abuse disorders. Am J Psychiatry 1996;153:1598–606.
[53] Rosenthal MZ, Cheavens JS, Lejuez CXW, et al. Thought suppression mediates the relationship between negative affect and borderline personality disorder symptoms. Behav Res Ther 2005;43:1173–85.
[54] Campo J, Nijman H, Merckelbach H, et al. Psychiatric comorbidity of gender identity disorders: a survey among Dutch psychiatrists. Am J Psychiatry 2003;160:1332–6.
[55] Wilkinson-Ryan T, Westen D. Identity disturbance in borderline personality disorder: an empirical investigation. Am J Psychiatry 2000;157:528–41.
[56] Golier JA, Yehuda R, Bierer LM, et al. The relationship of borderline personality disorder to posttraumatic stress disorder and traumatic events. Am J Psychiatry 2003;160:2018–24.
[57] Zittel Conklin C, Westen D. Borderline personality disorder in clinical practice. Am J Psychiatry 2005;162:867–75.
[58] Sar V, Akyüz G, Kundakci T, et al. Prevalence of trauma-related disorders in Turkey: an epidemiological study. Presented at the 14th Annual Meeting of the International Society for Traumatic Stress Studies. Washington, November 20–22, 1998.
[59] Yee L, Korner AJ, McSwiggan S, et al. Persistent hallucinosis in borderline personality disorder. Compr Psychiatry 2005;46:147–54.
[60] Zanarini MC, Ruser T, Frankenburg FR, et al. The dissociative experiences of borderline patients. Compr Psychiatry 2000;41:223–7.

[61] Zanarini MC, Frankenburg FR, Dubo ED, et al. Axis I comorbidity of borderline personality disorder. Am J Psychiatry 1998;155:1733–9.

[62] Zanarini MC, Frankenburg FR. Attainment and maintenance of reliability of axis I and II disorders over the course of a longitudinal study. Compr Psychiatry 2001;42:369–74.

[63] Bernstein ME, Reich DB, Zanarini MC, et al. Late-onset borderline personality disorder: a life unraveling. Harv Rev Psychiatry 2002;10:292–301.

[64] Brodsky BS, Cloitre M, Dulit RA. Relationship of dissociation to self-mutilation and childhood abuse in borderline personality disorder. Am J Psychiatry 1995;152:1788–92.

[65] Moskowitz A. Dissociation and violence: a review of the literature. Trauma Violence Abuse 2004;5:21–46.

[66] Lewis DO, Yeager CA, Swica Y, et al. Objective documentation of child abuse and dissociation in 12 murderers with dissociative identity disorder. Am J Psychiatry 1997;154:1703–10.

[67] Ystgaard M, Hestetun I, Loeb M, et al. Is there a specific relationship between childhood sexual and physical abuse and repeated suicidal behavior? Child Abuse Negl 2004;28:863–75.

[68] Yen S, Shea MT, Sanislow CA, et al. Borderline personality disorder criteria associated with prospectively observed suicidal behaviour. Am J Psychiatry 2004;161:1296–8.

[69] Koenigsberg HW, Harvey PD, Mitropoulou V, et al. Characterizing affective instability in borderline personality disorder. Am J Psychiatry 2002;159:784–8.

[70] Bernstein EM, Putnam FW. Development, reliability, and validity of a dissociation scale. J Nerv Ment Dis 1986;174:727–35.

[71] Coid J, Petruckevitch A, Chung WS, et al. Abusive experiences and psychiatric morbidity in women primary care attenders. Br J Psychiatry 2003;183:332–9.

[72] Sagduyu A, Rezaki M, Kaplan I, et al. Saglik ocagina basvuran hastalarda dissosiyatif (konversiyon) belirtiler [Prevalence of conversion symptoms in a primary health care center]. Turkish J Psychiatry 1997;8:161–9.

[73] Bowman ES, Markand ON. Psychodynamics and psychiatric diagnoses of pseudoseizure subjects. Am J Psychiatry 1996;153:57–63.

[74] Pribor EF, Yutzy SH, Dean JT, et al. Briquet's syndrome, dissociation, and abuse. Am J Psychiatry 1993;150:1507–11.

[75] Leavitt F, Katz RS. The dissociative factor in symptom reports of rheumatic patients with and without fibromyalgia. J Clin Psychol Med Settings 2003;10:259–66.

[76] Tezcan E, Atmaca M, Kuloglu M, et al. Dissociative disorders in Turkish inpatients with conversion disorder. Compr Psychiatry 2003;44:324–30.

[77] Nijenhuis ERS, Spinhoven P, Van Dyck R, et al. Degree of somatoform and psychological dissociation in dissociative disorder is correlated with reported trauma. J Trauma Stress 1998;11:711–30.

[78] Spitzer C, Spelsberg B, Grabe HJ, et al. Dissociative experiences and psychopathology in conversion disorders. J Psychosom Res 1999;46:291–4.

[79] Spitzer RL, Williams JBW, Gibbon M, et al. User's guide for the Structured Clinical Interview for DSM-III-R. Washington: American Psychiatric Press; 1990.

[80] Arvantis LA, Miller BG. Multiple fixed doses of seroquel (quetiapine) in patients with acute exacerbation of schizophrenia: a comparison with haloperidol and placebo. Biol Psychiatry 1997;42:233–46.

[81] Ross CA. A proposed trial of dialectical behavior therapy and trauma model therapy. Psychol Rep 2005;96:901–11.

[82] Goldberg JF, Garno JL. Development of posttraumatic stress disorder in adult bipolar patients with histories of severe childhood abuse. J Psychiatr Res 2005;39:595–601.

[83] Zanarini MC, Frankenburg FR, Hennen J, et al. Axis-I comorbidity in patients with borderline personality disorder. Am J Psychiatry 2004;161:2108–14.

[84] Evren C, Sar V, Karadag F, et al. Dissociative disorders among alcohol-dependent inpatients. Psychiatry Res, in press.

[85] Bremner JD, Krystal JH, Putnam FW, et al. Measurement of dissociative states with the Clinician-Administered Dissociative States Scale (CADSS). J Trauma Stress 1998;11:125–36.

[86] Nijenhuis ERS, Spinhoven P, Van Dyck R, et al. The development and psychometric characteristics of the Somatoform Dissociation Questionnaire (SDQ-20). J Nerv Ment Dis 1996; 184:688–94.

[87] Marmar CR, Weiss DS, Metzler T. Peritraumatic dissociation and posttraumatic stress disorder. In: Bremner JD, Marmar CR, editors. Trauma, memory and dissociation. Washington: American Psychiatric Press; 1998. p. 229–52.

[88] Ross CA, Heber S, Norton GR, et al. The Dissociative Disorders Interview Schedule: a structured interview. Dissociation 1989;2:169–89.

[89] Steinberg M. Structured Clinical Interview for DSM-IV Dissociative Disorders–Revised (SCID-D-R). Washington: American Psychiatric Press; 1994.

[90] Dell P. Multidimensional Inventory of Dissociation Inventory (MID): a comprehensive measure of pathological dissociation. J Trauma Dissociation, in press.

[91] Sar V, Öztürk E, Kundakci T. Psychotherapy of an adolescent with dissociative identity disorder: change in Rorschach patterns. J Trauma Dissociation 2002;3:81–95.

PSYCHIATRIC
CLINICS
OF NORTH AMERICA

Psychiatr Clin N Am 29 (2006) 145–168

Psychological Assessment of Patients with Dissociative Identity Disorder

Bethany L. Brand, PhD[a],[*], Judith G. Armstrong, PhD[b],
Richard J. Loewenstein, MD[c],[d]

[a]Towson University, 8000 York Road, Towson, MD 21252, USA
[b]University of Southern California, Los Angeles, CA, USA
[c]Sheppard Pratt Health Systems, Baltimore, MD, USA
[d]Department of Psychiatry, University of Maryland
School of Medicine, Baltimore, MD, USA

This article discusses how psychologic assessment can assist in the diagnosis of dissociative identity disorder (DID) and in planning treatment for patients who are dissociative. A battery of tests that can assess the extent of dissociation is outlined, the research on dissociation on various psychologic tests is reviewed, and new Rorschach data on severely dissociative patients that can be useful in planning treatment is presented.

Diagnosing DID is a complex process and requires assessors to have knowledge of the assessment and treatment literature on posttraumatic stress disorder (PTSD), dissociative disorders, and personality disorders. The literature provides excellent reviews of assessment of posttraumatic states [1–4]. In addition to the complexity of assessing PTSD itself, assessment of DID requires the patient to reveal what is often a private, hidden world to a powerful stranger [5]. These challenges may be further compounded because many of the measures, particularly the projective tests, can open up emotional wounds and stir potentially painful memories, triggering dissociation and switching among dissociated states during the testing itself [5,6]. Clinicians must develop a collaborative relationship with patients who have DID before beginning the assessment to make the experience therapeutic rather than retraumatizing. A collaborative relationship will also help yield meaningful, rather than defended, test results.

* Corresponding author.
E-mail address: bbrand@towson.edu (B.L. Brand).

0193-953X/06/$ - see front matter © 2005 Elsevier Inc. All rights reserved.
doi:10.1016/j.psc.2005.10.014

The assessment battery

People who have PTSD can present in testing as flooded with intense affect or emotionally numb and constricted [1,2,4]. DID is even more variable and complex, partially because PTSD is almost always a comorbid condition, and partially because of the complexity found in patients who have severe dissociative psychopathologies [7–9]. No specific recipe for "smoking out" DID exists, although a consistent finding across tests and researchers is that many individuals who have DID experience a wide variety of severe symptoms. Researchers believe this is because of disturbances in many different dimensions of functioning, including problems with affect tolerance (eg, severe anxiety and mood and state instability); dissociativity; interpersonal difficulties; impaired self functions such as an inability to self-soothe; disturbances of body image and somatization; and posttraumatic cognitive distortions [10]. In addition, individuals who have DID often experience various comorbid conditions, including mood disorders; PTSD and other anxiety disorders; eating disorders; substance abuse disorders; and personality disorders [7,11]. These fluctuating comorbid conditions, compounded by the shifting personality states found in DID, ensure that no one set of signs will be found for all individuals who have DID. Armstrong [12] suggests that the ability to dissociate during sustained childhood maltreatment allows for an atypical developmental pathway, a pathway in which contradictions and complexities can coexist. This pathway helps the person preserve intellectual skills and emotions, such as humor, hope, and joy, and maintain the capacity for attachment despite the abuse. The following review of the literature shows that the dissociative developmental pathway results in personality strengths and weaknesses that are important considerations in planning treatment.

The authors typically use a battery of tests tailored to the individual, designed to capture developmental strengths and weaknesses. Assessment usually begins with a phase of rapport-building and a thorough psychosocial history, including a trauma history. This step is followed by a cognitive test, a structured and objective personality test with validity scales (eg, the Minnesota Multiphasic Personality Inventory [MMPI]-2), projective personality tests, a self-report measure of dissociation, and a structured interview for dissociation. The authors then review the findings regarding dissociation for each of these types of tests, with emphasis placed on those considered most useful. However, limited research exists on DID patients on many measures.

Cognitive assessment

Cognitive testing is useful because it often provides important information about differential diagnosis. Intelligence tests such as the Wechsler Adult Intelligence Scale-III (WAIS-III) can clarify if a patient who hears voices is psychotic, or if their psychotic-like phenomena are actually of a dissociative nature. In contrast to a patient who is thought-disordered, the results of an intelligence quotient (IQ) test of a patient who is DID should not show signs of psychotically illogical thinking or impaired reality [13].

Although popular books about DID suggest that these patients are unusually bright, their IQ results are, in fact, "remarkably unremarkable" [5]. In a sample of 100 patients who had DID and dissociative disorder not otherwise specified (DDNOS), Armstrong [5] found that the average IQ in the sample was 100, with a range from mildly retarded to superior. No subtest or ability exists that seems particularly strong or weak for this group. Dissociation may, however, lead to a puzzling pattern of inconsistent performance within subtests. For example, a client may give some very concrete and some abstract responses within a single item or a subtest, which may reflect learning deficits in areas such as social skills or switching among different personalities.

Another potential benefit of cognitive testing is that it can provide information about seemingly conflict-free cues that may briefly evoke cognitive disorganization in an individual patient. For example, one patient became fearful and somewhat disoriented when asked to complete arithmetic problems. After the patient completed the subtest, the assessor asked her to share her experience. The patient reported being terrified by numbers. She connected this to having been ridiculed and sometimes beaten by her father when she was not able to complete her math assignments during grade school. After she began to break the unspoken bond between numbers and humiliation, she showed no subsequent lapses in attention on the WAIS-III, which clarified that she did not have attention deficit disorder.

Structured personality tests

Personality tests that have a true/false format are termed *objective* or *structured* personality tests. They often assess various domains and include validity scales that are useful in detecting response sets, such as exaggerating or minimizing symptoms. Broadband measures of psychopathology, such as the MMPI, the Millon Clinical Multiaxial Inventory (MCMI), and the Rorschach, can provide information about the personality context in which dissociation occurs, thus providing valuable insight regarding treatment recommendations [3]. New research indicates that many individuals who have DID give technically invalid profiles on various personality tests, and may be labeled as *feigning* by clinical and forensic interviews [14,15]. These findings show that to provide valid and ethical assessment, assessors must be well-informed about the impact of dissociation and severe trauma on testing.

Multiphasic Minnesota Personality Inventory-2

The MMPI-2 yields 10 clinical scales, including schizophrenia, depression, paranoia, four validity scales, and numerous subscales. It consists of

567 true/false questions, often making it a challenging test for patients who have DID to complete. Many patients who have DID report strong internal conflict about how to answer the questions because different aspects of their personalities can feel, think, and behave differently. If the assessor allows them to answer what is mostly true most of the time and not deliberate for too long about any one item, most of these patients can tolerate the MMPI-2. This direction does not deviate from the standard administration. Assessors must interpret the MMPI-2 carefully for their clients who are traumatized and dissociative because the computerized scoring programs for the MMPI-2 typically do not incorporate information about trauma, although trauma and dissociation have a large bearing on a patient's profile.

Probably the most consistent and important finding for people who are traumatized, and in particular those who have DID, is the elevation in the F scale [2]. The F scale is a validity scale that is traditionally interpreted as the *fake bad*, or exaggeration of symptoms scale. It includes items that patients who are dissociative might endorse because they experience voices of dissociated alters and severe family conflict. Many researchers have found that trauma exposure results in an elevated F scale and elevations in several clinical scales [2].

Research on MMPI-2 profiles of patients who have DID has not found a single diagnostic pattern, although numerous elevations have been described among validity and clinical scales [11,16]. The most common findings are elevations on F and 8 (Schizophrenia [Sc]) scales, which contain many trauma- and dissociation-linked items. Patients who are DID typically endorse so many items on the F scale that their profiles are often technically invalid [17]. The F(p) scale, which was created to remove the influence of trauma from the F scale, is not typically highly elevated in patients who have DID [18]. Clinicians should consider other MMPI validity scales, especially F(p) (Infrequency Psychopathology Scale); other test results; and the context of the testing to clarify whether the results are indicative of extreme distress, a cry for help, exaggeration, or malingering. Only a few items on scale 8 (Sc) are indicative of hallucinations and delusions. Many of the items reflect difficulties with attention and memory; negative attitudes toward oneself; feelings of alienation from and being unloved by others; dysphoria; and unusual sensorimotor experiences, including feeling unreal, being frightened by family members, and amnesia for one's behaviors. Such experiences are commonplace for most patients who have DID because of their traumatic and disorganizing childhood experiences [8,19]. Thus, the elevation on scale 8 is not surprising. Whether the elevation on scale 8 is caused by psychosis rather than trauma can often be clarified by questions about critical items. For example, a patient who is dissociative might endorse seeing visions, yet later report that the visions are of herself as a young child being molested by her father.

Scales 4 (Psychopathic Deviate [Pd]), 2 (Depression [D]), 6, (Paranoia [Pa]), 7 (Psychasthenia [Pt]), and 1 (Hypochondriasis [Hs]) are also often elevated among individuals who have DID [16,20]. These elevations on DID profiles are consistent with 30 years of research on the MMPI profiles of sexual abuse survivors, which have found elevations on scales 4 (Pd) and 8 (Sc) often with associated lesser elevations on 2 (D), 7 (Pt), or 6 (Pa) [2]. Although a traditional interpretation of this profile might be that the client has sociopathic or schizophrenic traits, subscale analysis can clarify the nature of these elevations. Individuals who are dissociative tend to be elevated on subscales, indicating family discord (Pd1), social alienation (Pd4), and a lack of self-awareness (Pd5), rather than having authority problems (Pd2) or bizarre sensory experiences (Sc6). However, even the bizarre sensory experiences subscale contains items that may reflect dissociative rather than truly psychotic experiences (eg, engagement in activities without recall), so item analysis is also helpful in clarifying the nature of elevations.

Like other psychologic tests, the MMPI-2 cannot yield a diagnosis of DID. Three attempts have been made to create a dissociative index based on its items [21], but none of these scales have sufficient sensitivity or specificity to justify their use.

Millon Clinical Multiaxial Inventory-II

Assessing personality disorders among people who are traumatized is difficult because highly emotional and dramatic, and emotionally restricted and avoidant presentations can result from PTSD and dissociation, rather than borderline, histrionic, or obsessive personality traits. However, the presence of PTSD or DID does not preclude a coexisting personality disorder [1,2]. Some researchers have proposed alternative classifications to account for long-term personality maladaptations to trauma, or have described a mixed personality disorder subsequent to early maltreatment that might be termed *posttraumatic personality disorder* [22,23]. In the last decade, the authors have seen a rise in cases of true co-morbid, severe personality disorders in dissociative patients brought for assessment. Although the projective tests, especially the Rorschach, have been most useful in clarifying the presence of a personality disorder (see later discussion), the MCMI-II can also provide helpful information [24]. (Researchers have yet to study patients who have DID using the MCMI-III.)

Research on the MCMI-II has shown that patients who have DID experience elevations on Axis I scales, including anxiety, depression, somatoform disorders, substance abuse, and personality disorders, with avoidant, self-defeating, and borderline personality disorders being the most severe [7,25]. Although similarities exist between individuals who have borderline personality disorder and DID on the MCMI-II, patients who had DID were more than 200 base rate points higher than Millon's borderline norms on schizoid, avoidant, and schizotypal scales [7]. In contrast to general adult psychiatric outpatients, patients who have DID have been found to be higher on all scales except compulsive, narcissistic, and histrionic [7]. These findings are consistent with Rorschach studies (see later discussion) that demonstrate that individuals who have DID are not histrionic; instead, they tend to avoid emotion and use an intellectualized coping style coupled with a traumatic thought disorder [26].

Dissociation specific measures

The two tests of dissociation that the authors use most are the Dissociative Experiences Scale (DES) and the Structured Clinical Interview for DSM-IV Dissociative Disorders–Revised (SCID-D-R) [27,28]. Several other useful self-report measures of dissociation now exist, including the Multidimensional Inventory of Dissociation (see the article by Dell elsewhere in this issue), which contains validity scales, and the Dissociative Disorders Interview Schedule, which is another structured interview for dissociation [29]. Because there are extensive reviews of the DES and SCID-D-R, the role of these measures is only briefly described [14,15]. As noted by Briere and Armstrong [3], testing is most helpful when it clarifies not only whether patients dissociate, "but also *how* they dissociate."

The DES is the most used, but probably also the most misunderstood, self-report measure of dissociation. Patients can easily complete the 28-item measure in a few minutes. The items are rated according to the frequency with which they are experienced, from 0% to 100%. The total score is the average item score. A multicenter study of the DES found that a cutoff score of 30 correctly identified 74% of individuals who had DID and 80% of those who did not have DID [30]. The DES assesses amnestic dissociation; depersonalization and derealization; and absorption. This test is popular because it is brief and easy to score. However, it is also easy to misuse. Because it is a screening test and not a diagnostic inventory, a high score does not mean that a person necessarily has DID. A score above the cutoff may raise the index of suspicion for a dissociative disorder. Further clinical or psychologic assessment is required to make a diagnosis, regardless of the DES score. For example, items that are endorsed can serve as a starting point for the interviewer to request concrete examples related to these items. The authors have found that patients who are nondissociative and questioned about their responses had not been thinking of truly dissociative experiences or had overrated the frequency with which they occur. This finding is important because the authors have seen many cases where clinicians erroneously assumed that a very high DES score meant that the person had DID. On the other hand, some patients who are truly dissociative may minimize responses on the DES, and on the clinical interview may describe far more frequent and profound dissociative experiences. In summary, the DES is best used as an initial screen for dissociation, which then may lead to further interviewing and possibly administration of a more rigorous measure, such as the SCID-D-R.

Current research suggests that dissociation is not unidimensional, and therefore the assessment of dissociation should be multidimensional [3].

Treatment recommendations will likely be different according to the type and severity of dissociation experienced. The SCID-D-R is recognized as the most useful of the structured interviews for dissociative disorders because it is the only one to provide exact diagnoses from the *Diagnostic and Statistical Manual of Mental Disorders, Fourth Edition* (DSM-IV) and because of its semistructured format [2,28]. Furthermore, it assesses five domains of pathologic dissociation: amnesia, depersonalization, derealization, identity confusion, and identity alteration. It is generally considered the gold standard measure for diagnosing dissociative disorders, partially because it has good interrater reliability and has shown promise in differentiating between factitious and malingered cases of DID [20,31]. The SCID-D-R is limited because there are few data on its sensitivity, specificity, or discriminative validity, and it does not have validity scales to measure defensiveness or malingering [3]. Although it can take more than 90 minutes to administer the more than 250-item interview, the authors have found it extremely useful in complicated diagnostic cases. Because the interviewer asks for concrete, detailed examples of each symptom, and must be convinced that these experiences are dissociative in nature, the interview provides some protection against overdiagnosing DID. Furthermore, interviewers observe carefully for dissociative behaviors to this anxiety-provoking interview, such as ongoing amnesia for test questions and eye rolls (often associated with entering a hypnotic state or change in dissociative state). Most patients who have genuine DID will feel ambivalent about reporting their symptoms on the SCID-D-R, so outward signs of internal conflict are also common, such as giving contradictory answers or briefly spacing out.

Projective tests

The authors have found that projective tests are particularly useful in assessing severe dissociative disorders because the ambiguity of the tests requires that individuals project their own ways of organizing reality onto the tests. Only the projective tests that have well-validated, reliable scoring systems are reviewed. The projective tests' validated scoring systems numerically capture the areas of a person's narrative that are disrupted or preserved by dissociation. These tests are not used to establish the diagnosis of DID; instead, they can confirm it and give a great deal of information about the person's conflicts; views of themselves and others; and personality strengths and weaknesses. Armstrong and Kaser-Boyd [1] review the findings regarding trauma and projective tests in detail. They identify an important role of projectives: that people who are traumatized sometimes convey information about their trauma on the projectives that they do not talk about directly.

Thematic Apperception Test

The Thematic Apperception Test (TAT) consists of 20 black-and-white drawings that depict people and scenes. Individuals are asked to tell stories that describe the characters' thoughts and feelings. The TAT particularly provides a method for describing how clients expect people to interact—internally in their alter world and externally in the social world [5]. Individuals who are severely traumatized and have DID typically tell stories with themes of danger, trauma, refuge, and dissociation. For example, using Westen and colleagues' [32] object relations scoring method, the Social Cognition and Object Relations Scale, adolescents who are traumatized have been found to tell TAT stories that are characterized by negative affect, have characters who are malevolent and self-centered, and have themes of violence [1]. Similar results were found with a small sample of adult patients who had DID [33]. However, the stories of participants who had DID had fewer extremely self-absorbed characters than did those of girls who were sexually abused [34]. This finding may reflect aspects of the alternative path of development that dissociation provides to those who are abused early in life. Individuals who have DID are able to compartmentalize some of their memories of traumatic life events or aspects of caregivers' malevolent behavior. Accordingly, despite experiences in which important people gratified themselves at the expense of the dissociative person's well-being, these patients are able to retain some aspects of self that can still view relationships as potentially supportive [12]. The ability of dissociative individuals to see others as supportive is consistent with the authors' DID Rorschach findings.

The Rorschach

People who are highly dissociative chronically avoid painful feelings and recollections. The Rorschach is particularly useful with them because it requires that they "delve into their internal store of associations, the very thing that dissociation has been helping them avoid" [26]. Another benefit of the Rorschach is that it can be helpful when someone endorses so many symptoms on the self-report measures that the validity of their profile is questionable [14,15]. It is not obvious what a "pathological" response would be on the Rorschach, so people who are attempting to exaggerate symptoms often do not know how to look extremely ill. The Rorschach is also helpful in clarifying the extent of difficulties with perception and thinking. For example, a client may respond to the MMPI-2 and MCMI-II in a way that suggests a thought disorder. If a person's reality testing is basically intact until they begin to report traumatic stimuli on the Rorschach, and only then do they respond with distorted, inaccurate perceptions that distort the blot or involve illogical combinations of ideas, they may have a traumatic thought disorder rather than a psychotic disorder [26]. The Rorschach is also useful because it provides a broad view of a person's cognition and problem solving; affective style; and representation of self and others, including what stimuli precipitate cognitive and emotional breakdown and how, if at all, the person can recover. The complexities, strengths, and vulnerabilities that result from these individuals developing along an atypical pathway are most clearly seen on the Rorschach.

The following interpretations are based on Exner's Rorschach scoring system (see Appendix A for an alphabetical listing of Rorschach variables) [35,36]. A recent review of trauma and the Rorschach concluded that individuals who are traumatized may show signs of avoidance (low R, pure form R, low Afr, low blends, low EB), flooding of intense and painful affect (CF + C > FC), high traumatic content, high shading (especially Y and V), hyperarousal (high m and positive HVI), and impaired reality testing (low X+, high Xu, high WSum6) [1].

Earlier studies of dissociative patients used small samples and often different scoring systems [13,37–39]. Despite these weaknesses, studies have shown that patients who have DID consistently exhibit a complexity of internal experiences that are unique, and a tendency to be flooded by traumatic material while paradoxically having defenses that permit distancing and detachment from their experience.

Rorschach profiles of 100 inpatients who are severely dissociative

The authors conducted the first study of a large group of patients who had dissociative disorders (DDs) and compared the results with published data of clinical and nonclinical groups to highlight issues of differential diagnosis and the strengths and weaknesses these patients. The authors collected Rorschachs on 100 inpatients (78 DID and 22 DDNOS) at Sheppard Pratt Health System. The patients who were DD were mostly young adult to middle-aged Caucasian women with some college education (see Table 1 for demographics). No significant differences between the DDNOS and DID groups were found on 17 important Rorschach variables, so the groups were collapsed. The patients were diagnosed as having a severe DD by senior psychiatrists and psychologists who were experienced in the assessment and treatment of patients who are dissociative. All participants met *Diagnostic and Statistical Manual of Mental Disorders, Revised Third Edition* (DSM-III-R) or DSM-IV diagnostic criteria for PTSD. Assessment included review of medical and psychiatric records, DES scores, and a detailed semistructured interview that assessed the presence or absence of dissociative amnesia, autohypnotic symptoms, somatoform symptoms, PTSD symptoms, mood disorder symptoms, and dissociative process symptoms such as the presence of alter self-states, passive influence, inner voices, and switching phenomena [19].

The authors make comparisons between their sample of 100 inpatients who had DD and published norms for 41 inpatient Vietnam veteran men who had chronic PTSD [40], 30 non–treatment seeking Desert Storm veterans who exhibited acute stress caused by recent exposure to war [41], 193 depressed inpatients [35], and 175 nonpatient adults ("normals") [42]. Most of the DD group was hospitalized because of an acute exacerbation of a combination of disorders, including DD, PTSD, and mood disorders. The clinical groups were chosen to contrast patients whose primary disorder was depression, acute stress, or chronic PTSD to patients who had DID/DDNOS comorbid with PTSD and mood disorders. Highlighting the commonalities and differences between the groups helps clarify the unique role that dissociation plays.

Two masters-level psychology technicians who worked as full-time assessors in the psychology department of the hospital administered and scored the Rorschachs. The technicians were trained in administration and scoring of the Rorschach by the second author. Of the protocols, 30 were randomly selected and scored by the second assessor to evaluate reliability. The agreement between the two assessors was acceptable and ranged from 82% to 100%, with an average agreement of 94.4%.

The Rorschach is generally the most challenging but most informative test used with this population because it opens up intense emotions and conflicts that patients who have DD habitually "turn off." As a result, patients who have DD often become flooded with emotions and bothersome percepts while completing the Rorschach. They sometimes become frightened of the cards, literally pushing them away as if they could be harmful. Sometimes the cards trigger switching of alters or intrusive PTSD symptoms such as flashbacks. Within the Exner Rorschach scoring system, patients must give at least 14 responses for the interpretations to be considered valid. It is commonplace for patients who have DD to give fewer responses than other patients. In this sample, 43 of the 100 patients gave fewer than 14 responses, which is also commonplace in the authors' clinical experience. The authors interpret this response as the patient's attempt to limit and escape painful associations. Because low responses are so common, the authors chose not to discard these low response profiles, believing that accurately summarizing a large sample of patients who have DD is more likely to help clinicians who are attempting to interpret brief protocols from these patients. Furthermore, Exner and Weiner (personal communication, 1993), advised that brief records may be potentially useful if they do not have signs of defensiveness (eg, high Lambda, high X+, low blends, brief responses) [43]. The authors' sample did not show these signs of defensiveness. In fact, the responses tended to be lengthy because of a high number of blends and special scores. Nonetheless, the following interpretations must be made cautiously because of the potential decreased validity of the 43 brief protocols.

Descriptive statistics were calculated for each variable in Exner's "structural summary" (see Tables 1 and 2 for a complete listing of these variables) [35,36]. Appendix B provides the percentages, means, and standard deviations for important structural variables for the DD group. The horizontal bars in Figs. 1 through 3 represent the 95% CI computed around each group's mean score. The vertical line within each bar indicates the group's mean score. If a sample's CI overlaps another sample's by less than a fourth of the length of the line, the samples are statistically different (p < .05).

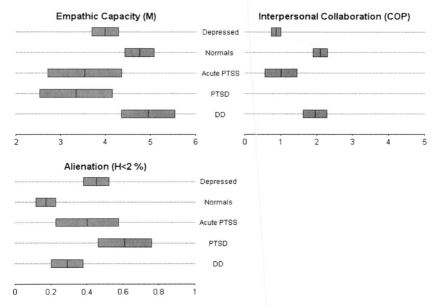

Fig. 1. Confidence intervals by group related to capacity for therapeutic alliance. "Depressed" from N = 193 depressed inpatients [26]; "Normals" from N = 175 nonpatient adults [27]; "Acute PTSS" from N = 30 non–treatment seeking Desert Storm veterans who have acute post-traumatic stress symptoms [46]; "PTSD" from N = 41 inpatient male Vietnam veterans who have chronic PTSD [33]; "DD" from N = 100 DDNOS/DID inpatients.

Capacity for therapeutic alliance

For patients who have DD, the dissociative pathway appears to provide some, yet not total, protection to their views of others. On the positive side, the DD group displayed an ability for collaborative give-and-take in relationships that was comparable to the normals, and greater capacity for collaboration than did patients who were depressed and veterans who had acute stress (eg, COP = 1.95 for DD versus 1.0 in veterans who had acute stress [41]) (see Fig. 1). (COP scores were not available in the report by Hartman and colleagues [40].) The DD group showed as much interest in others as the normals, and considerably less alienation (ie, lower percentages of H <2; see Fig. 1) than the patient groups. The DD group also showed a trend toward desiring more closeness to others than the chronic and acute PTSD groups (T > 1).

Many studies find that DID protocols tend to have a high number of total movement responses, which reflects a heightened ability to fantasize [38,44]. When human movement responses are not distorted, they also suggest empathic capacity. Unlike the acute and chronic PTSD and depressed groups, which showed reduced human movement (M), the patients who had DD were able to use imagination and show empathic capacity at a level comparable to normals (see Fig. 1). The ability to dissociate may have

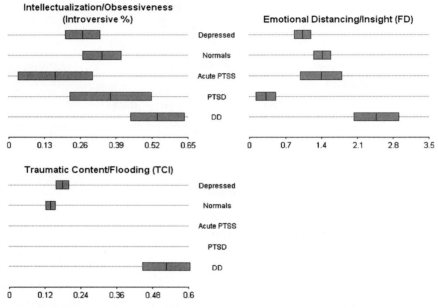

Fig. 2. Confidence intervals by group related to dissociative distancing. "Depressed" from N = 193 depressed inpatients [26]; "Normals" from N = 175 nonpatient adults [27]; "Acute PTSS" from N = 30 non–treatment seeking Desert Storm veterans who have acute posttraumatic stress symptoms [46]; "PTSD" from N = 41 inpatient male Vietnam veterans who have chronic PTSD [33]; "DD" from N = 100 DDNOS/DID inpatients.

allowed the DD group to develop a normal capacity for fantasy and empathy despite early, chronic trauma. Again, this hypothesis suggests a developmentally protective, preservative role of dissociation.

However, in contrast to these positive findings, except for patients who had chronic PTSD, patients who had DD also had more distorted views of others (M-; see below and Fig. 3) than the patient groups and normals. That the patients who had DD wanted to be close to others and could be collaborative indicates a resiliency, especially in light of the withdrawal from others that the individuals who were nondissociative and traumatized exhibited. These findings help explain why patients who have DD can often develop a working alliance with therapists, despite their frequently distorted views of others. Their social misperception paired with their elevated FD scores (see later discussion) speaks to the uncanny clinical experience that patients who have DD may seem to simultaneously misperceive and accurately perceive the intentions of others, depending on the alter that is accessed and the intensity of posttraumatic reactivity at a given time.

Dissociative distancing

The DD group showed a highly ideational, obsessive style of managing stress (ie, "introversive" or "highly introversive"; see Fig. 2) that is

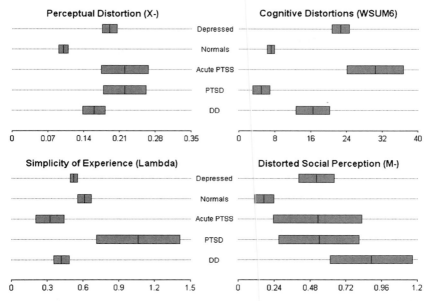

Fig. 3. Confidence intervals by group related to cognitive disorganization. "Depressed" from N = 193 depressed inpatients [26]; "Normals" from N = 175 nonpatient adults [27]; "Acute PTSS" from N = 30 non–treatment seeking Desert Storm veterans who have acute posttraumatic stress symptoms [46]; "PTSD" from N = 41 inpatient male Vietnam veterans who have chronic PTSD [33]; "DD" from N = 100 DDNOS/DID inpatients.

consistent with other research [13,37]. The DD group was significantly more introversive than the patient and normal groups. Because this style of coping is not common among individuals who have nondissociative PTSD, this intellectualized style may be directly related to dissociation. It may reflect the ability to disconnect from painful experiences by using fantasy and thinking. The introversive style of patients who have DD also differentiates them from people who have borderline personality disorder (BPD) who show a highly emotional style of coping (ie, "extratensive" [45]), and from hysterics who have more dramatic, yet fleeting and shallow, emotional displays [43].

Patients who have DD showed greater capacity for emotional distance and insight (high FD) compared with the other four groups (see Fig. 2). High FD suggests an ability to use insight-oriented psychotherapies because of the ability to be introspective [13]. BPDs do not show a similar elevation on scores, indicating the capacity for detached self-reflection [44]. Additionally, the DD group avoided emotional experiences (low Afr) as much as the three patient groups and more than the normals. The heightened unemotional self-introspection (elevated FD) combined with affective numbing (low Afr) allows the patient who has DD to avoid emotional pain.

The authors' DD group was not elevated on situational helplessness (high m), which contradicts the consistent finding of high m among patients

Table 1
Frequencies for 36 variables for adult DID/DDNOS inpatients (N = 100)

Demography variables

Marital status			Age			Race		
Single	38	37%	18–25	19	19%	White	91	91%
Lives w/SO	3	3%	26–35	39	39%	Black	9	9%
Married	36	36%	36–45	33	33%	Hispanic	0	0%
Separated	13	13%	46–55	6	6%	Asian	0	0%
Divorced	7	7%	56–65	0	0%	Other	0	0%
Widowed	3	3%	Over 65	0	0%			
			Education					
Sex			Under 12	5	5%			
Male	3	3%	12 y	23	22%			
Female	97	97%	13–15 y	45	45%			
			16+ y	29	29%			

Ratios, percentages and special indices

EB style			Form quality deviations		
Introversive	54	54%	X+ % > 0.89	1	1%
Super-introversive	33	33%	X+ % < 0.70	96	96%
Ambient	37	37%	X+ % < 0.61	88	88%
Extratensive	9	9%	X+ % < 0.50	63	63%
Super-extratensive	3	3%	F+ % < 0.70	82	82%
EA - es differences: D-scores			Xu% > 0.20	91	91%
D score > 0	13	13%	X-% > 0.15	41	41%
D score = 0	38	38%	X-% > 0.20	28	28%
D score < 0	49	49%	X-% > 0.30	11	11%
D score < −1	26	26%	FC: CF + C Ratio		
Adj D score > 0	19	19%	FC > (CF + C) + 2	12	12%
Adj D score = 0	52	52%	FC > (CF + C) + 1	27	27%
Adj D score < 0	29	29%	(CF + C) > FC + 1	26	26%
Adj D score < −1	9	9%	(CF + C) > FC + 2	11	11%
Zd > + 3.0 (Overincorp)	37	37%	S-constellation positive	19	19%
Zd < −3.0 (Underincorp)	12	12%	HVI positive	13	13%
			OBS positive	1	1%

SCZI = 6	9	9%	DEPI = 7	7	7%	CDI = 5	3	3%
SCZI = 5	2	2%	DEPI = 6	19	19%	CDI = 4	15	15%
SCZI = 4	7	7%	DEPI = 5	25	25%			

Miscellaneous variables

Lambda > 0.99	7	7%	(2AB + Art + Ay) > 5	15	15%
Dd > 3	39	39%	Populars < 4	30	30%
DQv + DQv/+ > 2	9	9%	Populars > 7	4	4%
S > 2	32	32%	COP = 0	22	22%
Sum T = 0	52	52%	COP > 2	29	29%
Sum T > 1	17	17%	AG = 0	35	35%
3r + (2)/R < 0.33	29	29%	AG > 2	23	23%
3r + (2)/R > 0.44	45	45%	MOR > 2	62	62%
Fr + rF > 0	25	25%	Level 2 Sp. Sc. > 0	62	62%
PureC > 0	27	27%	Sum 6 Sp. Sc. > 6	20	20%
PureC > 1	13	13%	Pure H < 2	29	29%
Afr < 0.40	43	43%	Pure H = 0	6	6%
Afr < 0.50	69	69%	p > a + 1	11	11%
(FM + m) < sum shading	47	47%	Mp > Ma	14	14%

Abbreviations: SO, significant other, (Also, see Appendix A).

who were nondissociative and traumatized [1]. Given how little control the patients who were hospitalized with DD had over many aspects of their immediate life (eg, not being able to control basics, such as when to go outside, eat, and smoke) and their life in general (eg, involvement in problematic relationships, financial struggles), one would expect a good deal of situational helplessness, even without exposure to chronic trauma. These patients' lack of helplessness about their external life may have been caused by dissociation, which involves focusing attention to one's inner world and an increased absorption in fantasy (high Ms and being introversive). Perhaps the DD group focused more on their internal world, specifically their distressing trauma-related intrusions (see later discussion) and their imaginative world of dissociative self states. In doing so, they may have become so enveloped in their inner world that they were less aware of their outer world. This response may be protective during abuse and allow for resiliency. However, it may leave the patient who is dissociative detached from the apperception of outer danger and at risk for re-victimization [46].

Despite their ability to distance themselves from emotions, the DD group showed signs of traumatic flooding. Armstrong's Traumatic Content Index (TCI) [37] is the sum of all sex, blood, anatomy, aggression, and morbid responses, divided by the number of responses. Four studies, including the present one, have found that DD protocols are very high on the TCI [13,37,44]. In the authors' DD sample, the average score on TCI was 0.50. Elevations on these variables suggest intense somatic preoccupation, a sense of being damaged, and a concern about physical integrity. The DD group was higher on TCI than the normal and depressed groups (see Fig. 2; data was not available for the TCI from either trauma sample). Another way that trauma may intrude into a Rorschach protocol is through biphasic responses within the content of responses themselves. For example, a woman who had DID who reported a history of severe early sexual abuse saw "a bloody vagina" on card 2, which made her extremely anxious. Immediately afterwards, she reported a dissociative-sounding percept of a "far away castle, surrounded by clouds." She disconnected from the discomfort aroused by a traumatic intrusion by immediately switching to a pleasant, fanciful image of a place of refuge, which is a classic example of the defensive role of dissociation. After she completed the Rorschach and the results were processed, she realized that she had switched alters after seeing the sexual image, illustrating that dissociation protected her from fully knowing and feeling the impact of trauma.

Cognitive disorganization

Patients who had DD and veterans who had acute stress showed thinking that was complex (high blends) and overly involved in the nuances and complexities of experience (low L). Consistent with other research, the DD group was lower on L than the normals and the patient groups, except

Table 2
Descriptive statistics for inpatient DID/DDNOS patients (N = 100)

Variable	Mean	SD	Minimum	Maximum	Frequency	Median	Mode	SK	KU
Age	32.77	8.23	15.00	54.00	100	33.00	25.00	0.11	−0.26
Years education	6.77	7.35	0.00	19.00	47	0.00	0.00	0.22	−1.85
R	17.47	7.52	10.00	40.00	100	15.00	10.00	1.02	—
W	8.81	3.81	1.00	23.00	100	8.00	6.00	1.06	2.12
D	5.44	5.19	0.00	21.00	89	4.00	1.00	1.22	0.73
Dd	3.22	[3.60]	0.00	17.00	73	2.00	0.00	1.52	2.32
S	2.27	[2.27]	0.00	10.00	80	2.00	1.00	1.37	1.47
DQ+	6.61	3.35	1.00	17.00	100	6.00	5.00	0.93	0.69
DQo	9.98	6.59	2.00	31.00	100	8.00	8.00	1.14	0.70
DQv	0.73	[0.87]	0.00	3.00	48	0.00	0.00	0.83	−0.45
DQv/ +	0.15	[0.44]	0.00	2.00	12	0.00	0.00	3.02	8.84
FQx+	0.41	0.87	0.00	4.00	25	0.00	0.00	2.52	6.40
FQxo	6.87	3.39	1.00	18.00	100	6.00	4.00	0.87	0.59
FQxu	7.05	4.24	1.00	20.00	100	6.00	6.00	1.05	0.74
FQx-	2.83	2.43	0.00	12.00	88	2.00	1.00	1.27	1.79
FQxNone	0.31	[0.58]	0.00	2.00	25	0.00	0.00	1.73	2.00
MQ+	0.25	0.58	0.00	3.00	19	0.00	0.00	2.53	6.66
MQo	1.80	1.50	0.00	6.00	84	1.00	1.00	1.12	1.02
MQu	1.96	1.60	0.00	8.00	84	2.00	1.00	1.24	2.23
MQ-	0.89	[1.39]	0.00	7.00	45	0.00	0.00	2.13	5.10
MQNone	0.05	[0.22]	0.00	1.00	5	0.00	0.00	4.19	15.90
SQual-	0.87	[1.28]	0.00	6.00	48	0.00	0.00	1.94	3.81
M	4.95	2.99	0.00	15.00	99	4.00	3.00	1.05	1.09
FM	2.73	1.74	0.00	8.00	93	3.00	2.00	0.69	0.33
m	2.20	1.77	0.00	8.00	84	2.00	2.00	1.00	1.06
FC	1.78	1.55	0.00	6.00	72	2.00	0.00	0.60	−0.30
CF	1.36	1.24	0.00	6.00	72	1.00	1.00	1.01	1.35
C	0.42	[0.77]	0.00	3.00	27	0.00	0.00	1.70	1.88
Cn	0.01	[0.10]	0.00	1.00	1	0.00	0.00	10.00	100.00
Sum Color	3.57	2.19	0.00	10.00	94	3.00	2.00	0.69	0.42
WSumC	2.88	1.92	0.00	7.50	94	2.50	2.00	0.75	0.01
Sum C'	1.99	[2.21]	0.00	12.00	71	1.00	0.00	1.88	4.81
Sum T	0.79	[1.09]	0.00	5.00	48	0.00	0.00	1.70	2.81
Sum V	0.91	[1.28]	0.00	8.00	51	1.00	0.00	2.41	8.98
Sum Y	2.40	[2.82]	0.00	22.00	83	2.00	1.00	3.89	23.49
Sum Shading	6.09	5.29	0.00	35.00	98	4.00	3.00	2.26	8.27
Fr+rF	0.40	[0.83]	0.00	5.00	25	0.00	0.00	2.71	9.56
FD	2.47	[2.21]	0.00	14.00	85	2.00	1.00	1.91	6.73
F	4.87	3.46	0.00	17.00	97	4.00	3.00	1.28	1.43
(2)	6.46	3.85	0.00	17.00	99	6.00	6.00	0.77	0.05
Lambda	0.42	0.32	0.00	2.00	97	0.35	0.25	1.98	6.25
FM+m	4.93	2.81	0.00	15.00	98	4.00	3.00	0.82	0.97
EA	7.83	4.06	1.00	20.50	100	7.00	6.00	1.05	0.93
es	11.02	6.85	1.00	42.00	100	9.00	8.00	1.53	3.59
D Score	−1.03	2.06	−11.00	2.00	62	0.00	0.00	−1.80	5.23
AdjD	−0.09	1.31	−6.00	4.00	48	0.00	0.00	−0.24	4.88
a (active)	6.41	3.48	0.00	16.00	98	6.00	5.00	0.74	0.24
p (passive)	3.72	2.60	0.00	13.00	96	3.00	2.00	1.20	1.45

Table 2 (*continued*)

Variable	Mean	SD	Minimum	Maximum	Frequency	Median	Mode	SK	KU
Ma	3.52	2.29	0.00	10.00	97	3.00	2.00	0.84	−0.01
Mp	1.57	1.73	0.00	8.00	71	1.00	1.00	1.62	2.70
Intellect	1.58	1.85	0.00	8.00	60	1.00	0.00	1.31	1.35
Zf	11.70	4.06	3.00	26.00	100	11.00	10.00	0.87	1.09
Zd	2.07	4.34	−7.00	14.50	96	2.00	4.50	0.24	0.16
Blends	6.49	3.79	0.00	19.00	99	6.00	6.00	0.99	0.98
Blends/R	0.39	0.18	0.00	0.82	99	0.40	0.50	0.19	−0.59
Col-Shd Blends	1.08	[1.26]	0.00	6.00	58	1.00	0.00	1.48	2.62
Afr	0.47	0.18	0.25	1.20	100	0.43	0.43	1.38	2.19
Populars	4.75	1.68	2.00	8.00	100	5.00	3.00	0.04	−1.03
X + %	0.43	0.15	0.17	0.92	100	0.42	0.50	0.71	0.64
F + %	0.51	0.27	0.00	1.00	91	0.50	0.50	0.16	−0.15
X-%	0.16	0.11	0.00	0.46	88	0.13	0.00	0.77	0.15
Xu%	0.39	0.14	0.07	0.67	100	0.40	0.50	−0.12	−0.67
S-%	0.26	[0.33]	0.00	1.00	48	0.00	0.00	1.05	−0.04
Isolate/R	0.16	0.16	0.00	0.58	80	0.11	0.00	1.33	1.15
H	2.99	2.25	0.00	10.00	94	2.50	1.00	1.13	0.89
(H)	1.22	1.36	0.00	7.00	62	1.00	0.00	1.38	2.45
HD	1.93	2.14	0.00	10.00	72	1.00	0.00	1.49	1.90
(Hd)	0.38	0.68	0.00	3.00	29	0.00	0.00	1.93	3.67
Hx	0.55	[1.05]	0.00	6.00	33	0.00	0.00	2.76	9.15
H + (H) + Hd + (Hd)	6.52	4.12	0.00	18.00	99	5.00	4.00	0.88	0.11
A	6.14	3.02	0.00	16.00	99	6.00	4.00	0.94	1.31
(A)	0.66	[0.89]	0.00	4.00	45	0.00	0.00	1.43	1.82
Ad	1.56	[1.52]	0.00	8.00	72	1.00	0.00	1.32	2.50
(Ad)	0.14	[0.49]	0.00	3.00	9	0.00	0.00	3.93	16.12
An	1.12	[1.21]	0.00	7.00	64	1.00	0.00	1.72	5.20
Art	0.49	0.94	0.00	5.00	30	0.00	0.00	2.47	6.93
Ay	0.49	[0.82]	0.00	4.00	33	0.00	0.00	1.86	3.55
Bl	0.89	[1.33]	0.00	6.00	44	0.00	0.00	1.77	2.90
Bt	0.68	0.92	0.00	5.00	47	0.00	0.00	1.87	5.11
Cg	1.68	1.59	0.00	6.00	75	1.00	1.00	0.99	0.27
Cl	0.20	[0.55]	0.00	3.00	15	0.00	0.00	3.41	13.09
Ex	0.24	[0.47]	0.00	2.00	22	0.00	0.00	1.80	2.46
Fi	0.41	[0.73]	0.00	3.00	30	0.00	0.00	1.93	3.53
Food	0.23	[0.58]	0.00	3.00	16	0.00	0.00	2.72	7.25
Ge	0.04	[0.24]	0.00	2.00	3	0.00	0.00	6.68	47.66
Hh	0.45	0.69	0.00	3.00	35	0.00	0.00	1.42	1.41
Ls	0.49	0.73	0.00	3.00	36	0.00	0.00	1.29	0.73
Na	0.56	[1.02]	0.00	6.00	37	0.00	0.00	3.02	11.57
Sc	0.40	[0.71]	0.00	4.00	31	0.00	0.00	2.34	7.21
Sx	1.42	[1.88]	0.00	12.00	61	1.00	0.00	2.49	9.68
Xy	0.12	[0.41]	0.00	3.00	10	0.00	0.00	4.50	25.37
Idiographic	1.99	1.75	0.00	9.00	80	2.00	1.00	1.36	2.88
DV	0.26	[0.58]	0.00	3.00	20	0.00	0.00	2.45	6.23
INCOM	0.62	[0.86]	0.00	3.00	42	0.00	0.00	1.30	0.91
DR	0.43	[0.89]	0.00	5.00	27	0.00	0.00	2.79	9.21
FABCOM	0.37	[0.68]	0.00	4.00	29	0.00	0.00	2.38	7.86

Table 2 (*continued*)

Variable	Mean	SD	Minimum	Maximum	Frequency	Median	Mode	SK	KU
DV2	0.09	[0.29]	0.00	1.00	9	0.00	0.00	2.90	6.59
INC2	0.53	[0.97]	0.00	5.00	31	0.00	0.00	2.22	5.49
DR2	0.36	[0.82]	0.00	5.00	22	0.00	0.00	3.01	11.13
FAB2	0.90	[1.40]	0.00	6.00	40	0.00	0.00	1.70	2.37
ALOG	0.15	[0.41]	0.00	2.00	13	0.00	0.00	2.83	7.86
CONTAM	0.10	0.30	0.00	1.00	10	0.00	0.00	2.70	5.44
Sum 6 Sp Sc	3.81	3.91	0.00	18.00	85	2.50	1.00	1.58	2.66
Lvl 2 Sp Sc	1.88	[2.51]	0.00	12.00	62	1.00	0.00	2.04	4.51
WSum6	16.48	18.89	0.00	95.00	85	11.00	0.00	1.76	3.32
AB	0.30	[0.69]	0.00	3.00	20	0.00	0.00	2.55	6.27
AG	1.57	1.78	0.00	7.00	65	1.00	0.00	1.42	1.81
CFB	0.00	0.00	0.00	0.00	0	0.00	0.00	—	—
COP	1.95	1.65	0.00	6.00	78	2.00	2.00	0.65	−0.53
CP	0.04	[0.24]	0.00	2.00	3	0.00	0.00	6.68	47.66
MOR	3.66	[2.71]	0.00	11.00	91	3.00	3.00	0.89	0.36
PER	2.12	2.35	0.00	10.00	67	1.00	0.00	1.32	1.42
PSV	0.16	[0.42]	0.00	2.00	14	0.00	0.00	2.67	6.92

Abbreviations: SK, skewness value; KU, Kurtosis value; (Also, see Appendix A).

for the veterans who had acute stress (see Fig. 3) [44]. The patients who had DD and the veterans who had acute stress were unable to back away from stimuli, distinguishing them from veterans who had chronic PTSD who defensively oversimplified their involvement with stimuli. Weiner [43] noted that low L occurs in "multifaceted individuals" who can become "cognitively scattered, easily distractible, and painfully aware of distressing aspects of their lives." Simply, patients who have DD have difficulty "seeing the forest for the trees."

The patients who had DD blatantly misperceived reality less than the other patient groups (lower X-; see Fig. 3). However, the patients who had DD showed more distorted and illogical thinking (WSum6) than the normals and patients who had chronic PTSD, yet less illogical thinking than the patients who were depressed and the veterans who had acute stress (see Fig. 3). Despite thinking that was often illogical, the DD group did not show frank psychosis. These findings on the Rorschach mirror the findings on the MMPI-2 of an elevation of scale 8 (Sc) and together portray the disorganizing impact of traumatic intrusions on cognition. The patients who had DD often experienced the most distorted perceptions and illogical thought on trauma-related percepts (eg, "two people pulling a baby apart"), and these often involved humans (see earlier discussion of M- and Fig. 3). Armstrong [26] suggests that people who are severely traumatized have a "traumatic thought disorder" stemming from exposure to a world in which others behaved inconsistently and violently. From that perspective, the illogical, idiosyncratic thinking of the patients who had DD is an accurate reflection of the chaos they have experienced. This idiosyncratic perception and tendency to put together unrelated ideas may facilitate their ability to experience themselves as being a combination of self-states, rather than existing as a conventional and cohesive self [44]. Patients who have DD also fail to put together ideas that are related, leaving them vulnerable to lapses in logic and, perhaps, judgment (eg, "My mother abused me," "I allow my mother to take care of my children").

Summary

The authors' Rorschach study is consistent with the research on objective and other projective measures. Patients who have DD can be differentiated from other patients who have other trauma-based disorders and depression, particularly in their greater use of imagination, cognitive complexity, ideational coping style, avoidance of emotion, greater capacity for self-reflection, and mixed interpersonal functioning [13,37,44]. Individuals who have DD are also distinguishable from patients who have other trauma-based disorders and depression and individuals who are not in treatment because they are flooded with traumatic content. The patients who had DD were preoccupied by a sense of their bodies being damaged and the world being filled with aggression. Veterans who have chronic PTSD live a life dictated by avoidance, overly simplified "tunnel vision," and withdrawal from others. In contrast, dissociation permitted patients who had DD to remain psychologically "alive" despite their chronic trauma. Although the individuals who were dissociative, like the veterans who had acute stress, experienced more distress, neither group was living as emotionally and socially diminished as the chronic PTSD group. Nonetheless, patients who had DD showed a pronounced traumatic thought disorder characterized by failing to integrate ideas logically and an impaired ability to perceive conventional reality. These findings are consistent with the trauma-based model of dissociation that suggests dissociation is an ideational defense employed to ward off overwhelming, intrusive, traumatic material. Armstrong [12] suggests that the ability to dissociate has the benefit of allowing for an atypical developmental pathway, a pathway in which contradictions and complexities, and vulnerabilities and strengths, can coexist. Within this pathway, individuals who are dissociative can show interest in others yet misunderstand them; they can be overinvolved in, yet reflective about, their experience; and they can avoid emotion yet be flooded with traumatic material. These seemingly contradictory findings among the DD Rorschach profiles support Armstrong's theory that dissociation is a factor that promotes resiliency in the midst of trauma by helping to preserve essential human intellectual and emotional capacities.

These findings point to important treatment implications. Most patients who have DD are capable of building a therapeutic alliance because of their interpersonal strengths. However, the alliance may be tested repeatedly because of their proclivity to misunderstand others. Patients who have DD can work through misunderstandings if therapists address these sensitively.

Similarly, assessors should be prepared to facilitate the processing of any misperceptions that involve them and the assessment process. In the authors' experience, giving feedback about assessments to patients who have DD can be therapeutic if the assessor emphasizes the person's strengths and shares information about the extent to which the patient avoids affect, what prompts them to become flooded and disorganized, and what they can do to recover from being flooded.

Acknowledgements

The authors would like to thank John Exner, PhD, for generously providing additional data on his previously published samples of normals and depressed patients; Rebecca Reiger, PhD, for her thoughtful contributions to this manuscript; and Scot McNary, PhD, for his assistance with the figures.

References

[1] Armstrong J, Kaser-Boyd N. Projective assessment of psychological trauma. In: Hilsenroth M, Segal D, editors. Comprehensive handbook of psychological assessment, vol. 2. Objective and projective assessment of personality and psychopathology. New York: Wiley; 2004. p. 500–12.
[2] Briere J. Psychological assessment of posttraumatic states: phenomenology, diagnosis, and measurement. 2nd edition. Washington (DC): American Psychological Association; 2004.
[3] Briere J, Armstrong G. Psychological assessment of posttraumatic dissociation. In: Vermetten E, Spiegel D, Dorahy M, editors. Traumatic dissociation: neurobiology and treatment. Washington (DC): American Psychiatric Press; in press.
[4] Wilson JP, Keane TM. Assessing psychological trauma and PTSD. 2nd edition. New York: Guilford Press; 2004.
[5] Armstrong JG. Psychological assessment. In: Spira JL, editor. Treating dissociative identity disorder. San Francisco (CA): Jossey-Bass; 1996. p. 3–37.
[6] Carlson EB, Armstrong JG. Diagnosis and assessment of dissociative disorders. In: Lynn SJ, Rhue JW, editors. Dissociation: theoretical, clinical, and research perspectives. New York: Guilford Press; 1994. p. 159–74.
[7] Ellason JW, Ross CA, Fuchs DL. Assessment of dissociative identity disorder with the Millon Clinical Multiaxial Inventory-II. Psychol Rep 1995;76:895–905.
[8] Loewenstein RJ, Putnam FW. The dissociative disorders. In: Sadock BJ, Sadock VA, editors. Posttraumatic stress disorder: DSM-IV and beyond. 8th edition. Baltimore (MD): Williams & Wilkins; 2004. p. 1844–901.
[9] Vermetten E, Loewenstein RJ, Zdunek C, et al. Cortisol, memory and the hippocampus in PTSD and DID. Biol Psychiatry 2002;51S:114S–45S.
[10] Putnam FW. Dissociation in children and adolescents: a developmental perspective. New York: Guilford Press; 1997.
[11] Coons PM, Bowman ES, Milstein V. Multiple personality disorder: A clinical investigation of 50 cases. J Nerv Ment Dis 1988;176:519–27.
[12] Armstrong JG. Reflections on multiple personality disorder as a developmentally complex adaptation. Psychoanal Study Child 1994;49:349–64.
[13] Armstrong JG, Loewenstein RJ. Characteristics of patients with multiple personality and dissociative disorders on psychological testing. J Nerv Ment Dis 1990;178:448–54.

[14] Brand B, McNary SW, Dell P, et al. Malingered DID: preliminary results of psychological tests and a structured interview. Presented at the 21st Fall International Society for the Study of Dissociation Conference. New Orleans, November 19, 2004.

[15] Brand BL, McNary SW, Loewenstein RJ, et al. Assessment of genuine and simulated dissociative identity disorder on the structured interview of reported symptoms. J Trauma Dissociation, in press.

[16] Coons PM, Stern AL. Initial and follow-up psychological testing of a group of patients with multiple personality disorder. Psychol Rep 1986;58:43–9.

[17] Coons PM, Fine CG. Accuracy of the MMPI in identifying multiple personality disorder. Psychol Rep 1990;66:831–4.

[18] Arbisi PA, Ben-Porath YS. An MMPI-2 infrequent response scale for use with psychopathological populations: the infrequency Psychopathology Scale, F(p). Psychol Assess 1995;7: 424–31.

[19] Loewenstein RJ. An office mental status examination for chronic complex dissociative symptoms and multiple personality disorder. Psychiatr Clin North Am 1991;14:567–604.

[20] Welburn KR, Fraser GA, Jordan SA, et al. Discriminating dissociative identity disorder from schizophrenia and feigned dissociation on psychological tests and structured interview. J Trauma Dissociation 2003;4:109–30.

[21] Leavitt F. The development of the Somatoform Dissociation Index (SDI): a screening measure of dissociation using MMPI-2 items. J Trauma Dissociation 2001;2:69–80.

[22] Herman JL. Sequelae of prolonged and repeated trauma: evidence for a complex posttraumatic syndrome (DESNOS). In: Davidson JR, Foa EB, editors. Posttraumatic stress disorder: DSM-IV and beyond. Washington (DC): American Psychiatric Press; 1993. p. 213–28.

[23] Fink D. The co-morbidity of multiple personality disorder and DSM-III-R Axis II disorders. Psychiatr Clin North Am 1991;14:547–66.

[24] Millon T. Manual for the MCMI-II. 2nd edition. Minneapolis (MN): National Computer Systems; 1987.

[25] Fink D, Golinkoff M. Multiple personality disorder, borderline personality disorder, and schizophrenia: a comparison of clinical features. Dissociation 1990;3:127–34.

[26] Armstrong JG. Deciphering the broken narrative of trauma: signs of traumatic dissociation on the Rorschach. Rorschachiana 2002;25:11–27.

[27] Bernstein EM, Putnam FW. Development, reliability, and validity of a dissociation scale. J Nerv Ment Dis 1986;174:727–34.

[28] Steinberg M. Structured Clinical Interview for DSM-IV Dissociative Disorders-Revised (SCID-D-R). Washington (DC): American Psychiatric Press; 1994.

[29] Ross CA, Heber S, Norton GR, et al. The Dissociative Disorders Interview Schedule: a structured interview. Dissociation 1989;2:169–89.

[30] Carlson EB, Putnam FW, Ross CA, et al. Validity of the Dissociative Experiences Scale in screening for multiple personality disorder: a multicenter study. Am J Psychiatry 1993;150: 1030–6.

[31] Draijer N, Boon S. The imitation of dissociative identity disorder: patients at risk, therapists at risk. J Psychiatry Law 1999;27:423–58.

[32] Westen D, Lohr N, Silk KR, et al. Object relations and social cognition in borderlines, major depressives, and normals: A TAT analysis. Psychol Assess 1990;2:355–64.

[33] Brand B, Couacaud K, Mattanah J, et al. Object relations and social cognition of severely dissociative patients: A TAT analysis. Presented at the meeting of the International Society for the Study of Dissociation. Baltimore, November 12, 2002.

[34] Ornduff SR, Kelsey RM. Object relations of sexually and physically abused female children: a TAT analysis. J Pers Assess 1996;66:91–105.

[35] Exner JE. A Rorschach workbook for the comprehensive system. 5th edition. Ashville (NC): Rorschach Workshops; 2001.

[36] Exner JE. The Rorschach: a comprehensive system. Volume 1: Basic foundations. 4th edition. New York: Wiley; 2003.

[37] Armstrong J. The psychological organization of multiple personality disordered patients as revealed in psychological testing. Psychiatr Clin North Am 1991;14:533–45.

[38] Leavitt F, Labott SM. Rorschach indicators of dissociative identity disorders: clinical utility and theoretical implications. J Clin Psychol 1998;54:803–10.

[39] Young GR, Wagner EE, Finn RF. A comparison of three Rorschach diagnostic systems and use of the hand test for detecting multiple personality disorder in outpatients. J Pers Assess 1994;62:485–97.

[40] Hartman WL, Clark ME, Morgan MK, et al. Rorschach structure of a hospitalized sample of Vietnam veterans with PTSD. J Pers Assess 1990;54:149–59.

[41] Sloan P, Arsenault L, Hilsenroth M, et al. Rorschach measures of posttraumatic stress in Persian Gulf War veterans. J Pers Assess 1995;64:397–414.

[42] Exner JE. A new nonpatient sample for the Rorschach Comprehensive System: a progress report. J Pers Assess 2002;78:391–404.

[43] Weiner IB. Principles of Rorschach interpretation. Mahwah (NJ): Lawrence Erlbaum Associates; 1998.

[44] Scroppo JC, Drob SL, Weinberger JL, et al. Identifying dissociative identity disorder: a self-report and projective study. J Abnorm Psychol 1998;107:272–84.

[45] Exner JE. Some Rorschach data comparing schizophrenics with borderline and schizotypal personality disorders. J Pers Assess 1986;50:455–71.

[46] Kluft RP. Dissociation and revictimization: a preliminary study. Dissociation 1990;3(2):167–73.

Appendix A. Alphabetical Abbreviations for Rorschach Variables

3r + (2)/R = Egocentricity Index
AB = abstract content
Adj D = stress tolerance with situational stress removed
Afr = affective ratio; a measure of willingness to process emotions
AG = aggression
Art = art response
Ay = anthropology response
C = pure color response with no form
CDI = Coping Deficit Index
CF = chromatic color where form is secondary to color
COP = cooperative movement
D score = scaled score based on EA - es; measure of stress tolerance
Dd = unusual detail response
DEPI = Depression Index
DQv = vague developmental quality
EA - es = EA (available resources) minus es (experienced stimulation)
EB = Erlebnistypus; compares human movement to weighted color responses
FC = chromatic color where form is primary to color
FD = form dimension response
FM = animal movement
Fr = reflection response in which form dominates over symmetry
H = human response
HVI = Hypervigilance Index
L = Lambda
Lambda = L = a measure of economizing resources
M- = distorted human movement
M = human movement
m = inanimate movement
Ma = active human movement
MOR = morbid response with damaged object or dysphoric characteristic
Mp = passive human movement
OBS = Obsessive Style Index
p = passive movement
Pure C = pure color response with no use of form
R = number of responses
r = reflection response
rF = reflection response in which symmetry is primary to form
S = space response
SCZI = Schizophrenia Index
Sp Sc = Special Scores; reflect problems with perception or thinking
T = shading-texture
TCI = Anatomy + Sex + Blood + Morbid + Aggression/R
V = shading-dimension
WSum6 = weighted sum of six special scores; measures logical thinking
X- = distorted from
X+ = conventional form
Xu = unusual form
Y = shading-diffuse
Zd = processing efficiency

Appendix B. Rorschach percentages, means, and standard deviations for patients who have dissociative disorder (N = 100)

	Percentage (%)	Mean (SD)
Capacity for therapeutic alliance		
Low alienation		
Pure H < 2	29	
Pure H = 0	6	
Capable of collaboration		
COP = 0	22	
COP > 2	29	
Often experience a need for closeness		
Sum T = 0	52	
Sum T > 1	17	
Heightened empathy and fantasy (M)		4.95 (2.99)
Dissociative distancing		
Highly ideational		
Introversive	54	
Super-introversive	33	
Ambitent	37	
Extratensive	9	
Avoid, yet can express, modulated emotion		
FC > (CF + C) + 2	12	
FC > (CF + C) + 1	27	
Afr < 0.40	43	
PureC > 0	27	
Flooded with traumatic images		
Aggression (AG)		1.57 (1.78)
Anatomy (An)		1.12 (1.21)
Blood (Bl)		0.89 (1.33)
Sex (Sx)		1.42 (1.88)
Morbid (MOR)		3.66 (2.71)
Self-reflective (FD)		2.47 (2.21)
Not helpless (m)		2.20 (1.77)
Cognitive disorganization		
Distorted perception		
Xu% > 0.20	91	
X-% > 0.20	28	
Distorted thinking (WSum6)		16.48 (18.89)
Overly involved in experience (L)		0.42 (0.32)
Complex thinking (Blends/R)		0.39 (0.18)
Distorted views of others (MQ-)		0.89 (1.39)

PSYCHIATRIC
CLINICS
OF NORTH AMERICA

ELSEVIER
SAUNDERS

Psychiatr Clin N Am 29 (2006) 169–184

The Forensic Evaluation of Dissociation and Persons Diagnosed with Dissociative Identity Disorder: Searching for Convergence

A. Steven Frankel, PhD, JD[a,b,]*,
Constance Dalenberg, PhD[c]

[a]*Golden Gate University School of Law, Lafayette, CA, USA*
[b]*University of Southern California, Los Angeles, USA*
[c]*Alliant International University, San Diego, CA, USA*

The concept of dissociation in general and the diagnosis of dissociative identity disorder (DID), formerly multiple personality disorder, more specifically have achieved increasing attention in the linked worlds of scientific research and psychiatric and psychologic forensic evaluations. The most dramatic increase in state and federal cases and legal commentary has occurred since the publication of an issue of *Psychiatric Clinics of North America* in June of 1991 devoted to DID (Table 1). This is paralleled by an increase in research attention (Table 2) in published journal articles, shown by the increase in number of articles published and by the percentage of these articles that use empiric methods. Increased empiric attention also has been given to recovered memories of abuse, but the area of false memories is dominated by opinion. Because the forensic material in the June 1991 *Psychiatric Clinics of North America* issue was divided into several articles, none of which sought to cover the general territory of the forensic evaluation of dissociative disorders, this article assumes the daunting task of reviewing the current knowledge base in the field as it applies to the general forensic context to provide brief empirically supportable conclusions.

This article addresses: (1) the role of the forensic mental health professionals in the context of court-related evaluations of claims of dissociative

---

* Corresponding author. Golden Gate University School of Law, 3527 Mt. Diablo Boulevard, #269, Lafayette, CA 94549.
E-mail address: drpsylex@earthlink.net (A.S. Frankel).

0193-953X/06/$ - see front matter © 2005 Elsevier Inc. All rights reserved.
doi:10.1016/j.psc.2005.10.002

Table 1
Frequency of state and federal cases involving multiple personality disorder or dissociative identity disorder

Time interval[a]	State and federal cases	Law reviews and journal articles[b]
1971–1981		
Lexis	3	0
Westlaw	1	0
1981–1991[c]		
Lexis	38	10
Westlaw	34	19
1991–2001		
Lexis	223	167
Westlaw	247	296
2001–2005		
Lexis	72	305
Westlaw	83	345

[a] The time periods run from June to June, as this article was written in June of 2005.

[b] The two primary legal search engines may cover different subsets of legal periodicals, accounting for some discrepancies in the totals.

[c] The most recent prior issue of *Psychiatric Clinics of North America* devoted to DID was published in June 1991.

Table 2
Articles published on dissociative disorders and percentage classified as empiric using the PsychLit database

Time interval[a]	Articles published	Empiric articles
1971–1981		
Diss disord	96	31 (32.3%)
FMS	0	0
RM	0	0
1981–1991		
Diss disord	605	337 (55.7%)
FM	0	0
RM	5	4 (80%)
1991–2001		
Diss disord	1648	998 (60.56%)
FM	118	24 (20.3%)
RM	317	86 (27.1%)
2001–2005		
Diss disord	550	349 (63.5%)
FM	14	1 (7.1%)
RM	54	22 (40.7%)

Abbreviations: Diss disord, search terms (dissociative + disorder*) or multiple personality; FMS, search terms false memory syndrome or (false mem* and (dissoci* or abuse); RM, search terms (recovered memor* or repressed memor*) and abuse.

[a] The time periods run from June to May, paralleling the Lexis and Westlaw tables.

disorders; (2) the possible relationships between such claims and the issues to be decided by the trier of fact; (3) research developments that may bear on the forensic evaluation of DID from (a) biologic, (b) psychologic, and (c) social data sources; and (4) a checklist of issues about which forensic evaluators should be prepared to respond on direct and cross-examination (Box 1).

The role of forensic evaluators when dissociation is an issue

There are a few guiding professional and ethical principles that are well settled in forensic mental health disciplines.

Forensic evaluators versus treaters

There are qualitative differences between forensic evaluation and clinical treatment, such that treaters are ill advised to offer forensic evaluations of patients for whom they provide treatment [1–8].

Commitment to impartiality and freedom from bias

Forensic evaluators strive for objectivity and freedom from personal and professional biases in their reports to the court. In service of this goal, opinions of forensic evaluators should be data based and present the data that do and do not support hypotheses offered [1–8]. As noted by the best-known reviews of clinical judgment, impartiality and accuracy also are served best by reliance on instrumentation, collateral data, and interview rather than interview alone [9,10].

Commitment to a broad range of data

Forensic evaluations should be based on a broad range of data, including collateral sources, as available [1–8]. As noted by Coons [11] regarding cases in which DID is an issue, "[t]he need for collateral material cannot be overemphasized...".

Commitment to competence

Forensic evaluators should be competent in the domains in which they provide services. Evaluators who agree to provide forensic services when DID is an issue should provide diagnostic, treatment, or forensic services to persons claiming dissociative symptoms sufficient to claim such competence [1–8]. Professional surveys that establish that the position that DID "does not exist" or that there is "no evidence" for the diagnosis are minority opinions, particularly among those who have any experience with alleged dissociative symptoms [12,13]. The related belief that traumatic memories cannot be forgotten is held by fewer than 10% of experimental psychologists and fewer than 5% of clinical psychologists [14]. Areas of contention

Box 1. Preparation for cross-examination of a forensic evaluator when dissociative identity disorder is at issue

1. Describe the evaluee's psychologic treatment history.
2. How much experience did past treaters have with DID?
3. Were patients of the treaters involved in litigation? If so, describe.
4. Was this patient in litigation regarding psychiatric and psychologic issues? If so, describe.
5. Did the treaters indicate that they believed the patient's reports of child abuse?
6. Did the evaluee remember his or her abuse history before entering treatment?
7. Describe the circumstances under which the evaluee came to believe she or he was abused.
8. Did the issue of corroboration of abuse come up in treatment? If so, how was it handled?
9. Were there attempts to corroborate abuse memories? If so, describe.
10. How much exposure did the evaluee have to DID literature, groups, and so forth?
11. How was the diagnosis of DID made? Was there any formal assessment?
12. Were there any comorbid disorders diagnosed? On what bases?
13. Review the assessment measures you administered to the evaluee and those formally given. What reliability and validity data exists for each measure?
14. Were symptoms reported by the evaluee on interview consistent with symptoms reported on formal assessment measures you administered?
15. Did you ask the evaluee to describe his or her life story, from the earliest point in time she or he could remember? Describe.
16. Did the evaluee display a wide range of affect during the evaluation, including intense anger?
17. Did the evaluee discuss his or her abuse history without clear experience of shame or guilt? Describe.
18. How did the evaluee's performance on any measure compare with the performances of persons who do and do not have DID and to those who do and do not have other competing or comorbid diagnoses?

19. Are there other disorders, conditions, or reasons that may account for the evaluee's symptoms? Describe and indicate how each was included as a comorbid diagnosis, included as an alternative hypothesis, or ruled out.
20. If the evaluee has DID, how does that disorder relate to the legal questions before the trier of fact?
21. Be prepared to show that "belief" in DID or dissociation is the mainstream professional opinion.
22. Be prepared to show that the majority of mainstream professionals support the concept of recovered memory.
23. Be prepared to offer support for your knowledge base on dissociation through publications, attendance of relevant professional meetings, or other relevant education.

concern the mechanisms involved in the occurrence of dissociative symptoms and the bearing of the existence of such symptoms on questions of fact, such as criminal culpability, *mens rea*, parenting and custody decisions, consent to sexual activity, capacity to contract, and so forth. *In extremis*, opining that a particular evaluee's dissociative symptoms cannot be relevant to a psycholegal question solely because the evaluator has never seen a case, is indefensible. (This is not to say that an opinion that DID does not exist has no place in court. Given that such testimony is held to be relevant and helpful to a trier of fact and that it survives Daubert and Kumho [15,16] or Frye scrutiny [17], it may be admitted into evidence.)

In any given instance, it may be true that an evaluee who claims dissociative symptoms is malingering or otherwise inaccurate; ruling out this hypothesis and providing other options for the trier of fact to consider should be made based on relevant forensic findings, rather than put forth as the position to take by fiat [18–27]. Further, as discussed later, a forensic evaluator who agrees to work on a dissociation or dissociative disorder case should be familiar with a range of theory, research, and assessment instruments, including attachment, hypnotic capacity, suggestibility, memory, other cognitive functions, and neurophysiology. The depth and diversity of knowledge requisite for forensic specialization in evaluating dissociative phenomena are formidable. As attorneys become better educated about the nature of dissociation and its manifestations, variations, and assessment approaches, and so forth, those forensic evaluators who have the requisite level of expertise are more likely to find work in this growing and developing arena [28–32].

Commitment regarding testifying to the "ultimate issue"

There are few forensic issues that require opinions that address the legal questions directly before a court. Forensic professionals may be asked to testify as to competency for execution, competency to be tried, or even the "...issue of whether or not the accused actually formed a required specific intent, premeditated, deliberated, or harbored malice aforethought, when a specific intent crime is charged" [33]. Such opinions are rare, however. Most frequently, forensic evaluators are asked to offer information that helps the trier of fact reach a legal conclusion in a case. A professional does not opine as to a conclusion, but rather lays out the dots that can then be connected by the trier of fact. This principle is addressed in many ways by the ethics codes of forensic mental health organizations and also is addressed in the law. For example, California Penal Code §29 states:

> In the guilt phase of a criminal action, any expert testifying about a defendant's mental illness, mental disorder, or mental defect shall not testify as to whether the defendant had or did not have the required mental states, which include, but are not limited to, purpose, intent, knowledge, or malice aforethought, for the crimes charged. The question as to whether the defendant had or did not have the required mental states shall be decided by the trier of fact.

Research developments that may bear on forensic assessment of dissociation: a biopsychosocial approach

In the authors' view, the biopsychosocial model that has come to characterize psychiatric training in general also provides a helpful model for a review of data that may be brought to bear on forensic evaluations of dissociative disorders [34,35]. Thus, discussion begins with data relating to the biologic aspects of DID.

Biologic

Arguably, some of the most interesting developments in the biology of DID come from brain imaging studies using positron emission tomography, MRI, and hexamethylpropyleneamine oxime single photon emission CT. Although many such studies concern single case presentations [36–38], an increasing number of studies examines larger cohorts of patients diagnosed with DID [39–41] and compares patients diagnosed with DID to simulators [40]. Results of these studies suggest that cerebral blood flow may vary for DIDs as a function of alternate personalities and that the reported cerebral blood flow differences may discriminate between DIDs and normal controls or simulators. Hypothesized blood flow differences in the temporofrontal cortex and structural differences in the hippocampus are reported [36–40].

Neurobiologic studies of DIDs versus controls or simulators also demonstrate differential findings regarding alternate personalities [36–41], "switching" between personalities [38], and amnesia between alternate personalities [42–47]. In addition, there are studies of neurobiologic anomalies (eg, electroencephalogram abnormalities [48] and hypnotic capacity using the eye-roll technique [49]). Finally, neurobiologic studies have discriminated successfully between DID, seizures, and pseudoseizures [50,51].

Dissociative experiences theoretically are associated with dampened autonomic output and inhibited amygdala functioning. Recent research supports this model, noting lower heart rates, suppressed physiologic activity, or lowered startle reaction during dissociative states [52–54]. A corticolimbic disconnection model of dissociation [55] is the mechanism cited most frequently .

Although neurobiologic assessment for these purposes still is in an early stage of development [56], it may be that such assessments will be a centerpiece of the forensic evaluation protocol of the future. Given recent advances in user-friendly technology for measuring heart rate and skin conductance continuously over the course of an interview, these evaluative tools soon will be available more widely to forensic professionals.

Psychologic

Advances in the psychologic assessment of DID include developments in attachment theory, cognition and memory, hypnotic capacity, suggestibility, malingering and deception, screening interviews and instruments, and diagnostic interviews and instruments.

Attachment

Using research protocols implemented and validated worldwide, the attachment literature increasingly points to disorganized and disoriented attachment patterns in patients who have dissociative disorders [56–58]. Data from prospective studies are particularly strong [57]. In nonclinical samples, attachment insecurity also repeatedly is linked to dissociation [59]. Training in the assessment protocols for attachment increasingly is available [58], providing more accessibility of instruments for inclusion in forensic batteries.

Cognition and memory

Because memory impairments or cognitive impairments are central features of DID and other dissociative disorders [43,60–63], the area of cognition and memory has received a great deal of research interest. Extreme statements that delayed recall does not occur now are rare in the scientific literature, but the precise nature of the link between dissociation and amnestic experiences remains controversial [26,40,43,61–65]. Research by Brewin and associates [66–69] on repressive coping style shows that repressors recall fewer negative childhood memories and fewer younger negative memories than do nonrepressors. With directed forgetting tasks, repressors show an enhanced capacity for using retrieval inhibition [69], as do those who have dissociative disorders [70]. Freyd [71–73] and associates postulate that amnesia may at times be adaptive, demonstrating that high dissociators have impaired memory for traumatic words (relative to neutral words) and, thereby, can selectively ignore their betrayal at the hands of a caregiver to rely on this attachment figure in other ways.

Considerable research effort addresses the issue of interidentity amnesia [61,74], although clinical reports emphasize that amnestic barriers between personalities rarely, if ever, are impermeable. In sum, there is evidence to suggest that patients diagnosed with DID do demonstrate elevated interidentity amnesia compared with simulators, but much information is shared across personalities [60,74–76].

Research efforts investigating the validity of delayed recall of abuse also have been fruitful, with corroboration of abuse memories occurring in 40% to 60% of the cases when it is sought [30,77–79]. Failure to corroborate is not taken to mean that the memories are definitively inaccurate, as childhood abuse is a private matter.

Hypnotic capacity

Given that it is well-established that patients who have DID score higher in hypnotic capacity than the general population, it is not surprising that assessments of hypnotic capacity are shown to aid in the discrimination between patients who have DID, schizophrenics, and those who feign DID, and that efficient use of the eye-roll sign can be of significant aid to forensic evaluators [48,80].

Suggestibility

Suggestibility is an important dimension in the forensic contex [80–82]. Some investigators offer the possibility that retractors—patients who remember being abused in childhood and later retract those assertions—are influenced by suggestive elements, first accusing a parent and then suing a therapist (gaining approval and sympathy for victim status at both stages) [82]. Currently, there are only two empirically developed measures of suggestibility: for adults, the Gudjonsson Scale of Interrogative Suggestibility [83], and for children, the newly developed Video Suggestibility Scale [84]. Because the Gudjonsson measure has been in use since the mid 1980s, evaluators are cautioned to assess for the likelihood that evaluees are familiar with the measure. Because concerns regarding suggestibility are reported commonly in clinical literature (and may be at the heart of a given case, if the dissociative client is pursuing a case involving misuse of influence), however, the related concepts of social desirability [85], conscious and unconscious deception [79,80,85], fantasy proneness [86,87], and psychopathy [88,89] should be explored.

Malingering and deception

In the forensic context, the possibility of malingering and deception must be addressed [79,80,90–96]. In addition to the types of evaluations of malingering and deception that are available for psychiatric and psychologic disorders in general [96], there are several categories of assessments that can assist forensic evaluators with these questions as they apply to evaluees claiming DID. These include neurobiologic assessments (eg, hypnotic capacity via the eye-roll test [48,80]), screening instruments [79], structured clinical interviews [80] (discussed later), and availability of corroboration of either premorbid symptoms [97] or memories.

Screening interviews and instruments

Informed professionals' capacity to screen for the presence of dissociative disorders reliably has increased substantially in recent years, largely because of the newly validated semistructured interviews for dissociation that may be used with psychometrically sound objective or projective assessment instruments. In terms of semistructured interviews, the two formats used most frequently in the field are Loewenstein's office mental status examination [98] and Ross' Dissociative Disorders Interview Schedule (DDIS) [99,100]. Both formats provide a thorough list of questions, with the Loewenstein measure linked to known qualities of dissociative disorders and the DDIS linked to the *Diagnostic and Statistical Manual of Mental Disorders* model of psychodiagnosis.

In terms of assessment instruments used to screen (rather than make diagnoses definitively), there are many that have appeared over the years [101,102], but the two instruments that appear most frequently are the Dissociative Experiences Scale (DES) [101,103,104] and the Somatoform Dissociation Questionnaire (SDQ) [105–108]. Both instruments yield cut-off scores that maximize the likelihood that evaluees have a dissociative disorder. Taxonic analysis of the DES yields a "pathologic" taxon versus a "nonpathologic" continuum [109,110], although both forms of dissociation seem related to relevant clinical phenomena [111,112]. The DES purports to screen for "psychoform" dissociation, whereas the SDQ purports to screen for "somatoform" dissociation. Administration and scoring are efficient and inexpensive. The DES, in particular, has appeared in more than 1100 research studies and is a staple in the armamentarium of clinical and forensic evaluators. A newer related measure, the DCS [113], is available for use with populations that may show high levels of "nonpathologic" dissociation. The DCS has a greater number of nontaxon items, a different metric, and a more normal distribution. Evaluee responses to screening instrument items also provide helpful questions for follow-up during evaluations.

Diagnostic interviews and instruments

Although there is considerable research on dissociation with projective tests, such as the Rorschach test [114–116] and thematic apperception test [92], and objective tests, such as the Minnesota Multiphasic Personality Inventory (MMPI) and MMPI-2 [117–119], there is one structured interview that has earned top billing as a diagnostic instrument and two newly developed "objective" devices that may share the top billing spot in future years. The Structured Clinical Interview for Dissociative Disorders—Revised

(SCID-D-R) [120–123] has earned the premiere position as a structured diagnostic interview and is used routinely in clinical and forensic evaluations. The SCID-D requires the examiner to cover common dissociative symptoms thoroughly and provides for a follow-up for each question, which often can lead to examples of the pathology emerging in the interview itself. The SCID-D-R yields scores along five dimensions of dissociative disorder: amnesia, depersonalization, derealization, identity confusion, and identity alteration [122].

The Multidimensional Inventory of Dissociation (MID) [124,125] is a 218-item, self-administered, multiscale instrument that assesses the domain of dissociation and diagnoses the dissociative disorders comprehensively (see the article by Dell elsewhere in this issue). It measures 14 major facets of dissociation and has 23 dissociation diagnostic scales that operationalize (1) the subjective and phenomenologic domain of dissociation and (2) 23 hypothesized dissociative symptoms of dissociative identity disorder. Briere's Multiscale Dissociation Inventory (MDI) [126,127] explores six domains of dissociation in a 30-item self-report format and offers a profile of dissociative symptoms that can be compared to clinical and nonclinical samples. The MID gives a more comprehensive profile of DID clients who actively report alter states, whereas the MDI is the better choice for more general dissociative phenomena. At present, only the MDI has published norms on a large standardization sample and a published administration and interpretation manual. The MDI, therefore, is more defensible forensically, although the MID provides supplemental data in a DID-specific case.

Social

The assessment of DID in the social domain includes history of exposure to DID literature, groups and treatment, corroboration of reports of abuse, past medical records, school records, employment records, and litigation history (including depositions) [26,50,79,92]. Evaluators should attempt to map the social context in which dissociative symptoms emerged, to make a determination of the role of suggestibility or social desirability (eg, if the symptoms appear only with a therapist) and to chart the context-specific changes in clients' personality, knowledge, and presentation.

Screening for alternative and comorbid diagnoses

The comorbidity of DID with personality disorders, substance abuse, and axis I disorders is well established [120,128]. A forensic evaluation for a purported dissociative disorder always should include more general screening devices to examine alternative hypotheses for behavior and symptoms. The evaluation thus should include a broad axis I screener (such as the MMPI) and a broad neuropsychologic screening tool (eg, subtests of the Wechsler Adult Intelligence Scale or Luria-Nebraska Neuropsychological Battery) to provide data that might produce alternative explanations for findings attributed to dissociation.

Summary and conclusions

The authors believe that the forensic evaluation of DID and the dissociative disorders requires expertise in the assessment and treatment of those disorders and that it requires an integration of data gathered from biologic psychologic, and social domains.

References

[1] Goldstein A. Handbook of psychology, vol. 11: forensic psychology. Hoboken (NJ): John Wiley & Sons; 2003.
[2] Greenberg SA, Schuman DW. Irreconcilable differences between therapeutic and forensic roles. Prof Psychol Res Pr 1997;28:50–7.
[3] Hess AK, Weiner IB. The handbook of forensic psychology. New York: John Wiley & Sons; 1999.
[4] Melton GB, Petrila J, Poythress NG, et al. Psychologicevaluations for the courts. New York: Guilford Press; 1997.
[5] Rosner R, editor. Principles and practice of forensic psychiatry. 2nd edition. London: Arnold Publishers; 2003.
[6] American Academy of Psychiatry & the Law. Available at: www.aapl.org. Accessed October 15, 2005.
[7] American Board of Forensic Psychology. Available at: www.abfp.org. Accessed October 15, 2005.
[8] National Organization of Forensic Social Work. Available at: www.nofsw.org. Accessed October 15, 2005.
[9] Dawes R, Faust D, Meehl P. Clinical versus actuarial judgment. Science 1989;243: 1668–74.
[10] Meehl P. Clinical versus statistical prediction: a theoretical analysis and review of the evidence. Northvale (NJ): Jason Aronson; 1996.
[11] Coons PM. Iatrogenesis and malingering of multiple personality disorder in the forensic evaluation of homicide defendants. Psychiatr Clin North Am 1991;14:757–68.
[12] Dunn G, Paolo A, Ryan J. Belief in the existence of multiple personality disorder among psychologists and psychiatrists. J Clin Psychol 1994;50:454–7.
[13] Cormier J, Thelen M. Professional skepticism of multiple personality disorder. Prof Psychol Res Pr 1998;29:163–7.
[14] Dammeyer M, Nightingale N, McCoy M. Repressed memory and other controversial origins of sexual abuse allegations: beliefs among psychologists and clinical social workers. Child Maltreat 1997;2:252–63.
[15] Daubert v. Merrell Dow Pharmaceuticals, Inc., 509 US 579 (1993).
[16] Kumho Tire Co. v. Carmichael 000 US 97–1709 (1999).
[17] Frye v. United States 293 F. 1013 (DC Cir. 1923).
[18] Hartocollis L. The making of multiple personality disorder: the role of experts in the production of psychiatric knowledge. Dissertation Abstr Int Sect A Humanities Soc Sci 1999; 60(5-A):1767.
[19] James D. Multiple personality disorder in the courts: a review of the North American experience. J Forensic Psychiatry 1998;9:339–61.
[20] Kanovitz JR, Kanovitz BS, Bloch JP. Witnesses with multiple personality disorder. 23 Pepp L Rev 387, 1996.
[21] Kennet K, Matthews S. Identity, control and responsibility: the case of dissociative identity disorder. Philos Psychol 2002;15:509–26.
[22] Moskowitz AK. Dissociative pathways to homicide: clinical and forensic implications. J Trauma Dissociation 2004;5:5–32.

[23] Noonan JR. Dissociative identity disorder and criminal intent: an approach to determining responsibility. Am J Forensic Psychol 2000;18:5–26.

[24] Owens SM. The multiple personality disorder (MPD) defense. 8 Md J Contemp L Issues, 237, 1997.

[25] Owens SM. Conducting medical research on the decisionally impaired: note: diagnostic evidence admissibility and the multiple personality disorder defense. J Health Care Law Policy 1998;236.

[26] Pope K, Brown L. Recovered memories of abuse: assessment, therapy, forensics. Washington, DC: American Psychological Association; 1996.

[27] Saks ER. Jekyll on trial: multiple personality disorder and criminal law. New York: New York University Press; 1997.

[28] Armstrong J. The case of Mr. Woods: psychological contributions to the legal process in defendants with multiple personality disorder/dissociative identity disorder. 10 S. Cal Interdis. L.J. 205, 2001.

[29] Behnke S. Assessing the criminal responsibility of individuals with multiple personality disorder: legal cases, legal theory. J Am Acad Psychiatry Law 1997;25:391–9.

[30] Chu J, Frey LM, Ganzel BL, et al. Memories of childhood abuse: dissociation, amnesia, corroboration. Am J Psychiatry 1999;156:749–55.

[31] Dawson J. The alter as agent: multiple personality and the insanity defence. Psychiatry Psychol Law 1999;6:203–6.

[32] Vesper JH. Consulting with attorneys on dissociative disorders and recovered memories. Am J Forensic Psychol 1996;14:19–36.

[33] California Penal Code §28(a).

[34] Dilts S Jr. Models of the mind: a framework for biopsychosocial psychiatry. New York: Brunner-Routledge; 2001.

[35] Engel GL. The clinical application of the biopsychosocial model. Am J Psychiatry 1980; 137:535–44.

[36] Hughes JR, Kuhlman DT, Fichtner CG, et al. Brain mapping in a case of multiple personality. Clin Electroencephalogr 1990;21:200–9.

[37] Mathew RJ, Jack RA, West WS. Regional cerebral blood flow in a patient with multiple personality. Am J Psychiatry 1985;142:504–5.

[38] Tsai GE, Condie D, Wu MT, et al. Functional magnetic resonance imaging of personality switches in a woman with dissociative identity disorder. Harv Rev Psychiatry 1997;7: 119–22.

[39] Reinders AA, Nijenhuis ERS, Paans AM, et al. One brain, two selves. Neuroimage 2003;20: 2119–25.

[40] Sar V, Unal SN, Kiziltan E, et al. HMPAO SPECT study of regional cerebral blood flow in dissociative identity disorder. J Trauma Dissociation 2001;2:5–25.

[41] Saxe GN, Vasile RG, Hill TC, et al. SPECT imaging and multiple personality disorder. J Nerv Ment Dis 1992;180:662–3.

[42] Allen JB, Iacono WG. Assessing the validity of amnesia in dissociative identity disorder: a dilemma for the DSM and the Courts. Psychol Public Policy Law 2001;7:311–44.

[43] Allen JG, Console DA, Lewis L. Dissociative attachment and memory impairment: reversible amnesia or encoding failure? Compr Psychiatry 1999;40:160–71.

[44] Allen JJ, Movius HL 2nd. The objective assessment of amnesia in dissociative identity disorder using even-related potentials. Int J Psychophysiol 2000;38:21–41.

[45] Marinos JM. Laterality and dissociative identity disorder: perceptual asymmetries in host and alter personalities on tests of dichotic listening and global-local processing. Dissertation Abstr Int Sect B Sci Engineering 1998;58(8-B):4506.

[46] Stone JJ. A neuropsychological investigation of memory functioning in dissociative identity disorder. Dissertation Abstr Int Sect B Sci Engineering 1997;58(3-B):1548.

[47] Braun BG, Schwartz DR, Kravitz HM, et al. Frequency of EEG abnormalities in a large dissociative population. Dissociation Prog Dissociative Disord 1997;10:120–4.

[48] Torem MS, Egtvedt BD, Curdue KJ. The eye-roll sign and the PAS Dissociation Scale. Am J Clin Hypn 1995;38:122–5.

[49] Bowman ES, Coons PM. The differential diagnosis of epilepsy, pseudoseizures, dissociative identity disorder and dissociative disorder not otherwise specified. Bull Menninger Clin 2000;64:164–80.

[50] Brown RJ, Trimble MR. Dissociative psychopathology, non-epileptic seizures and neurology. J Neurol Neurosurg Psychiatry 2000;69:286–8.

[51] Hersh J, Chan Y-C, Smeltzer D. Identity shifts in temporal lobe epilepsy. Gen Hosp Psychiatry 2002;24:185–7.

[52] Ebner-Priemer W, Badeck S, Beckmann C, et al. Affective dysregulation and dissociative experience in female patients with borderline personality disorder: a startle response study. J Psychiatric Res 2005;39:85–92.

[53] Griffin M, Resick P, Mechanic M. Objective assessment of peritraumatic dissociation: Psychophysiological indicators. Am J Psychiatry 1997;154:1081–8.

[54] Koopman C, Carrion V, Butler L, et al. Relationships of dissociation and childhood abuse and neglect with heart rate in delinquent adolescents. J Trauma Stress 2004;17:47–54.

[55] Sierra M, Berrios G. Depersonalization: neurobiological perspectives. Biol Psychiatry 1998;44:898–908.

[56] Cicchetti D, Walker EF, editors. Neurodevelopmental mechanisms and psychopathology. New York: Cambridge University Press; 2004.

[57] Lyons-Ruth K. Dissociatiation and the parent-infant dialogue: a longitudinal perspective from attachment research. J Am Psychoanal Assoc 2003;3:883–911.

[58] Solomon J, George C, editors. Attachment disorganization. New York: Guilford Press; 1999.

[59] Crowell JA, Treboux D. A review of adult attachment measures: implications for theory and research. Soc Dev 1995;4:294–327.

[60] Dorahy MJ. Dissociative identity disorder and memory dysfunction: the current state of experimental research and its future directions. Clin Psychol Rev 2001;21:771–95.

[61] Dorahy MJ, Irwin HJ, Middleton W. Assessing markers of working memory function in dissociative identity disorder using neutral stimuli: a comparison with clinical and general population samples. Aust N Z J Psychiatry 2004;38:47–55.

[62] Dorahy MJ, Middleton W, Irwin HJ. The effect of emotional context on cognitive inhibition and attentional processing in dissociative identity disorder. Behav Res Ther 2005;43:555–68.

[63] Dalenberg C. Accuracy, timing and circumstances of disclose in therapy of recovered and continuous memories of abuse. J Psychiatry Law 1996;24:229–75.

[64] Goodman GS, Ghetti S, Quas JA, et al. A prospective study of memory for child sexual abuse: new findings relevant to the repressed memory controversy. Psychol Sci 2003;14:113–8.

[65] DiTomasso MJ, Routh DK. Recall of abuse in childhood and three measures of dissociation. Child Abuse Negl 1994;18:885–7.

[66] Andrews B, Brewin C, Ochera K, et al. Characteristics, context and consequences of memory recovery among adults in therapy. Br J Psychiatry 1999;175:141–6.

[67] Brewin CR, Andrews B. Recovered memories of trauma: phenomenology and cognitive mechanisms. Clin Psychol Rev 1998;18:949–70.

[68] Myers LB, Brewin CR. Recall of early experience and the repressive coping style. J Abnorm Psychol 1994;103:288–92.

[69] Myers LB, Brewin CR, Power MJ. Repressive coping and the directed forgetting of emotional material. J Abnorm Psychol 1998;107:141–8.

[70] Elzinga BM, Phaf RH, Ardon AM, van Dyck R. Directed forgetting between, but not within, dissociative personality states. J Abnorm Psychol 2003;112:237–43.

[71] DePrince AP, Freyd JJ. Forgetting trauma stimuli. Psychol Sci 2004;15:448–92.

[72] Goldsmith R, Barlow MR, Freyd JJ. Knowing and not knowing about trauma: implications for therapy. Psychother Theory Res Practice Training 2004;41:448–63.

[73] Sivers H, Schooler J, Freyd J. Recovered memories. Encyclopedia of the Human Brain 2002;4:169–84.

[74] Eich E, Macaulay D, Loewenstein RJ, et al. Implicit memory, interpersonality amnesia and dissociative identity disorder: comparing patients with simulators. In: Read JD, Lindsay DS, editors. Recollections of trauma: scientific evidence and clinical practice. New York: Plenum Press; 1997. p. 469–74.

[75] Huntjens RJ, Postma A, Peters ML, et al. Interidentity amnesia for neutral, episodic information in dissociative identity disorder. J Abnorm Psychol 2003;112:290–7.

[76] Nissen MJ, Ross JL, Willingham DB, et al. Evaluating amnesia in multiple personality disorder. In: Klein RM, Doane BK, editors. Psychological concepts and dissociative disorders. Hillsdale (NJ): Lawrence Erlbaum Associates; 1994. p. 259–82.

[77] Cheit R. The recovered memory project. Available at: www.recoveredmemory.org. Accessed October 16, 2005.

[78] Kluft RP. The confirmation and disconfirmation of memories of abuse in DID patients: a naturalistic clinical study. Dissociation Prog Dissociative Disord 1995;8:243–8.

[79] Thomas A. Factitious and malingered dissociative identity disorder. J Trauma Dissociation 2001;2:59–77.

[80] Welburn KR, Fraser G, Jordan SA, et al. Discriminating dissociative identity disorder from schizophrenia and feigned dissociation on psychological tests and structured interview. J Trauma Dissociation 2003;4:109–30.

[81] Eisen ML, Quas JA, Goodman GS. Memory and suggestibility in the forensic interview. Mahwah (NJ): Lawrence Erlbaum Associates; 2001.

[82] Scheflin AW, Brown D. The false litigant syndrome: "nobody would say that unless it was the truth." J Psychiatry Law 1999;27:649–705.

[83] Gudjonsson CH. A new scale of interrogative suggestibility. Pers Individ Dif 1984;5: 303–14.

[84] Scullin M, Ceci S. A suggestibility scale for children. Pers Individ Dif 2001;30:843–56.

[85] Paulhus D. Two-component models of socially desirable responding. J Pers Soc Psychol 1984;46:596–609.

[86] Pekala R, Angelini F, Kumar V. The importance of fantasy- proneness in dissociation: A replication. Contemp Hypnosis 2001;18:204–14.

[87] Waldo T, Merritt R. Fantasy Proneness, dissociation and DSM- IV Axis II symptomatology. J Abnorm Psychol 2000;109:555–8.

[88] Barone N. The Hare Psychopathy Checklist revised. J Psychiatry Law 2004;32:113–4.

[89] Gacono C. Clinical and forensic assessment of psychology: a practitioner's guide. Mahwah (NJ): Lawrence Erlbaum; 2000.

[90] Armstrong J. False memories and true lies: the psychology of a recanter. J Psychiatry Law 1999;27:519–47.

[91] Brandsma JM, Hobson DP. Somatoform, dissociative and factitious disorders. In: Morrison RL, Bellack AS, editors. Medical factors and psychological disorders: a handbook for psychologists. New York: Plenum Press; 1987. p. 115–39.

[92] Draijer N, Boon S. Validity of Dissociative Experiences Scale vs. Structured Clinical Interview for DSM-III-R Dissociative Disorders, differential diagnosis, psychiatric patients with vs without dissociative disorders. Dissociation Prog Dissociative Disord 1993;6:28–37.

[93] Draijer N, Boon S. The limitations of dissociative identity disorder: patients at risk, therapists at risk. J Psychiatry Law 1999;27:423–58.

[94] High JR. Deception through factitious identity. J Psychiatry Law 1999;27:483–518.

[95] Putnam FW. Fabrications of things past: factitious identities and fictional life histories. J Psychiatry Law 1999;27:639–47.

[96] Rogers R, editor. Clinical assessment of malingering and deception. 2nd ed. New York: Guilford Press; 1997.

[97] Gleaves DH, Hernandez E, Warner MS. Corroborating premorbid dissociative symptomatology in dissociative identity disorder. Prof Psychol Res Pr 1999;30:341–5.

[98] Loewenstein RJ. An office mental status examination for complex chronic dissociative symptoms and multiple personality disorder. Psychiatr Clin North Am 1991;14:567–605.

[99] Ross CA, Heber S, Anderson L. The dissociative disorders interview schedule. Am J Psychiatry 1990;147:1698–9.

[100] Ross CA, Heber S, Norton GR, et al. The dissociative disorders interview schedule: a structured interview. Dissociation Prog Dissociative Disord 1989;2:169–89.

[101] Carlson EB. Trauma assesements: a clinician's guide. New York: Guilford; 1997.

[102] Briere J. Psychological assessment of adult posttraumatic states. 2nd ed. Washington, DC: American Psychological Association; 2004.

[103] Carlson EB, Putnam F. An update on the Dissociative Experiences Scale. Dissociation Prog Dissociative Disord 1993;6:16–27.

[104] Carlson EB, Putnam F, Ross CA, et al. A validity study of the Dissociative Experiences Scale in screening for multiple personality disorder: a multicenter study. Am J Psychiatry 1993;150:1030–6.

[105] Nijenhuis ERS. Somatoform dissociation. Assen (the Netherlands): Van Gorcum; 1999.

[106] Nijenhuis ERS, Spinhoven P, van Dyck R, et al. The development and psychometric characteristics of the Somatoform Dissociation Questionnaire (SDQ-20). J Nerv Ment Dis 1996; 184:688–94.

[107] Nijenhuis ERS, Spinhoven P, van Dyck R, et al. Dissociative pathology discriminates between bipolar mood disorder and dissociative disorder. Br J Psychiatry 1997;170:581.

[108] Nijenhuis ERS, Spinhoven P, van Dyck R, et al. Psychometric characteristics of the Somatoform Dissociation Questionnaire: a replication study. Psychother Psychosom 1998;67: 17–23.

[109] Waller N, Putnam FW, Carlson EB. Types of dissociation and dissociative types: a taxometric analysis of dissociative experiences. Psychol Methods 1996;1:300–21.

[110] Waller N, Ross CA. The prevalence and biometric structure of pathological dissociation in the general population: taxometric and behavior genetic findings. J Abnorm Psychol 1997; 106:499–510.

[111] Allen J, Fultz J, Huntoon J, et al. Pathological dissociative taxon membership, absorption, and reported childhood trauma in women with trauma-related disorders. J Trauma Dissociation 2002;3:89–110.

[112] Levin R, Spei E. Relationships of purported measures of pathological and nonpathological dissociation to self-reported psychological distress and fantasy immersion. Assessment 2004;11:160–8.

[113] Coe M, Dalenberg C, Aransky K. Adult attachment style, reported childhood violence history and types of dissociative experiences. Dissociation Prog Dissociative Disord 1995;8: 14254.

[114] Armstrong J. Psychological assessment. In: Spira, J, editor. Treating dissociative identity disorder. San Francisco: Jossey-Bass; 1996. p. 3–38.

[115] Labott SM, Wallach HR. Malingering dissociative identity disorder: objective and projective assessment. Psychother Psychosom 1998;6717–23.

[116] Leavitt F, Labott SM. Rorschach indicators of dissociative identity disorders: clinical utility and theoretical implications. J Clin Psychol 1998;54:803–10.

[117] Coons PM. Use of the MMPI to distinguish genuine from factitious multiple personality disorder. Psychol Rep 1993;72:401–2.

[118] Coons PM, Fine CG. Accuracy of the MMPI in identifying multiple personality disorder. Psychol Rep 1990;66(3 Pt 1):831–4.

[119] Phillips DW. Initial development and validation of the Phillips Dissociation Scale (PDS) of the MMPI. Dissociation Prog Dissociative Disord 1994;7:92–100.

[120] Steinberg M. Handbook for the assessment of dissociation. Washington, DC: American Psychiatric Press; 1995.

[121] Steinberg M. Advances in the clinical assessment of dissociation: the SCID-D-R. Bull Menninger Clin 2000;64:146–63.

[122] Steinberg M, Bancroft K, Buchanan J. Multiple personality disorder in criminal law. Bull Am Acad Psychiatry Law 1993;21:345–56.
[123] Steinberg M, Hall P, Lareau C, Cicchetti DV. Recognizing the validity of dissociative symptoms using the SCID-D-RL guidelines for clinical and forensic evaluations. 10 S Cal Interdis L J 2001;225.
[124] Dell PF. The Mulidimensional Inventory of Dissociation (MID): a comprehensive measure of pathological dissociation. J Trauma Dissociation, in press.
[125] Dell PF. Dissociative phenomenology of dissociative identity disorder. J Nerv Ment Dis 2002;190:10–5.
[126] Dietrich A. Characteristics of child maltreatment, psychological dissociation, and somatoform dissociation of Canadian inmates. J Trauma Dissociation 2003;4:81–100.
[127] Briere J. Multiscale dissociation inventory. Odessa (FL): Psychological Assessment Resources; 2002.
[128] Ellason J, Ross C, Fuchs D. Lifetime axis I and II comorbidity and childhood trauma history in dissociative identity disorder. Psychiatry Interpersonal Biol Proc 1996;59:255–66.

ELSEVIER
SAUNDERS

PSYCHIATRIC
CLINICS
OF NORTH AMERICA

Psychiatr Clin N Am 29 (2006) 185–211

Why Conversion Seizures Should Be Classified as a Dissociative Disorder

Elizabeth S. Bowman, MD[a,b,*]

[a]Indiana University Epilepsy Clinic, Indianapolis, IN, USA
[b]Indiana University School of Medicine, Department of Neurology, Indianapolis, IN, USA

Conceptions from the past blind us to facts which almost slap us in the face.
William Stuart Halsted

*In psychiatry there are forms of illness with names going back two and a half
millennia, which have had the sentence of death passed upon them more than
once, yet they obstinately survive.... Hysteria is indeed an extreme case... in
any case a tough old word like hysteria dies very hard... It tends to outlive its
obituarists.*

Sir Aubrey Lewis

The Bible reports that the ancient Israelites wandered 40 years in the wilderness of the Sinai between escaping slavery and finding a home in the land of Canaan [1]. The diagnostic wanderings of pseudoseizures (conversion disorder, seizure type in the *Diagnostic and Statistical Manual of Mental Disorders, Fourth Edition [DSM-IV]*) [2] have lasted 40 centuries. Both journeys began in Egypt. Pseudoseizures are a hallmark of the ancient illness, hysteria. The symptoms of hysteria now are classified as dissociative and somatoform disorders in the *DSM-IV* and the *International Statistical Classification of Diseases, 10th Revision (ICD-10)* [3], but conversion seizures are in the somatoform section of *DSM-IV* and in the dissociative disorders section of *ICD-10*.

The written journey of hysteria began in Egypt in approximately 1900 BCE, when the *Kahun Papyrus* and the extensive Egyptian medical text, *Papyrus Ebers* (approximately 1800 BCE), attributed it to the effects of uterine dysfunction [4]. Hippocrates [4] introduced the name, hysteria, from *hystera*, the Greek word for uterus. Plato's *Timaeus* connects hysteria with uterine

---

* Indiana University Hospital, 550 North University Boulevard, Suite 1711, Indianapolis,
IN 46202.

E-mail address: ebowman@iupui.edu

0193-953X/06/$ - see front matter © 2005 Elsevier Inc. All rights reserved.
doi:10.1016/j.psc.2005.10.003   *psych.theclinics.com*

wandering: "When it [the womb] remains barren too long after puberty, it is distressed and sorely disturbed, and straying about in the body and cutting off the passages of breath, it impedes respiration and brings the sufferer into the extremest anguish and provokes all manner of diseases besides" [4].

Since the identification of dissociation with conversion seizures in the nineteenth century, modern psychiatry has been unable to agree on the classification of hysteria or its relationship to somatization or dissociative mechanisms, leaving conversion's diagnostic classification to wander like the ancient Israelites. This article joins a rising chorus [5–10] advocating for returning to Pierre Janet's view of conversion seizures as dissociative disorders. It proposes that American psychiatry should reclassify conversion in the *DSM* [11–14] as a dissociative disorder, in line with the *ICD-10* [3]. I base my argument that conversion seizures are a dissociative disorder on historical, theoretical, research, clinical, and taxonometric grounds. With the remainder of the world using the *ICD-10* [3], which classifies conversion seizures as dissociative seizures, it is a scientific embarrassment for American psychiatry to continue to deny the dissociative nature of pseudoseizures. It is time to let clinical observations and research facts on conversion seizures slap us in the face.

Historical data and theoretic arguments

Why is a discussion of dissociation and the ancient concept of hysteria needed in the twenty-first century? Despite what Sir Aubrey Lewis [15] wrote (see introductory quotation), isn't hysteria really a dead term? This discussion uses the term, hysteria, for conversion/dissociation/somatization combined, because this is the term used in nearly all writings on conversion seizures until the late twentieth century. I dislike the term, because it associates conversion symptoms solely with women, but hysteria is a name that "dies very hard" [15] and continues to be used because of "the difficulty finding a substitute for it" [16]. I use the terms, pseudoseizures and conversion seizures, interchangeably to denote the conversion type of psychgenic or nonepileptic seizures. I understand that not all nonepileptic seizures are psychological and not all psychogenic seizures are conversion seizures (those somatically symbolizing unconscious material) but use the terms interchangeably for simplicity [17]. Extensive discussion of the problems of names for nonepileptic seizures is beyond the scope of this article.

Historical data

The association of hysteria (and its seizures) with the uterus began approximately 4000 years ago and anchored the association between hysteria and sexuality, especially inappropriate early sexual experiences, in the medical imagination. The fierce loyalty of medical writers across the centuries to the uterine theory of revered ancients, such as Hippocrates and Galen, blinded them to perceiving hysteria as a mental symptom or heeding those who noted by the first century CE that it occurred in men [4]. The belief that hysterical conversion was related to uterine displacement declined gradually as a result of anatomic study but not before it spawned a spate of creative and bizarre physical treatments of hysteria designed to lure the wayward uterus back to the pelvis [4].

Medical theories about hysteria took a turn from physical to mental when Thomas Sydenham first recognized the emotional nature of hysteria in 1697 [4]. Recognition of the mental, dissociative and traumatic nature of hysteria blossomed in the nineteenth century in response to interest in hypnosis, with which hysteria was strongly associated. Briquet's original *Treatise on Hysteria* [18] reports sensory, motor, and seizure conversion symptoms as the "core of the illness" [15,18]. He did not describe dissociative amnesia in hysteria but noted an association with psychologic and sexual trauma [19]. The dissociative nature of conversion seizures was first specified in medical writings in 1845 by French physician Moreau de Tours [20], who used the term, *désagrégation* (translated as dissociation), to describe the isolation of ideas in hysterics [21]. In nineteenth-century literature, conversion hysteria and dissociation were associated heavily with hypnosis. Taine [22] described the *dédoublement* (splitting) of the ego and of consciousness during hypnosis in hysterical subjects [4]. Gilles de la Tourette and others began to use the concept of dissociated consciousness in the latter half of the nineteenth century [4].

Charcot's study of hysterical women at the Hôpital Salpêtrière in Paris in the nineteenth century enabled Janet and Freud to observe the connection between sexuality, hypnotic trance, suggestibility, and hysterical conversion. Charcot, following theorists of prior centuries who noted the central role of seizures in hysteria [4], referred to hysterical seizures as major hysteria and all other conversion symptoms as minor hysteria. Charcot pointed subsequent theorists to the suggestibility of hysterical patients.

Janet's dissociative theory of hysteria

The theory of French neuropsychologist Pierre Janet [23] laid a theoretical foundation for understanding the dissociative nature of conversion disorder that remains firm and valid today. Janet studied with Charcot and developed his theory of dissociation from clinical observations of hysterical patients. Charcot and Janet each posited involvement of body and mind in hysteria, but Janet felt conversion was solely mental in origin and did not include the physical lesion hypothesized by Charcot. The two conceptual pillars of Janet's dissociative theory of hysteria were the clinical characteristics of retraction of the field of consciousness and dissociation [9]. Janet noted that the perceptions of hysterics are not integrated into normal consciousness and personality but that they do not simply disappear. They escape the normal control of consciousness and may start to lead a life of their own, influencing a person from outside of conscious awareness. Janet observed that dissociated processes express themselves somatically in disturbances of vision, hearing, speech, movement, and sensation and psychologically in alterations of consciousness, memory, and identity. He noted how psychological, physical, and sexual traumas were relived unconsciously and expressed in all types of conversion.

Janet is responsible for bringing the term, dissociation, into general psychiatric awareness. He recognized that dissociation was described but not recognized in the literature on hysteria of nineteenth-century authors: "...they always speak of localized amnesias, of alternating memory, which in reality are only to be met among hysterical somnambulisms [state of hypnosis]...of total modifications of the personality divided into two successive or simultaneous persons, which is again the dissociation of consciousness in the hysteric" [21].

Janet defined dissociation as exclusion from consciousness and inaccessibility of voluntary recall of mental events of varying degrees of complexity, including mental and somatic aspects [8]. The core of his dissociation theory was that memories and emotions that are unavailable to conscious awareness had not been obliterated but are held in another separate state of consciousness and subsequently can be recalled. He noted that separated states of consciousness could influence patients without them being aware of it. He termed this phenomenon, psychologic automatism, an idea and emotion bound together in consciousness and able to influence behavior from outside consciousness. For Janet, psychologic automatisms were the basic element of mental life [23]. He believed they were split off (dissociated) from conscious control under conditions of trauma. In this way, he explained involuntary repetition of forgotten traumatic experiences in conversion symptoms.

Janet summarized his dissociative theory in his major works, *L'Automatisme Psychologique* [23,50] and *The Major Symptoms of Hysteria* [24], which are replete with cases of persons who had dissociative amnesia, dissociated ego states, and dissociated personalities. Using hypnosis, he discovered several personality states in hysterical patients. He noted that the personality who had conversion symptoms often suffered one-way amnesia for the altered state that was free of conversion [25]. Janet emphasized the connection between dissociated trauma, fixed ideas related to trauma, and the representation of trauma in conversion symptoms. For example, in a case of motor conversion, his patient "He." was frightened by a lioness in a zoo and then spent a week running about on all fours, biting people, and devouring food like a lion [24]. When in her ordinary state, she was amnestic for her trauma at the zoo. Janet [10,23] documented monocular blindness and hemifacial anesthesia from psychological trauma in his patient, Marie, who was amnestic for being traumatized by being forced to sleep with a disfigured child who lay by the side of Marie's face that exhibited symptoms. Another patient re-enacted the manner of the traumatic death of her niece hysterically [24]. One hundred years before modern research statistically demonstrated the significant association of dissociative disorders with childhood trauma, Janet linked psychological, sexual, and physical traumas to dissociation and conversion symptoms decisively. The traumas he described often were recent and corroborated.

This brilliant clinician described the dissociative core of conversion symptoms at approximately the same time that Freud was repudiating belief in the incest reports of his patients that resulted in their conversion symptoms [26]. Janet noted that conversion symptoms remitted when patients could recall their traumas. His patients' symptoms and traumas and their relationship to dissociative states bear striking resemblance to my twenty-first century conversion patients and other modern reports of dissociative disorders in conversion disorder [8,10]. Janet's theories laid the foundation for modern theories of dissociation and conversion.

Freud's theory of hysteria

Because of Janet's efforts, conversion seizures and other conversion symptoms became identified with trauma and dissociation in the late nineteenth and early twentieth centuries, but as Freud's repression-based theory held sway, Janet's dissociation-based theory faded from prominence. The concept of dissociation fell into disuse after Freud abandoned his sexual seduction theory of hysteria [26–29]. Freud initially believed hysteria was the result of the sexual traumas reported by his patients, then repudiated this theory, proposing instead that sexual fantasy and forbidden wish fulfillment led to repression of the incestuous wish and transformation to a somatic expression via the mechanism of conversion. Freud's infantile sexuality theory gave us the term "conversion" for transformation of a psychological conflict into a somatic expression.

Janet's "mental function deficit" model of hysteria posited a weak ego that was unable to control symptoms. In contrast, Freud's psychoanalytic model of hysteria featured an ego strong enough to repress unacceptable material that returned in hysterical somatic symptoms [30]. The triumph of Freud's psychoanalytic theory led to loss of interest in Janet's theory of dissociation of trauma until late twentieth-century research again found connections between trauma, dissociative disorders, and conversion seizures. Only a few clinicians, such as Morton Prince [31], retained interest in dissociation, and published on conversion symptoms in patients who had multiple personality disorder (MPD). Reports of dissociative disorders in patients who had conversion became less frequent until late twentieth-century researchers rediscovered them and conducted research that gave clinical support to Janet's dissociative theory of conversion. In the past 30 years, since the advent of videotaped electroencephalography (VEEG), research on conversion seizures has flourished as neurologists have discovered that psychogenic seizures are more common than had been suspected.

Modern theories of dissociation and conversion: Nijenhuis and Hilgard

Janet laid the groundwork for the modern research and theory of somatoform dissociation of Dutch psychologist, Sir Ellert Nijenhuis. Nijenhuis' research has validated Janet's theory that dissociation is somatic and psychological and that somatoform and psychological expressions of dissociation are found together in patients who have modern conversion disorder, somatization disorder, and *DSM-IV* dissociative disorder. Nijenhuis proposed the construct of somatoform dissociation (contrasted with psychological dissociation) [9] and developed two instruments to measure somatoform dissociation: the Somatoform Dissociation Questionnaire-20 (SDQ-20) and a 5-item screening version, the SDQ-5 [32] (these instruments are discussed later). Nijenhuis and Dutch psychiatrist Onno van der Hart [21] have revived interest in Janet's theories of somatoform and psychological trauma and of the connection of trauma to dissociation and conversion. Nijenhuis [9] has demonstrated that modern conversion disorder patients show the same symptoms as Janet's nineteenth-century hysterics.

A later twentieth-century theory, Ernest Hilgard's neodissociation theory, posits that people shift psychic material to other forms rather than struggle with difficulty suppressing it [33]. Hilgard believed that unity of consciousness is an illusion and that consciousness is partial and divided. People can (and do) alternate the aspects of their consciousness that they use, as when people absorbed in a cell phone conversation do not attend completely to driving a vehicle until the brake lights of the vehicle in front of them signal an impending accident. Then, their attention switches quickly from auditory and verbal attention to their visual and motor systems. Another common example of neodissociation theory is the person who focuses on one conversation at a party, tuning out the din of other conversations until executing a rapid switch of attention after hearing her own name mentioned in a nearby conversation.

Hilgard proposes that the mind operates in a modular fashion, with each module of mental content having the capability of consciousness. He believed that the modular structure of the brain (a concept supported by the modern theory of parallel neural networks in the brain) leads people to shift material to other modules rather than struggle with repressing it. Neodissociation theory is completely compatible with the clinical presentation of dissociative identity disorder (DID) and of conversion seizures.

I believe Hilgard's neodissociation theory can be combined with Nijenhuis' somatoform dissociation theory to understand conversion seizures. Conversion seizures (and other conversion) can be viewed as a shifting of consciousness to a module of mental content that includes the somatosensory aspects of a memory (often traumatic) or a conflict that the seizure expresses.

I often observe that the dissociated mental module that exhibits the seizure also is aware of the affect or conflict that the patient's ordinary state cannot tolerate in conscious awareness. If it is posited that some dissociated mental modules contain primarily somatic aspects of conscious awareness, whereas others contain primarily psychologic aspects, there is a the basis for somatoform and psychological dissociation as proposed by Nijenhuis. A combination of Hilgard's and Nijenhuis' theories fits my clinical observation of conversion seizure patients well, as the cases in this article demonstrate.

Research data

Observations of dissociation in nineteenth-century cases of conversion hysteria do not prove conclusively that current conversion seizure patients have dissociation. The presentation of hysteria always has been shaped by cultural norms, so it needs to be asked if research on modern conversion seizure patients supports an association with dissociative disorders. I find it most definitely does. Late twentieth-century research shows that patients diagnosed with dissociative disorders frequently display somatization disorder and conversion symptoms, including conversion seizures [34,35]. Conversely, patients diagnosed with conversion seizures are characterized by high rates of dissociative symptoms and disorders [36]. Patients who have another aspect of hysteria, somatization disorder, exhibit robust rates of trauma and dissociative symptoms [37]. The two-way association of dissociation and conversion does not prove that dissociation is the mechanism of conversion seizures but suggests this possibility. In addition, both conversion seizure subjects and dissociative disorder subjects have high rates of childhood trauma, a condition commonly linked to dissociation.

Studies of patients who have dissociative disorders

Somatoform and conversion symptoms, including seizures, are reported in many of the historical cases of MPD, including Mary Reynolds' conversion seizures, blindness, and deafness in 1817 [38,39]; severe headaches in one personality of Prince's Miss Beauchamp [31]; and Sybil's "psychological seizures," numbness, and alternating hemiplegia [40]. If dissociation and conversion truly are linked, modern cases of dissociation also should exhibit conversion and other somatic symptoms. Indeed they do.

Sixteen studies (14 on DID or MPD) report high rates of occurrence of somatic symptoms in patients who have dissociative disorder. In five [35,41–44] of nine studies [35,41–48] that report somatization disorder in subjects who have MPD/DID, the rate of somatization is above 50%. (The term, MPD/DID, is used, because the same illness, termed MPD in *Diagnostic and Statistical Manual, Third Edition [DSM-III]* and *DSM, Revised Third Edition [DSM-III-R]*, is called DID in *DSM-IV*. Research studies often include patients diagnosed under both diagnostic categorizations.) These nine studies came from cultures in North America, Puerto Rico, the Netherlands, Turkey, and Australia. Somatization disorder also occurs frequently in less severe dissociative disorders: 44% in dissociative disorder not otherwise specified (DDNOS) [49] and 26% in subjects who have dissociative amnesia [50]. *DSM-IV* criteria for somatization disorder include conversion symptoms. Accordingly, studies of patients who have MPD/DID that report somatization disorder usually do not report specifically on conversion disorders, so fewer data are available on conversion in DID/MPD. It is unclear in many studies if systematic inquiry on conversion was conducted or if lifetime symptoms or only symptoms currently present were recorded. Conversion is an episodic symptom that may be missed if patients are not exhibiting it at the time of evaluation or treatment. Accordingly, these data safely can be assumed to constitute a minimum occurrence.

Six studies [35,41,42,46,51,52] report that various types of conversion disorder in subjects who have MPD/DID occur in 10% to 57% of subjects. Two reports note 10 [35] and 12 [34] types of conversion in patients who have MPD. All types of conversion combined in DDNOS [49] and dissociative amnesia [50] are less frequent (14% and 24%, respectively) but still considerable. Traditionally, hysteria also included symptoms of conversion pain. One symptom shared by persons who have conversion seizures and dissociative disorders is severe headaches, found in a minimum of 61% of patients who have conversion seizure [36,53] and in more than 75% of patients who have MPD/DID on four continents [35,41–43,45,48,54]. Reports of seizures in MPD/DID are difficult to interpret, because neurologic evaluations of patients are not undertaken in most studies and few subjects have ictal EEG recordings. Seizures are reported in 11% [34], 14% [35], 18% [14], 26% (seizure type unclear) [42], and 67% ("bizarre seizures") [41] of subjects who have MPD/DID. In the absence of systematic studies that include ictal VEEG recordings, the actual occurrence of conversion seizures and epileptic seizures in MPD/DID remains unknown. Patients who have MPD/DID may have epileptic and psychogenic seizures. Co-occurring epileptic seizures also are evident in 11% to 66% of patients who have conversion seizures [55]. Lifetime occurrence of nonseizure conversion symptoms is 19% to 93% [55] in persons who have conversion seizures. The occurrence of such high rates of other types of conversion in MPD/DID and the robust co-occurrence of conversion seizures with other types of conversion suggest that not all the seizures noted in DID are epileptic. The occurrence of seizures of any kind in DID far exceeds the world's general population prevalence of epilepsy is 1% [56]. In patients who have dissociative disorder, nonseizure types of conversion symptoms are reported at a considerably higher rate than reports of seizures. This may be because of the combining of reports of different types of conversion (eg, anesthesia, blindness, aphonia, paralysis, tremors, dystonias, and so forth) into a single category. The yearly prevalence of conversion disorder is 0.022% of the general population in the United States and 4.5% of psychiatric outpatients [57].

Conversion is associated with dissociative disorders at far higher than the expected rate if these conditions are independent of one another. This does not prove causality, but should cause consideration of conversion possibly as a somatic dissociative symptom. In summary, the literature on seizures in MPD/DID shows this population to have high rates of seizures. Although the characterization of these seizures is less certain, conversion seizures, considerable other conversion symptoms, and some epilepsy characterize patients who have MPD/DID.

How might the high rates of seizures in DID be explained? Are they conversion seizures, missed diagnoses of epilepsy, or both? It is possible that patients who have DID, like patients who have conversion seizure, have abnormal EEGs from head injuries sustained in childhood physical abuse, which is common in both groups [36]. Coons and colleagues [46] report abnormal paroxysmal EEGs (with a history of seizure behaviors) in 7 of 30 patients who had MPD. Three of these seven also had nonseizure conversion symptoms. Two studies [58,59] that compared subjects who had MPD and those who had epilepsy conclude that the dissociative symptoms of MPD patients differed significantly from persons who had epilepsy and that MPD does not have an ictal etiology, as suggested by earlier reports [39,60]. Abnormal EEGs are found in some patients who have DID, and some doubtless have comorbid epilepsy [61]. Three studies [49,58,62] report normal EEGs in male and female patients who have MPD. Lowenstein and Putnam's [58] review of the MPD literature concludes that the vast majority of patients who have MPD do not have detectable EEG abnormalities, but Cocores and colleagues [62] note previous reports of seizures and a normal EEG in Sybil [40] and EEG abnormalities in other MPD cases of the 1970s [52,63]. The overlap of conversion seizures or temporal lobe epilepsy with dissociative symptoms is an important consideration because of the well-known phenomena of organic depersonalization and derealization in persons who have electroencephalographic disturbances of the temporal lobe and postictal personality changes resembling MPD in persons who have epilepsy [64,65].

The literature on MPD reports higher than expected rates of seizures and somewhat higher than expected rates of abnormal EEGs. Research indicates that MPD and epilepsy are independent conditions but have overlapping symptoms of depersonalization, paroxysmal changes of behavior, and personality alterations. Studies regularly report conversion seizures in MPD and document the co-occurrence of epilepsy and MPD in a few cases. Overall, there is little support for epilepsy as the explanation for all the seizures of patients who have MPD or as the cause of MPD/DID.

In summary, the literature on dissociative disorder patients, especially patients who have MPD or DID, shows they have extremely high occurrences of conversion; 10% to 25% are diagnosed formally with conversion seizures and up to two thirds with some conversion symptom. They have high occurrences of somatization disorder and of medically unexplained pain. They share considerable clinical and diagnostic overlap with conversion seizure patients, suggesting the association of conversion seizures with dissociative mechanisms.

Studies of dissociation in patients who have conversion seizures or somatization disorder

Table 1 summarizes studies of dissociative symptoms and disorders in patients who have conversion seizures or mixed conversion disorder populations. These studies and other reports on dissociation in conversion seizures present odd findings. Dissociation (especially trance states) is described in patients who had conversion disorder from the nineteenth [23] to late twentieth centuries [8,36]. Many modern investigators refer directly or indirectly (using other terminology) to dissociation as a cause of conversion seizures [6,10,63,66–68,70–74]. Most modern reports are theory combined with descriptions of a few cases [6,8,10] Dissociation is widely assumed to explain the occurrence of the conversion type of pseudoseizures, but few studies systematically have collected data on actual dissociative disorders in conversion seizure subjects with valid instruments [36,74]. Why so few studies?

The few studies are not because of lack of studies assessing the psychiatric causes of conversion seizures. More than 24 such studies exist [55], but few of them assess dissociative disorders, which are omitted from most widely used structured psychiatric diagnostic interviews, such as the Structured Clinical Interview for *DSM-III-R* Axis I Disorders (SCID) [75] or the Symptom Checklist-90-Revised (SCL-90-R) [76]. Most patients who have conversion seizures do not volunteer their dissociative symptoms (which they view as evidence that they are "crazy") unless asked specifically, so studies of conversion seizures mostly are silent about dissociative disorders, unless the investigators studied them specifically. Neurologists generally are unfamiliar with dissociative disorders (beyond dissociative amnesia) so they tend to not report them in conversion seizure subjects. One example is neurologists Leis and colleagues [77], who report that the most common presentation of pseudoseizures in their series of 47 patients was unresponsive behavior in the absence of motor manifestations. This report describes but does not mention dissociation. A century after Janet coined the term, dissociation, nearly solely from clinical observation of conversion patients, modern researchers still manage to banish dissociation from their awareness.

Two studies [36,74] of dissociative disorders in groups of patients who have pseudoseizures used the SCID-D [60], a valid and reliable semistructured interview that makes *DSM-IV* dissociative disorder diagnoses. Bowman and Markand [36] studied American outpatients who had pseudoseizures in a university seizure clinic. Tezcan and coworkers [74] studied Turkish inpatients who had all types of conversion symptoms (44% had conversion seizures). Despite their different subject populations and cultural

Table 1
Dissociative disorder diagnoses or symptoms in conversion seizure patients

Study	Subjects, N	Percent with any dissociative disorder	Percent with MPD or DID	Percent with dissociative symptoms
Bowman and Markand, 1996 [36]	Conversion seizure, 45	91% (DDNOS with ego state: 49%)	16%	98% (amnesia)
Jawad et al, 1995 [97]	Conversion seizure, 46	11%	Not reported	Not reported
Kanner et al, 1999 [69]	Pseudoseizure, 45	22% (dissociation amnesia, not assessed systematically)	Not reported	≤45% (past dissociative disorder diagnosis)
Nash, 1993 [98]	Pseudoseizure, single case report	100% (DDNOS with ego states)	Not reported	100%
Ramchandani and Schindler, 1992 [99]	Pseudoseizure, 3 (case reports)	100% (depersonalization disorder)	Not reported	100%
Ramchandani and Schindler, 1993 [81]	Pseudoseizure, 11	36% (27% DDNOS; 9% dissociative amnesia)	0%	Not reported
Gross, 1983 [100]	Psychogenic seizure, 8	100% (dissociative amnesia)	Not reported	100%
Harden, 1997 [6]	Pseudoseizure, 2 (case reports)	100% (dissociative amnesia and fugue)	Not reported	100%
Alper et al, 1997 [66]	Not reported	Not reported	Not reported	Elevated DES depersonalization scale compared to CPE ($P = .005$)
Othmer and DeSouza, 1997 [101]	Somatization disorder, 45	Not reported	Not reported	49% (amnesia)
Tezcan et al, 2003 [74]	Conversion disorder, 59, (includes 26 with pseudoseizure)	30.5%	15% DID; 13.5% DDNOS	1.6% dissociative amnesia diagnosis
Torem, 1993 [10]	Pseudoseizure, four cases	100%	25% DID, 50% DDNOS, 25% amnesia	100% (four case examples)

Abbreviations: CPE, complex partial epilepsy subjects; DES, Dissociative Experiences Scale (*Data from* Bernstein EM, Putnam FW. Development, reliability, and validity of a dissociation scale. J Nerv Ment Dis 1986;174:727–35; Carlson EB, Putnam FW. An update on the dissociative experiences scale. Dissociation 1993;6:17–27.).

settings, these two studies report a consistent finding: 15% to 16% of patients who had conversion had DID. The similarity between findings ends there. Bowman and Markand [36] found dissociative disorders of some type in 91% of pseudoseizure subjects. These finding likely are related to the chronicity of their study population and to systematic inquiry about amnesia in childhood and adulthood. Tezcan and coworkers [74] found dissociative disorder diagnoses in 30% of their subjects—a much lower but notable proportion of patients. It is possible that the lower overall rates found by Tezcan and coworkers are the result of the diversity of their patients who had conversion disorder. Conversion seizures may be major hysteria and be characterized by more generalized dissociation than are other conversion symptoms. This field needs replication of these two studies and studies of dissociation in conversion seizures versus other conversion symptoms. These two studies clearly show, however, that conversion disorder patients have considerable dissociative pathology.

Other studies (see Table 1) show that dissociative symptoms of amnesia often are noted by researchers, regardless of whether or not they make a diagnosis of dissociative amnesia. Studies are inconsistent in mentioning if they evaluated dissociation systematically [10,36] or anecdotally noted it [69]. Even without systematic evaluation, the minimum proportion of pseudoseizure patients noted to have dissociative amnesia is approximately 10%. Systematic inquiry [36] reveals dissociative amnesia outside of seizures in up to 82% of pseudoseizure outpatients in adulthood and in up to 73% of them during childhood. Bowman and Markand [36] describe observing intrainterview amnesia in 44% of pseudoseizure subjects during emotionally intense discussions.

It is difficult to summarize the literature on dissociation in patients who have pseudoseizure because of lack of agreement of what characterizes conversion seizures and whether or not amnesia during the seizure should be diagnosed separately as dissociative amnesia or should be subsumed under the conversion seizure diagnosis [17,78]. The observation that dissociated ego states cause conversion seizures is evident in published cases [54,80] and is noted in 27% [81] to 49% [36] of cohorts of patients who have pseudoseizure. (Ego states are dissociated partial identities that fall short of having definite alter-identity formation or are separated incompletely from the usual state of consciousness. They are diagnosed as DDNOS, example 1 in *DSM-IV*.) Dissociated personalities are one underlying cause of pseudoseizures and of motor conversion [8].

Are seizures the only conversion symptom that is strongly associated with dissociation? Tezcan and colleagues [74] studied multiple types of patients who had conversion disorder and suggested the answer is "no." Nonseizure conversion symptoms are found concurrently with conversion seizures at the time of evaluation in 4% [36] to 21% [64] of subjects who have pseudoseizure. In four studies, the lifetime incidence of nonseizure conversion in subjects who have pseudoseizure ranges from 42% to 93% [55]. Conversion seizures seem to be one of many somatoform symptoms exhibited over a life-time by a highly traumatized dissociative population. The literature on dissociation in conversion patients speaks strongly to a robust overlap of the dissociative disorder and conversion disorder populations. It supports a close relationship between dissociation and conversion.

Specific studies of somatoform dissociation

Using Janet's theory, Nijenhuis [9] proposed dissociative and conversion disorders be viewed as psychological and somatoform types of dissociation. He and colleagues developed the first instrument to measure somatoform dissociation, SDQ, in a 20-item format (SDQ-20) [9] and a five-item screening format (SDQ-5) [82]. The SDQ-20 correlates highly (r = .76, *P* < .0001) [9] with the Dissociation Questionnaire (DIS-Q) [83] and the Dissociative Experiences Scale (DES) [84,85], which measure psychological dissociation. This demonstration that conversion symptoms correlate highly with psychological dissociation is strong evidence that conversion may be a somatic form of dissociation [9]. The SDQ-20 includes positive and negative conversion symptoms (including seizures). The SDQ-5 includes one pain symptom and four conversion symptoms: visual changes, analgesia, disappearance of the body, and aphonia/dysphonia [9].

Using somatoform items only, the SDQ-5 and SDQ-20 each have excellent positive predictive value in distinguishing patients who have dissociative disorder (DID and DDNOS) from other psychiatric outpatients [9,86], even after controlling for general levels of psychopathology. This demonstrates that somatoform dissociation is highly characteristic of DID and DDNOS and is not reflecting general psychopathology. Correlations with the SCL-90-R [76] show the SDQ-20 is not merely measuring a tendency to report somatic symptoms. The SDQ-20 has high convergent validity with the DIS-Q and good construct validity for the dimensional construct of somatoform dissociation. It demonstrates that somatoform dissociation correlates highly with psychological dissociation and supports the concept of conversion as somatic dissociation. From this work, Nijenhuis [9] proposed the term, somatoform dissociation, for the symptoms labeled hysteria in the nineteenth century.

Whether or not people who have dissociation are studied as subjects who have conversion seizures, other conversion symptoms, somatoform disorders, or dissociative disorders seems to depend on the collection methods of the researchers and the sheer timing of the co-occurrence of patients' conversion symptoms and a research study. Studies make clear that the dissociative disorders are highly associated with trauma [34,43,46,49] and that conversion seizures are highly associated with a history of trauma [6,36,66,67,69,74,79,87–89]. Conversion seizures and dissociative disorders have robust associations with each other and with co-occurring somatization disorder [37,68]. Association does not prove causality, but the multiple studies that consistently find dissociation co-occurring with conversion seizures strongly suggest this association is not accidental. I propose that the most logical approach to this literature is to agree with Nihjenhuis (and Janet) that conversion is a somatoform manifestation of dissociation.

Clinical case evidence

The strongest evidence for conversion seizures being a dissociative disorder comes from observing patients who have conversion seizures. When I first interviewed patients who had conversion seizures in the epilepsy clinic, I found that their life histories, symptoms, and mental status examinations appeared identical to those patients of mine in the psychiatry clinic who had dissociative disorders. Clinicians in the past 150 years have made similar clinical observations of dissociation in patients who had conversion seizures. Among the more famous are Janet's case reports of conversion hysteria resulting from dissociated traumas. The early twentieth-century American physician, Morton Prince [31], described the hysterical (neurasthenic) somatization of one personality of his female patient, B.C.A., in contrast to the lack of headaches, fatigue, or other symptoms when an alter personality was in evidence [8,31]; he documented how the alter personality caused conversion dystonia by influence from outside the awareness of the patient's neurasthenic personality. Nemiah [8] published a case of motor conversion that resulted from the alter state of a patient who had MPD. Janet [23,24] wrote at length about patients who had conversion symptoms (including seizures) related to dissociated traumatic experiences and who experienced remission after recalling their trauma. Janet's cases clearly demonstrate the re-enactment of dissociated trauma in conversion symptoms; he wrote: "The convulsions have all sorts of meanings..." [24].

Torem [10] and Nemiah [8] published case vignettes of patients whose non-epileptic seizures were re-enactments of dissociated trauma, expressions of dissociated anger, or manifestations of alter personalities abreacting trauma. Nemiah reported a dissociated alter personality of a patient that caused her conversion gait disturbance, weakness, and lower extremity paralysis. When the alter personality was in ascendance (in control of consciousness and the body), this patient had none of her usual conversion symptoms and seemed normal. The conversion symptoms recurred with a switch to the personality that usually was present. Nemiah's description of his patient closely fits my observations during clinical consultations of many conversion seizure patients.

During the past 14 years, I have evaluated approximately 800 patients in a tertiary care epilepsy clinic who had conversion seizures and have conducted structured research interviews on their axis I diagnoses, including dissociative disorders [36,67,80]. Patients who have conversion seizure are blatantly dissociative and nearly always have dissociative symptoms outside of their conversion seizures. I have observed many conversion seizures episodes provoked by discussion of past trauma or of the current life situation or emotional conflict that the seizures express. These patients often stare blankly and recurrently enter spontaneous trance states and have amnesia when topics of conflict are addressed. If these episodes of trance are not interrupted promptly, they often evolve into conversion seizures in the interview. Patients often exhibit amnesia for portions of the interview that address dissociation or childhood trauma. If asked, they often report depersonalization during and outside of conversion seizures. Many are unable to remember large portions of reportedly abusive childhoods or portions of domestic violence in adulthood. At times they spontaneously dissociate into frightened or angry ego states or other personality states when discussing emotionally evocative topics. Some declare spontaneously that they are more than one person (or their families volunteer this observation). Representative cases describe my patients who had conversion seizures with several dissociative conditions. They were treated by me to remission.

Case 1. Dissociated acute trauma

Mr. A. was a married middle-aged employed man who was referred by a neurologist who diagnosed his generalized shaking as nonepileptic with VEEG testing. Mr. A. initially reported onset of gross tremors of all extremities approximately 2 weeks after an auto accident 1 year previously in which his vehicle was violently rear-ended while at a stop sign beside a busy highway. His auto was propelled by the collision across the highway and was damaged severely. Mr. A. sustained soft tissue back and neck injuries but had no head injury. He remembered nothing between the initial impact and finding himself in an ambulance. He initially reported his symptom onset 2 weeks later during a medical test to assess his neck injuries but later recalled having symptoms in the ambulance ride to the hospital. His shaking occurred three to four times weekly and was interfering with his skilled labor job seriously. He reported diminished sensation from his shoulders downward since the accident and feeling "floaty" during his conversion movements. He was quite anxious about supporting his family and met criteria for major depression. He had been treated unsuccessfully with several anticonvulsants and a benzodiazepine and was on a seemingly adequate dose of an antidepressant. A previous attempt at treatment with hypnosis and relaxation training had not alleviated his tremors. He was extremely skeptical about psychotherapy and convinced he could not be hypnotized. He had filed a legal suit against the driver who had hit him. He reported a childhood of severe physical abuse by his father and witnessing the physical abuse of his mother and his siblings. He was unwilling to discuss his childhood, for which he reported considerable memory gaps. He indicated that he avoided anger and conflict because of their painful consequences in his childhood. He had been stressed in the past several years by anger about pressure in a previous job. His symptoms were threatening his childhood coping strategies of hard work and independence. He exhibited la belle indifférence with frequent smiling as he discussed emotionally painful topics. He exhibited mild to moderate hand and leg tremors when discussing his history and accident.

Mr. A. agreed reluctantly to hypnosis and achieved a deep trance rapidly. As muscle relaxation was suggested during induction, his right leg began to shake coarsely with forward kicking flexion and extension. This spread to his left leg, then to both arms in a nonphysiologic pattern. His right leg shook most vigorously. I had suggested before hypnosis that he might think about whether or not his accident was or was not related to his tremors. He began to remember the accident spontaneously during hypnosis and reported remembering being pushed helplessly across the four lanes of the high speed highway in his disabled auto, terrified that he would crash into the concrete barrier on the other side or be struck by cross traffic and killed. His forearms moved up and down repeatedly in coarse jerky movements and his right leg made forward pumping motions forward. He looked terrified and described the concrete abutment approaching while he tried helplessly to pump the brakes of his damaged car, to no effect. At the end of his memory, his right leg continued to move until I suggested that the accident was over and his brake foot had done its job and could stop now. This stopped his leg tremor. Outside of trance, he reported remembering this core part of the accident for the first time. He described seeing himself from outside his body as he flailed helplessly when his auto first was struck. He described watching himself from a viewpoint on the passenger side dashboard as he tried to steer and stop the car. In the subsequent 2 weeks after this hypnosis, the frequency and severity of his leg tremors diminished by 50% but his arm tremors worsened. He was seen for one more session of hypnosis during which he abreacted the accident again, focusing on his helpless horror as he tried to steer his auto with a broken steering mechanism. He spontaneously recalled neck pain and his bumpy ambulance ride in a cervical collar to the hospital, memories that had previously been unavailable to him. He had feared becoming quadriplegic and became partially numb from the neck down. I gave his arms permission to stop steering in the second hypnotic session and reminded him that he had not suffered a cervical fracture. After this session, he reported no more episodes of tremulousness when he was seen several weeks later. His sensory deficits cleared gradually. He remained in remission from conversion seizures for at least a year despite some severe family stresses. He was treated in five sessions.

This man had prior experience with dissociation from his child abuse experiences and automatically used a dissociative defense in the panic of a life-threatening accident. His dissociated memory of the accident was re-enacted in dissociative trance states until he recalled it during hypnosis. After he regained conscious control of his trauma and could discuss it, conversion into a somatic expression no longer was necessary. I observed him go into and out of spontaneous trances many times and exhibit anesthesia and tremors during these trances. His conversion clearly was dissociated trauma. The relationship of his current symptoms to his childhood was not explored at his request.

Case 2. Dissociative identity disorder and dissociated anger

Ms. B. ("Carol") was a college-educated employed woman who presented in her mid 30s, referred by her neurologist for conversion syncope and tremors that had recurred 6 months earlier. She reported first onset of syncope in adolescence with several episodes monthly. Her seizures consisted of syncope followed by generalized trembling, with amnesia for the entire seizure. At times, she presented with face lacerations from falling. She reported considerable childhood amnesia and several episodes of adulthood amnesia, including one fugue of nearly 10 miles. She reported that seizures and headaches had recurred after her recent divorce as memories of childhood sexual abuse increasingly bothered her. She had a major depression when evaluated. She was compulsively polite, studiously avoided anger or conflict, and was eager to please.

She lost brief amounts of time in spontaneously occurring trance states in treatment and often had a different affect as she stared angrily at the therapist. During psychotherapy for memories of childhood physical and sexual abuse and posttraumatic stress disorder (PTSD) symptoms, she dissociated into an angry-appearing personality who called herself "Ann" and who had a deeper voice and an irritated demeanor as she spoke derisively of the presenting personality as "she." Ann considered herself a different person from Carol and admitted to causing the syncope and seizures along with other angry personality states that Carol very faintly perceived as internal voices. Ann stated that Carol would not let herself feel any anger (I observed this as well) and dissociatively shunted her anger to the other ego states. They felt enraged at Carol, so they caused seizures to embarrass and punish her and to vent intolerable anger regarding childhood abuse. As Carol learned about Ann and her other personalities and began to share control of consciousness with them and allowed them to express feelings in therapy sessions, her seizures stopped for approximately 6 months. When she encountered her childhood abuser, seizures began again as Carol redissociated her anger and anxiety. When Carol struggled in psychotherapy with disbelief of her diagnosis, the seizures recurred as the disavowed alter personalities punished her for doubting their existence. Throughout the first 2 years of therapy, her seizures remitted when she accepted her dissociated alter states and recurred when she attempted to redissociate anger or dissociatively distance from awareness of her alter personalities. As she progressed to integration of her DID and resolved her PTSD, she recovered memories of her childhood abuse and achieved permanent remission of her syncope and seizures. Her seizures were dissociative episodes of the expression of anger by several alternate personalities formed during experiences of childhood sexual abuse. These personalities voiced anger at Carol for not stopping the abuse and at the abuser for his perpetration of rape and physical torture. She achieved full integration of her personality states and has remained free of seizures for more than a decade.

Ms. B.'s situation is common in conversion seizure patients who have DID. Alter personalities often create conversion seizures to express rage over childhood abuse that the host personality defensively dissociates from awareness. Another more common scenario, which I have insufficient space to demonstrate in this article, is patients who have affect-based ego states that abreact trauma (such as adulthood or childhood rapes or adult domestic violence) in conversion seizures. These patients often lapse into spontaneous trances and shake in interviews while expressing affect that the host ego state denies ever experiencing. In spontaneous trances, the ego states of these patients can describe the conflict or emotion that is producing the seizure. These ego states consider themselves the carriers of affect and trauma but they do not consider themselves separate entities. Patients whose conversion seizures are produced by dissociated ego states often come from families that create intense anger or conflict but severely punish any expression of anger in the patient. They dissociate their affect to survive emotionally.

Evidence from taxonomy

Do psychiatric classification systems support the dissociative nature of conversion seizures? That depends on which system is used. Since its inception, psychiatry has been unable to agree on classification of the somatic and psychological expressions of conversion, dissociation, and hysteria. The major problem with the *DSM* [2,11–14] classification of the offspring of hysteria is that it has ignored somatic expressions of dissociation in the dissociative disorders section and does not recognize the dissociative basis of conversion that is placed in the somatoform disorders section. From *DSM-III* [5] onward, the *DSM* has been out of step with the rest of the world, which uses the *ICD-10* [3], in which conversion is classified as a dissociative disorder. *ICD-10* states "the common theme shared by dissociative disorders is a partial or complete loss of the normal integration between memories of the past, awareness of identity and immediate sensations and control of bodily movements" [3]. In contrast, *DSM-IV* [2] defines dissociation as "a disruption in the usually integrated functions of consciousness, memory, identity, or perception of the environment." Somatic dissociative expressions are not mentioned in *DSM-IV*. In the *ICD-10* system, used in all the world except the United States, conversion has found a home in the dissociative disorders. *DSM* classification should take a hint from *ICD-10* about classifying conversion seizures. Following is a discussion of the details of this confused taxonometric situation.

The International Classification of Diseases classification

The *International Classification of Diseases, Ninth Revision* (*ICD-9*) [90] uses the term, hysterical neurosis, which includes conversion and alterations of consciousness and personality, but *ICD-9* makes no mention of the term, dissociation [91,92]. In moving from *ICD-9* to *ICD-10*, the term, neurosis, was dropped. *ICD-10* adds trance and possession states, dissociative stupor, and dissociative (conversion) convulsions, which are absent in *ICD-9* [91,92]. *ICD-10* also introduces organic conversion (dissociative) disorders. Each time conversion is mentioned in *ICD-10*, dissociation is included in the disease name.

I find the association of dissociation and conversion seizures in *ICD-10* welcome, but Coons [91] criticizes it for making conversion and dissociation seem synonymous. Nijenhuis [9] laments that *ICD-10* splits up the classification of positive and negative somatoform dissociation. In *ICD-10*, positive somatoform dissociation (additional sensations or movements) is grouped with somatoform disorders. In contrast, negative conversion symptoms (loss of or interference with sensations, identity, memory, or movement) are classified with the dissociative disorders. It is difficult to understand why positive symptom forms of conversion are somatoform and negative symptom forms are dissociative. *ICD-10* can use improvement in classification of conversion.

ICD-10 includes somatic dissociation (conversion) with psychological dissociative disorders in the section, "Neurotic, somatoform and other stress-related disorders." Section F44 of *ICD-10*, labels dissociative (conversion) disorders, which includes dissociative amnesia, fugue, stupor, dissociative type movement disorder (conversion movements other than seizures), dissociative convulsions, anesthesia and alteration of the senses of the dissociative type, mixed dissociative and conversion disorders, and others. There also is a "not characterized" dissociative disorder in F44. What is diagnosed as conversion seizures in *DSM-IV* might fall in *ICD-10* under dissociative convulsions (generalized movement), dissociative-type movement disorder (partial convulsive movements resembling complex partial epilepsy), or dissociative stupor (dissociative trance states resembling absence epilepsy). All three manifestations of dissociation have been diagnosed by neurologists as conversion seizures. The convulsive type was the type that was recognized by Charcot, Janet, and others as the classic symptom of hysteria. Unresponsive staring is the most common manifestation of conversion in Pakistan [94], the most common manifestation of "conversion seizures" in the United States [77], and extremely common in the conversion seizure population I see in an American epilepsy clinic.

I believe dissociative stupors without motor movements should not be diagnosed as conversion seizures, but they are diagnosed as such because neurologists who evaluate them are obligated to eliminate absence (petit mal) epilepsy as a cause. Depending on whether or not symptoms are evaluated first by a neurologist or a psychiatrist, a person who has unresponsive states might receive a *DSM-IV* conversion seizure diagnosis or a *DSM-IV* DDNOS diagnosis (or the "criteria set provided for further study" *DSM-IV* diagnosis of dissociative trance disorder) [2]. I propose that the *DSM* system should rename dissociative trance disorder as dissociative stupor in line with *ICD-10* and should include it with other dissociative disorders. This would help neurologists and psychiatrists to have dissociative stupor as a separate diagnosis from DDNOS, which is a hopelessly diverse collection of symptoms. Dissociative stupor would provide a more realistic alternative to conversion seizures for diagnosing many patients who have simple trance states.

The testimony of *ICD-10*, the world's most widely used classification system, is that conversion seizures are dissociative in their mechanism and are not somatoform disorders, as in *DSM-IV*. In moving from *ICD-9* to *ICD-10*, the World Health Organization partially restored the close relationship of conversion disorder and dissociation. The *DSM* system has yet to follow their lead and is out of step with the rest of the world's taxonomy.

The Diagnostic and Statistical Manual of Mental Disorders *system*

Modern American psychiatry has had herculean diagnostic struggles with the concept that conversion disorders are dissociative. In the early twentieth century, dissociation and conversion disorders were classified together as "conversion hysteria" [93]. The last three [2,13,14] of the five versions of the *DSM* [2,11–14] of the American Psychiatric Association have misled American psychiatry to see conversion in a somatic rather than a dissociative light. The first *DSM* (later known as *DSM-I*) [11] divided conversion and dissociation, listing them as separate categories (dissociative reaction and conversion reaction) of psychoneurotic disorders. Dissociative reaction included psychological dissociation, whereas conversion reaction designated somatic sensory and motor symptoms, deficits, and motor dyskinesias [93]. The *Diagnostic and Statistical Manual of Mental Disorders, Second Edition (DSM-II)* [12] dropped the term, reaction; retained the term, neurosis; and reintroduced the concept of hysteria. *DSM-II* used the term, hysterical neurosis, with subclassifications of conversion type (including pseudoseizures) and dissociative type. Fourteen categories of diagnoses related to hysteria emerged in *DSM-II*. The modern diagnostic shattering of hysteria had begun [93].

DSM-III [13] introduced drastic changes in American psychiatric nosology by attempting to shift from psychoanalytic and theoretically based classifications to descriptive diagnoses based on theory-neutral phenomena [8,93]. No taxonomy is divorced from the theoretic concepts of its authors, however [92], so the psychodynamic terms, conversion and dissociation, remained. In *DSM-III*, after more than 3800 years, "the traditional marriage of conversion and dissociative hysteria was annulled" [8]. *DSM-III* and its two successors placed conversion and other somatic manifestations of hysteria within the somatoform disorders; the psychological manifestations of hysteria became the five dissociative disorders. The placement of conversion disorder with the somatoform disorders emphasized its physical symptoms rather than their underlying cause. Conversion pain was separated from the other conversion manifestations as somatoform pain disorder in the somatoform disorders section of *DSM-III*. The terms, neurosis and hysteria, disappeared from the DSM nomenclature but did not die. The division of dissociation from conversion was not even-handed; dissociative disorders became an entire category of *DSM-III* diagnoses, whereas conversion became a subordinate diagnosis on a lower level of the taxonomy of somatoform disorders. This diagnostic scatter was logically consistent with *DSM-III*'s supposedly theory-free philosophy but was extremely shortsighted in light of the history of hysteria. Soma and psyche, always united in hysteria, were split asunder and the body was dissociated from dissociation.

DSM-III-R [15] preserved the diagnostic confusion about hysteria introduced by *DSM-III*. In *DSM-III-R*, conversion and dissociation remained in their respective separate *DSM-III* categories of disorders. *DSM-IV* [2] continued the separation of somatoform dissociation (conversion) and the psychological dissociative disorders. Somatoform pain (called simply pain disorder in *DSM-IV*) continued to be divided from other types of conversion in the somatoform disorders section. *DSM-IV* subdivided conversion into only four categories: conversion with (1) sensory symptom or deficit, (2) motor symptom or deficit, (3) seizures or convulsions, and (4) mixed presentation (more than one type of conversion symptom). Psychogenic "seizures" that present solely with unresponsive states (no motor movements) fall under example 5 of DDNOS in the *DSM-IV* rather than conversion disorder. This clinically is appropriate but is unhelpful to clinicians who see unresponsive patients who are suspected of having absence seizures and are diagnosed (I believe misdiagnosed) with conversion seizures.

DSM-IV's conversion subclassification is imprecise and results in patients who have conversion hemiplegia and those who have conversion thrashing receiving the same diagnosis. American psychiatric taxonomy has continued to be the world's only major classification system that ignores the dissociative nature of conversion. That needs to change.

Does classification matter?

Aside from the problems of having a dissociative disorder classification that works poorly in non-Western cultures [5,94] and the embarrassment of being the only system that does not recognize somatic expressions of dissociation, why does it matter that *DSM-IV* classifies conversion as a somatoform disorder rather than a dissociative disorder? The somatoform disorder classification of conversion in *DSM-IV* is important because it misleads clinicians in their view of conversion symptoms and the patients who have them. Names and classifications shape cognitions of the named phenomena. For example, policemen and firemen now are called police officers and firefighters to erase the gender expectations created by the former terms. Cognitions influence the treatments offered. Conversion seizure patients often report to me of being deeply hurt by physicians who have told them their seizures are not real or are faked, simply because they are called pseudoseizures. Categorizing conversion disorders with the somatoform disorders puts them in association with hypochondriasis and somatization disorders—disorders that raise negative feelings in physicians and sometimes are viewed as untreatable.

Classifying conversion as separate from dissociative disorders discourages physicians from exploring psychological dissociative symptoms in these patients. Patients who have pseudoseizure usually do not volunteer their psychologic dissociation (if they are aware of it), because they think it means they are "crazy" or they assume that "losing-time," for example, is completely normal. Physicians need to ask about dissociative symptoms, and they have to think of it to ask. Classification of pseudoseizures as a somatoform disorder matters because it encourages physicians to explore less fruitful avenues of etiology and does nothing to help mental health clinicians evaluate dissociative disorders in these patients. Studies show that patients who have pseudoseizure have substantial rates of dissociative symptoms [6,36,54,67,70] and of trauma experiences [36,66,67,79,87,95]. The *ICD-10* classification suggests clinicians look at trauma and dissociation in this population. *DSM-IV* does not. The success of these patients' treatment may be affected adversely by their dissociative disorders and trauma remaining undiagnosed and unaddressed [53]. I have witnessed many patients who have conversion seizures improve rapidly after discussing their trauma and learning how to avoid entering trance states that culminate in conversion seizures. Patients whose treatments are purely pharmacologic often continue to have frequent conversion seizures. Accurate diagnostic classification helps guide effective treatment. I cannot state it better than Janet: "You must be able quickly to recognize this disease, to foresee its evolution, to provide against its dangers, and immediately begin a rational treatment.... what is always very serious is to mistake a hysterical accident (symptom) for another one, and to treat it for what it is not" [24].

Summary

So where do these data and arguments leave us? Are there logical reasons to avoid recognizing conversion as a dissociative condition? The history of hysteria always has pointed to a link between conversion seizures and sexuality. Modern research shows the link often is sexual trauma and resulting dissociation. The history of conversion in the nineteenth century, via the clinical observations and theory of Janet, links conversion seizures to dissociation and psychological trauma. Janet provided a clear theoretical statement of the traumatic etiology of conversion and the link to dissociated ideas and emotions. The modern somatoform disorder theory of Nijenhuis [86], backed by solid research with the SDQ-20, provides evidence that today's conversion disorder patients are as dissociative as those of the Hôpital Salpêtrière. Hilgard's neodissociation theory [33] provides a construct for the modular structure of consciousness in conversion (as described by Janet). History points indirectly and theory points directly to conversion seizures as dissociative.

Modern research on the "diagnostic children" of hysteria is a messy melange of studies that points consistently to a large overlap of conversion symptoms, somatization, trauma, and dissociative symptoms in persons now diagnosed in *DSM-IV* with conversion disorder (all types), somatization disorder, dissociate identity disorder, DDNOS, and PTSD. Research supports the conclusion that persons who have conversion disorder have dissociation and persons who have psychological dissociative disorders often have conversion symptoms.

Clinical cases of persons who have conversion seizures provide the most striking evidence that conversion seizures are somatic dissociative episodes. My experience with 800 patients who have conversion seizure confirms this. Taxonometric evidence for the dissociative nature of conversion seizures is found in the *ICD-10* classification of them as dissociative (conversion) convulsions, within the dissociative disorders section. *DSM-IV* is out of step with the rest of the world in separating somatoform (conversion) dissociation from the rest of the dissociative disorders.

Conversion seizures have devastating effects on the lives of people who have them. They cannot drive, swim, or cook alone; they often cannot obtain or keep employment; they injure themselves; and they suffer many comorbid psychiatric illnesses [55]. The link between dissociation and conversion is important to understand because the lives and futures of patients who have conversion disorder hang in the balance between proper mental health evaluation and appropriate treatment. Conversion seizures are produced by lifetimes of unspeakable trauma and stress [36,80]. The best explanation of the link between dissociation, trauma, and conversion was penned by neurologist Andres Kanner: "We hypothesize, therefore, that patients with PPS (Psychogenic Pseudoseizures) and a prior history of abuse, initially make use of dissociation as a defense mechanism against the overwhelming trauma on its first occurrence. Over time, these patients learn (unconsciously) to dissociate in the presence of other traumatic as well as nontraumatic events. In this manner, dissociation becomes a pivotal coping device with stressful situations. Thus merely informing patients that their paroxysmal events are not epileptic may be meaningless to them, unless and until the process of dissociation is integrated in the explanation of their PPS occurrence" [69].

In closing, I wish to add that even a clinically untrained person can recognize the association of trance (dissociation) and conversion seizures. Poet Emily Dickinson [96], the astute nineteenth-century recluse of Amherst, Massachusetts, summed up the connection between women, trance, trauma, and conversion seizures in 1861:

> I like a look of Agony,
>
> Because I know it's true—Men do not sham Convulsion,
>
> Nor simulate a Throe—
>
> The Eyes glaze once—and that is Death—
>
> Impossible to feign
>
> The Beads upon the Forehead
>
> By homely Anguish strung.

References

[1] Exodus 16:35–6; Numbers 32:13. Holy Bible, contemporary English version. New York: American Bible Society; 1995.

[2] American Psychiatric Association. Diagnostic and statistical manual of mental disorders. 4th edition. Washington, DC: American Psychiatric Association; 1994. p. 477.

[3] World Health Organization. The ICD-10 classification of mental and behavioural disorders. Clinical descriptions and diagnostic guidelines. Geneva (Switzerland): World Health Organization; 1992. p. 151, 737–9.

[4] Veith I. Hysteria. The history of a disease. Chicago: University of Chicago; 1965. p. 2–10.

[5] Alexander PJ, Joseph S, Das A. Limited utility of IDC-!0 and DSM-IV classification of dissociative and conversion disorders in India. Acta Psychiatr Scand 1997;95:177–82.

[6] Harden CL. Pseudoseizures and dissociative disorder: a common mechanism involving traumatic experiences. Seizure 1997;6:151–5.

[7] Kihlstrom JF. Dissociative and conversion disorders. In: Stein DJ, Young J, editors. Cognitive science and clinical disorders. San Diego: Academic Press; 1992. p. 247–70.

[8] Nemiah JC. Dissociation, conversion, and somatization. In: American psychiatric association review of psychiatry, vol. 10. Washington, DC: American Psychiatric Association; 1991. p. 248–60.

[9] Nijenhuis ERS. Somatoform dissociation. Assen (The Netherlands): Van Gorcum; 1999. p. 26–39, 54, 66–81, 186.

[10] Torem M. Non-epileptic seizures as a dissociative disorder. In: Rowan AJ, Gates JR, editors. Non-epileptic seizures. Boston: Butterworth-Heinemann; 1993. p. 173–9.

[11] American Psychiatric Association. Diagnostic and statistical manual of mental disorders. Washington, DC: American Psychiatric Association; 1952.

[12] American Psychiatric Association. Diagnostic and statistical manual of mental disorders. 2nd edition. Washington, DC: American Psychiatric Association; 1968.

[13] American Psychiatric Association. Diagnostic and statistical manual of mental disorders. 3rd edition. Washington, DC: American Psychiatric Association; 1980.

[14] American Psychiatric Association. Diagnostic and statistical manual of mental disorders, 3rd edition, revised. American Psychiatric Association. Washington, DC: American Psychiatric Association; 1987.

[15] Lewis A. The survival of hysteria. Psychol Med 1975;5:9–12.

[16] Skey FC. Hysteria. London: Longmans & Co.; 1867.

[17] Parra J, Iriarte J, Kanner AM. Are we overusing the diagnosis of psychogenic non-epileptic events? Seizure 1999;8:223–7.

[18] Briquet P. Traité d'hysterie. Paris: Ballière et Fils; 1859.

[19] Ford CV, Folks DG. Conversion disorders: an overview. Psychosomatics 1985;26:371–83.

[20] Moreau de Tours JJ. De la folie hystérique et de quelques phénomènes nerveux propres à l'hystérie (convulsive), a l'hystérie- épilepsie et à épilepsie. Paris: Victor Masson et Fils; 1865.

[21] Van der Hart O, Horst R. The dissociation theory of Pierre Janet. J Trauma Stress 1989; 2(4):397–412.

[22] Taine H. De l'intelligence. 3rd edition. Paris: Librairie Hachette & Cie; 1878.

[23] Janet P. L'automatisme psychologique. Paris: Félix Alcan; 1889.

[24] Janet P. The major symptoms of hysteria. London/New York: Macmillan; 1907. p. 11, 22 [reprint of 1920 edition. New York: Hafner; 1965.]

[25] Janet P. Les actes inconscients et le dédoublement de la personalité. Rev Philos 1886;22: 212–23.

[26] Freud S. My views on the part played by sexuality in the etiology of the neuroses. In: Strachey J, editor. The standard edition of the complete works of Sigmund Freud, vol. 7. London: Hogarth; 1953. p. 269–79. [Strachey J, Trans.; original work published 1906.]

[27] Breuer J, Freud S. Studies in hysteria. In: Strachey J, editor. Standard edition of the complete works of Sigmund Freud, vol. 2. London: Hogarth; 1895. p. 80. [Strachey J, Trans.]

[28] Freud S. The etiology of hysteria, vol. 3. In: Strachey J, editor. The standard edition of the complete works of sigmund Freud. London: Hogarth; 1953. p. 189–221. [Strachey J, Trans.; original work published 1896.]

[29] Freud S. Three essays on the theory of sexuality. In: Strachey J, editor. The standard edition of the complete works of Sigmund Freud, vol. 7. London: Hogarth; 1953. p. 125–243. [Strachey J, Trans.; original work published 1905.]

[30] Ishikura R, Tashiro N. Frustration and fulfillment of needs in dissociative and conversion disorders. Psychiatry Clin Neurosci 2002;56:381–90.

[31] Prince M. The dissociation of a personality. New York: Longmans, Green & Co.; 1906. p. 13–6.

[32] Nijenhuis ERS. The development of the somatoform dissociation questionnaire (SDQ-5) as a screening instrument for dissociative disorders. In: Somatoform dissociation. Assen (The Netherlands): Van Gorcum; 1999. p. 41–53.

[33] Hilgard ER. Divided consciousness. Multiple controls in human thought and action. New York: John Wiley & Sons; 1977.

[34] Putnam FW, Guroff JJ, Silberman ED, et al. The clinical phenomenology of multiple personality disorder: review of 100 recent cases. J Clin Psychiatry 1986;47:285–93.

[35] Saxe GN, Chinman G, Berkowitz R, et al. Somatization in patients with dissociative disorders. Am J Psychiatry 1994;151:1329–34.

[36] Bowman ES, Markand ON. Psychiatric diagnoses and psychodynamics of pseudoseizure subjects. Am J Psychiatry 1996;153:57–63.

[37] Pribor EF, Yutzy SH, Dean JT, et al. Briquet's syndrome, dissociation and abuse. Am J Psychiatry 1993;150:1507–11.

[38] Greaves GB. Multiple personality 165 years after Mary Reynolds. J Nerv Ment Dis 1980; 168:577–96.

[39] Taylor WS, Martin MF. Multiple personality. J Abnorm Soc Psychol 1944;39:281–300.

[40] Schreiber F. Sybil. Chicago: Henry Regnery; 1973. p. 165–6.

[41] Martínez-Taboas A. Multiple personality in Puerto Rico: analysis of fifteen cases. Dissociation 1991;4:189–92.

[42] Middleton W, Butler J. Dissociative identity disorder: An Australian series. Aust N Z J Psychiatry 1998;32:794–804.

[43] Ross CA, Miller SD, Reagor P, et al. Structured interview data on 102 cases of multiple personality disorder from four centers. Am J Psychiatry 1990;147:596–601.

[44] Sar V, Yargiç I, Tutkun H. Structured interview data on 35 cases of dissociative identity disorder in Turkey. Am J Psychiatry 1996;153:1329–33.

[45] Boon S, Draijer N. Multiple personality disorder in the Netherlands: a clinical investigation of 71 cases. Am J Psychiatry 1993;150:489–94.

[46] Coons PM, Bowman ES, Milstein V. Multiple personality disorder. A clinical investigation of 50 cases. J Nerv Ment Dis 1988;176:519–27.

[47] Ellason JW, Ross CA, Fuchs DL. Lifetime axis I and II comorbidity and childhood trauma history in dissociative identity disorder. Psychiatry 1996;5:255–66.

[48] Ross CA, Norton GR, Wozney K. Multiple personality disorder: an analysis of 236 cases. Can J Psychiatry 1989;34:413–8.

[49] Coons PM. Dissociative disorders not otherwise specified: a clinical investigation of 50 cases with suggestions for treatment. Dissociation 1992;5:187–95.

[50] Coons PM, Milstein V. Psychogenic amnesia: a clinical investigation of 25 cases. Dissociation 1992;5:73–9.

[51] Bliss EL. Multiple personalities. Report of 14 cases with implications for schizophrenia and hysteria. Arch Gen Psychiatry 1980;37:1388–97.

[52] Cutler B, Reed J. Multiple personality: a single case study with a 15 year follow-up. Psychol Med 1975;5:18–26.

[53] Ettinger AB, Devinsky O, Weisbrot DM, et al. Headaches and other pain symptoms among patients with psychogenic non-epileptic seizures. Seizure 1999;8:424–6.
[54] Tutkun H, Sar V, Yargiç I, et al. Frequency of dissociative disorders among psychiatric inpatient in a Turkish university clinic. Am J Psychiatry 1998;155:800–5.
[55] Bowman ES. Psychopathology and outcome in pseudoseizures. In: Ettinger AB, Kanner AM, editors. Psychiatric issues in epilepsy. Philadelphia: Lippicott, Williams & Wilkins; 2001. p. 355–77.
[56] World Health Organization. Media Centre, Epilepsy, epidemiology. Available at: http://www.who.int/mediacentre/factsheets/fs165/en/. Accessed June 10, 2005. Geneva: World Health Organization.
[57] Stefánsson JG, Messina JA, Meyerowitz S. Hysterical neurosis, conversion type: clinical and epidemiological considerations. Acta Psychiatr Scand 1976;53:119–38.
[58] Loewenstein RJ, Putnam FW. A comparison study of dissociative symptoms in patients with complex partial seizures, MPD, and posttraumatic stress disorder. Dissociation 1988;1:17–33.
[59] Ross CA, Heber S, Anderson G, et al. Differentiating multiple personality disorder and complex partial seizures. Gen Hosp Psychiatry 1989;11:54–8.
[60] Steinberg M. The structured clinical interview for DSM-IV dissociative disorders (SCID-D). Washington, DC: American Psychiatric Press; 1993.
[61] Brende JO, Rinsley DB. A case of multiple personality with psychological automatisms. J Am Acad Psychoanal 1981;9:129–51.
[62] Cocores JA, Bender AL, McBride E. Multiple personality, seizure disorder, and the electroencephalogram. J Nerv Ment Dis 1984;172:436–8.
[63] Larmore K, Ludwig AM, Cain RL. Multiple personality—an objective case study. Br J Psychiatry 1977;131:35–40.
[64] Mesulam MM. Dissociative states with abnormal temporal lobe EEG: Multiple personality and the illusion of possession. Arch Neurol 1981;38:178–81.
[65] Schenk L, Bear D. Multiple personality and related dissociative phenomenon in patients with temporal lobe epilepsy. Am J Psychiatry 1981;138:1311–6.
[66] Alper K, Devinsky O, Perrine K, et al. Dissociation in epilepsy and conversion nonepileptic seizures. Epilepsia 1997;38:991–7.
[67] Bowman ES. The etiology and clinical course of pseudoseizures: Relationship to trauma, depression and dissociation. Psychosomatics 1993;34:333–42.
[68] Guz H, Doganay Z, Ozkan A, et al. Conversion and somatization disorders. Dissociative symptoms and other characteristics. J Psychosom Res 2004;56:287–91.
[69] Kanner AM, Parra J, Frey M, et al. Psychiatric and neurologic predictors of psychogenic pseudoseizure outcome. Neurology 1999;53:933–8.
[70] Kuyk J, Dunki Jacobs L, et al. Use of a dissociation questionnaire and a hypnotizability scaele in a population with pseudo- and epileptic seizures. Epilepsia 1995;36:S173.
[71] Kuyk J, Dunki Jacobs L, et al. Pseudo-epileptic seizures: hypnosis as a diagnostic tool. Seizure 1995;4:123–8.
[72] Kuyk J, Van Kyck RV, Spinhoven P. The case for a dissociative interpretation of pseudoepileptic seizures. J Nerv Ment Dis 1996;184:408–74.
[73] LaBarbera JD, Dozier E. Hysterical seizures: the role of sexual exploitation. Psychosomatics 1980;21:897–903.
[74] Tezcan E, Atmaca M, Kuloglu M, et al. Dissociative disorders in Turkish inpatients with conversion disorder. Compr Psychiatr 2003;44:324–30.
[75] Spitzer RL, Williams JBW, Gibbon M, et al. Structured clinical interview for DSM-III-R. Washington, DC: American Psychiatric Press; 1990.
[76] Derogatis LR. SCL-90: administration, scoring, and procedures manual-I for the R(evised) version and other instruments of the psychopathology rating scale series. Baltimore: Clinical Psychometric Research Unit of John Hopkins University School of Medicine; 1977.

[77] Leis AA, Ross MA, Summers AK. Psychogenic seizure: ictal characteristics and diagnostic pitfalls. Neurology 1992;42:95–9.

[78] Devinsky O. Nonepileptic psychogenic seizures: quagmires of pathophysiology, diagnosis, and treatment. Epilepsia 1999;39:458–62.

[79] Alper K, Devinsky O, Perrine K, et al. Nonepileptic seizures and childhood sexual and physical abuse. Neurology 1993;43:1950–3.

[80] Bowman ES, Markand ON. The contribution of life events to pseudoseizure occurrence in adults. Bull Menninger Clin 1999;63:70–88.

[81] Ramchandani D, Schindler B. Evaluation of pseudoseizures. A psychiatric perspective. Psychosomatics 1993;34:70–9.

[82] Nijenhuis ERS, Spinhoven P, Van Dyck R, et al. The development of the Somatoform Dissociation Questionnaire (SDQ-5) as a screening instrument for dissociative disorders. Acta Psychiatr Scand 1997;96:311–8.

[83] Bernstein EM, Putnam FW. Development, reliability, and validity of a dissociation scale. J Nerv Ment Dis 1986;174:727–35.

[84] Carlson EB, Putnam FW. An update on the dissociative experiences scale. Dissociation 1993;6:17–27.

[85] Nijenhuis ERS. Dissociatieve stoornissen en psychotrauma [Dissociative disorders and psychotrauma]. Houtem, Belgium: Bohn Stafleu Van Loghum; 1994. [in Dutch]

[86] Betts T, Boden S. Diagnosis, management and prognosis of a group of 128 patients with non-epileptic attack disorder. Part II. Previous childhood sexual abuse in the aetiology of these disorders. Seizure 1997;1:27–32, 49–50.

[87] Goodwin J. Pseudoseizures and incest. Am J Psychiatry 1979;135:1231.

[88] Gross M. Incestuous rape: a cause for hysterical seizures in four adolescent girls. Am J Orthopsychiatry 1979;49:704–9.

[89] Vanderlinden J, Van Dyck R, Vandereycken W, et al. The Dissociation Questionnaire: development and characteristics of a new self-reporting measure. Clin Psychol Psychother 1993;1:21–7.

[90] World Health Organization. Mental disorders glossary and guide to their classification in accordance with the ninth revision of the International Classification of Diseases (ICD-9). Geneva: World Health Organization; 1978.

[91] Coons PM. Commentary: ICD-10 and beyond. Dissociation 1990;3:216–7.

[92] Garcia FO. The concept of dissociation and conversion in the new edition of the International Classification of Diseases (ICD-10). Dissociation 1990;3:204–8.

[93] Kihlstrom JF. One hundred years of hysteria. In: Lynn SJ, Rhue JW, editors. Dissociation. Clinical and theoretical perspectives. New York: Guilford; 1994. p. 365–94.

[94] Syed EU, Atiq R, Effendi S, et al. Conversion disorder: difficulties in diagnosis using DSM-I. J Pakistan Med Assoc 2001;51:143–5.

[95] Snyder SL, Rosenbaum DH, Rowan AJ, et al. SCID diagnosis of panic disorder in psychogenic seizure patients. J Neuropsychiatry Clin Neurosci 1994;6:261–6.

[96] Dickinson E. Untitled poem, c. 1861. In: Johnson TH, editor. The complete poems of Emily Dickinson. Boston: Little, Brown; [original work written in 1861, but not published unedited until 1960]. p. 110.

[97] Jawad SSM, Jamil H, Clarke EJ, et al. Psychiatric morbidity and psychodynamics of patients with convulsive seizures. Seizure 1995;4:201–6.

[98] Nash JL. Pseudoseizures: etiologic and psychotherapeutic considerations. South Med J 1993;86:1248–52.

[99] Ramchandani D, Schindler BA. Distinguishing features of pseudocomplex partial seizures. Bull Menninger Clin 1992;56:479–86.

[100] Gross M. The clinical diagnosis of psychogenic seizures. In: Gross M, editor. Pseudoepilepsy: the clinical aspects of false seizures. Lexington (MA): Lexington Books; 1983. p. 79–86.

[101] Othmer E, DeSouza C. A screening test for somatization disorder (hysteria). Am J Psychiatry 1985;142:1146–9.

ELSEVIER
SAUNDERS

Psychiatr Clin N Am 29 (2006) 213–226

PSYCHIATRIC
CLINICS
OF NORTH AMERICA

Culture-Bound Dissociation:
A Comparative Analysis

Eli Somer, PhD[a,b,*]

[a]School of Social Work, University of Haifa, Mt. Carmel, Haifa 31905, Israel
[b]Maytal–Israel Institute for Treatment and Study of Stress, 5 David Pinski Street,
Haifa 34351, Israel

Pathologic dissociation has been defined as a "disturbance or alteration in the normally integrated functions of identity, memory or consciousness" [1] and as having a probable post-traumatic etiology [2,3]. The concept has generated considerable controversy that is centered on whether dissociative disorders (in particular, dissociative identity disorder) are valid clinical diagnoses [4,5] and on the import of the increased number of diagnosed cases in North America [6]. Some mental health investigators have claimed that Western clinicians inadvertently elicit these phenomena during therapy because of the allure of the dissociation model [7,8]. Others have implied that the notable increase in the diagnosis of dissociative identity disorder reflects a popular/professional North American trend that has developed into a form of social hysteria [9,10]. This article attempts to describe dissociation in the context of indigenous cultures and to resolve identified discrepancies in divergent idiom and classification systems. For this purpose, a broader, more inclusive, definition is called for. Dissociation is the experience of having a mind in which there can be at least two independent streams of consciousness flowing concurrently, allowing some thoughts, feelings, sensations, and behaviors to occur simultaneously or outside awareness. The cross-cultural perspective offered in this article aims to explore commonalities across cultural variations in phenomena involving these altered states of consciousness (ASC).

Colonial psychiatry espoused racially prejudiced ideas of biologic evolution and psychologic development to explain differences of experience and action between contemporary societies [11]. Current thought in comparative psychiatry recognizes that many non-Western illnesses should not be considered primitive varieties of universal taxonomic classes [12]. As a result of this

* School of Social Work, University of Haifa, Mt. Carmel, Haifa 31905, Israel.
E-mail address: somer@research.haifa.ac.il

0193-953X/06/$ - see front matter © 2005 Elsevier Inc. All rights reserved.
doi:10.1016/j.psc.2005.10.009   *psych.theclinics.com*

new, less ethnocentric approach, comparative, or cultural psychiatry has proposed a new class of mental illnesses unclassifiable in terms of Western psychiatry and termed "culture-bound syndromes" [13,14]. The notion that psychologic conditions that are unclassifiable by Western psychiatric nosology are "culture-bound" exceptions, to be contrasted with the "uninfluenced" Western medical standard, is unconvincing.

The occurrence of ASC and the belief in possession by discarnate entities has been documented throughout history and is present in most cultures of the world. Bourguignon [15,16] studied 488 societies and identified various forms of institutionalized ASC in 90%, possession beliefs in 74%, and possession trance in 52%. Lewis-Fernandez [17] argued that most non-Western cultures, which make up 80% of the world's total, exhibit culturally patterned dissociative syndromes, typically manifesting major discontinuities of consciousness, memory, identity, and behavior. In sum, dissociation ostensibly plays a significant role in the lives of billions of people outside North America. This finding could mean that in some cultures, dissociation might convey not only psychopathology but also more normative idioms of disavowing or distancing from certain experiences.

Ideas about the self, the soul, and the nature of reality influence the way society views the etiology of dissociative experiences, the way it shapes tolerance of these occurrences, and the way it determines attitudes to these phenomena and the need to treat or heal them. A culture that believes the self to be continuous but the relationship between what is internal and external to be distinct regards dissociation and psychologic multiplicity differently from a society that considers a continuous self illusory and self and universe one. The behavioral and medical sciences consider the human being an integrated biopsychosocial system, with all its experiences resulting from interaction of various subsystems within this integrated unit. The concept or theory of the soul is incompatible with this view. An alternative model assumes that humans consist of a shell that is occupied by an ethereal substance called a soul [18,19]. Among many non-Western cultures, the earthly casing, which we call self, yields to an alien entity whose character is culturally determined, resulting in an aboriginal dissociative presentation [15,17].

In contrast to psychiatry, which tends to inquire how mental disorders are alike across cultures, anthropology, the field most concerned with culture-bound syndromes, tends to study ethnic variance and cultural meaning in the expression of behavioral and experiential phenomena [20]. The present article is written from an etic perspective—one that rests on extrinsic concepts and categories with meaning for scientific observers. All the same, I will attempt to weave into my descriptions nonetiologic perspectives on some culturally determined ASC, also adopting the descriptive emic—the perspective with meaning derived from an insider's or native outlook. In doing so, I express my identity as a dissociation scientist-clinician whose interest in emic perspectives on cultural variants of dissociation is principally etic in its motivation.

Medical models of culture-bound ASC tend to view this mental experience as a form of disease that is universal, although colored by culture. A case in point would be Silverman's [21] description of shamans as hysterical and blatantly psychoticlike, and their shamanism as equivalent to acute schizophrenia. Interpreting native manifestations of ASC in terms of psychiatric classification systems could be an overextension of Western psychiatry and an unwarranted ethnocentric intimation of inherent pathology. Such pathologization is particularly dubious in light of empirically documented nonpathologic dissociative phenomena in the scientific literature (eg, nonvolition in hypnosis [22], hypnotic analgesia [23]). This article discusses native dissociation along two major classifications: nonpossession trance and possession trance.

Nonpossession trance

Uncritical assumptions that extraordinary states of mind are essentially pathologic are particularly unnecessary in cases in which trances are ritually induced in culturally sanctioned ceremonies. Under such circumstances, individuals often seek the rewarding effects of ASC.

Kinetically induced dissociation

Rhythmic music and dance are principal vehicles for religious and secular observance in many parts of the world. They provide a mechanism for communal coping—an expressive outlet with restorative advantages to ensure adaptive functioning, particularly under hard conditions [24]. It is believed that the communal ethos of tribal endurance and oneness with nature can generate a host of spiritual, affective, cognitive, and behavioral patterns based on a congruous relationship of nature, body, and mind [25–27]. In many indigenous communities, particularly in African cultures, kinetic expression is an important mode of symbolizing this ethos. Kelly and Locke [28] described the trance dances of the Kung bushmen and the role of the tribal shaman in inducing trances and possession trances in the dancing tribesmen. The Nigerian Tuareg were said to cure *tamazai*, "an illness of the heart and soul," through music and dance-induced healing rituals [29]. ASC among the Tuareg is not pathologic but is evoked for the purpose of easing distress of the body and the mind.

An ethnographic study by Somer and Saadon [30] described Stambali, a trance dance practiced in Israel by Tunisian-Jewish immigrants, as a prophylactic anxiolytic activity (eg, to deter the "evil eye") and as a healing ritual. Stambali is performed for the promotion of personal well-being or as a crisis intervention technique. The experience was described by informants as involving dissociated eroticism and aggression, and was said to often end in a convulsive loss of consciousness.

Elsewhere, self-induced trancelike states among indigenous folk dancers and their audiences were observed among American Indians [31], Australian

Aborigines [32], and Indonesian Balinese [33]. These ceremonies were said to serve as communal emotional outlets.

The quest of ASC, often through music and dance, seems universally pleasing. Becker-Blease [34] argued that although dance has been converted into recreation in our society, the potential for trance dance as a healing, meditative, and spiritual activity still exists. She maintains that new-age ambient and electronic trance music genres in modern Western culture have much in common with ancient styles of music produced for the same purpose.

Kinetically induced dissociation as devoutness

The wish to experience a discarnate feeling as an expression of spirituality and union with the Creator has been observed in many religions. Jewish learning and prayer often involves shut-eyed torso-rocking movements that are said to enhance the ability for enthralled focused attention. Jewish Hassidic chants and dance also involve practices that cultivate mind states that allow for ecstatic depersonalization or "dissolution of the fixed boundaries of self to achieve continuous awareness of God's Presence" (Rabbi Zalman, personal communication, June 16, 1985).

In Christianity, Charismatic and Pentecostal denominations encourage personal freedom of prayer style and spontaneity during their religious services that often involve rocking, singing, dancing, and various dissociative states. A major defining feature of Pentecostalism is the belief in glossolalia, or the ability to speak "in tongues" during ASC. This behavior is linked to "Baptism of the Holy Spirit" and was found to be unrelated to psychopathology [35].

In Islam, Sufism centers on the subconscious self (*nafs*) and its present and potentially more conscious relationship with divine Unity (Allah) as soul (*ruh*) [36]. Sufi practices promote what the twentieth-century Sufi, Hazrat Inayat Khan [37], called "the dissolution of the false ego in the real." Kennedy [38] described the *zikr*, a traditional form of chanting and movement ritual practiced in most Sufi orders, as an attempt to leave the material body to experience unity with God.

Reports from Southeast Asia the and Pacific rim nations illustrate similar processes. Simons and colleagues [39] described the festival of Thaipusam in Kuala Lumpur, Malaysia, in which devotees display their skill in achieving profound religious and spiritual experiences through specific trance-inducing dance patterns. Devotees demonstrate their spirituality by dissociating from physical pain: they spear their cheeks with long steel rods and pierce their chests and backs with small, hooklike needles.

In the Yoruba religion, brought to Cuba by African slaves, believers attempt to achieve spiritual power in which the individual's material self is said to "disappear," burned up by the passion and energy generated by liturgical drumming, chanting, and dancing [40]. African religions and culture were syncretized in Catholic Latin America to establish such cults as Candomble, Umbanda, Quimbanda, Macumba, and Voodoo. The institutions created within such Afro-Brazilian and Afro-Caribbean subcultures provide ritualized emotional release, based primarily on kinetically induced trances [41,42]. Akstein [43] claimed that through these ritual trances, participants of African descent in Brazil and the Caribbean find means of escape from daily worries, securing release of their blocked emotional tensions, liberating "primitive instincts and tendencies."

Other forms of nonpossession trance

Cross-cultural mental health scholars have described a variety of nonpossession dissociative syndromes, including amok, a dissociative episode characterized by a period of brooding followed by an outburst of aggressive behavior [1,44]; *latah* in Java, Indonesia [45], a condition characterized by an exaggerated motor startle response, often followed by hypersuggestibility and mimicry sometimes accompanied by obscene expressions [46]; and *pibloktoq* seen among the native people of the Arctic, an alteration of consciousness accompanied by erratic behaviors [47]. Anthropologic evidence suggests that many of these conditions are regarded as harmless. For instance, *latah* is often considered by Malays as undisruptive or even entertaining [48].

Much culture-bound dissociation in nonpossession trance states is considered normal. Inasmuch as it does not lead to distress or impairment, it often arises in willing subjects in appropriate (and frequently religious) contexts, and is commonly experienced as beneficial. Yet in some instances, nonpossession trance is strongly associated with potential psychopathology. In Latin America, a range of nonpossession somatoform and dissociative states have been portrayed over the years, including *susto,* a loss of soul from the body [49], and *ataque de nervios.* The latter is typically described among unmarried, undereducated Puerto Rican and Caribbean women following exposure to stressful events, with an estimated lifetime prevalence assessed to be 16% [50]. Common signs of *ataque de nervios* include headache, trembling, heart palpitations, amnesia, numbness of extremities, paralysis, pseudoseizures (see the article by Bowman elsewhere in this issue), and more [51].

A recent study on psychosocial stressors that precipitate dissociative trance disorder in Singapore revealed that 100% of the dissociative trance disorder group described at least one psychosocial stressor [52]. A common characteristic of indigenous ASC phenomena, mostly embedded in the context of conservative cultures, is apparently that they are sanctioned expressions of mostly disowned and disremembered aggression and sexuality. Could these behaviors represent the cultures' regulation of these conflict-ridden behaviors? In other words, is nonpathologic dissociation a distress-regulating mechanism?

Anthropologists have argued that nonpathologic indigenous dissociation often involves (1) ecstatic experiences in which subjects report a feeling of depersonalization (ex-stasis, meaning "standing outside") that mostly provided a temporary haven from anxiety, permitting the subject to view his or her distressing situation with composure; (2) aesthetic incidents in which subjects report derealization experiences of joyful distancing from the imperfections of the surrounding environs; and (3) hallucinatory experiences in which subjects feel they receive supernatural aid in handling severe life-stress often associated with conflicts [53]. Illustrations of these mechanisms can be found in many cultures. For instance, one of North and East Africa's oldest ASC rituals, the *zar*, was described by El-Guindy and Schmais [54] as mostly used by unhappily married housebound Egyptian women. A similar ritual was described by El-Islam [55] who studied 60 women participants in Qatar. The respondents were described as living under harsh social conditions and lacking a nuclear family because they were divorced or widowed. Over half [56] of the participants in these ritually induced ASC were described as hysterical, implying that they had attempted to cope with their somatized distress by using (kinetically induced) ASC. I maintain that dissociated expression of aggression and sexuality may be very adaptive in conservative societies because it provides relief for the oppressed while the traditional patriarchal social order continues to be respected. In many traditional communities, individuals are enmeshed in the collective identities of their families and tribes and see themselves as extensions of a collective core identity [57]. Many of these cultures are family and society directed. Conformity to a well-defined set of group norms is often expected of every individual. The personal struggle for a separate individual identity, one that may diverge from the values of the community, is often frowned on. In the Arab world, for example, individuality is said to be an illusion; emphasis and value are placed on affiliation [58]. Many traditional cultures are shame oriented, rather than more guilt-prone as the West appears to be. Thus, potential public shame or shunning can act as externalized superego and function as a powerful controlling factor within these societies. From a Western perspective, numerous aboriginal societies are characterized by authoritarian male hierarchies that are often repressive to women and children. Parental authority is rarely to be challenged or criticized. Hardship is often faithfully accepted as the will of God, as fate, or as the outcome of external agents such as spirits or demons. From early childhood, members of traditional societies are pressured to compromise their individuality and sacrifice it in exchange for the support and security provided by the family and the tribal community. As a result, many individuals become detached from their true emotions and needs. For example, Dwairy and Van Sickle [57] claimed that repression and disavowal of the self are inevitable consequences of traditional Arab society. The inability to focus on the self, to communicate about it, and to resolve intrapsychic conflicts can create not only somatoform dissociations such as hysterical paralyses or deafness but also psychoform dissociations. In these cases, traditional societies may offer culturally sanctioned dissociative means for the articulation and amelioration of emotional distress, without Western-style disclosure and self-exploration.

The inter-relationship between culture and idioms of illness was eloquently described by Geertz [59]. Commenting on the Javanese syndrome of *latah,* she noted that in this indigenous society, social etiquette has profound ethical importance. Conversely, obscenity (as often expressed during this culture-bound dissociative syndrome) in any form is deemed morally wrong and reproachable.

> It may be that here is a case in which the culture represents to a certain—as yet unspecifiable—category of disturbed persons, a coherent set of culturally meaningful behavior patterns, through which they find it possible to express their personal conflicts...Instead of creating their own idiosyncratic symptoms, they found a satisfying solution to their conflicts in the preexisting cultural pattern of latah.

Nonpossession trance such as ASC can therefore be seen as a sometimes-desired and socially sanctioned condition that can occur and dissolve under distinct regulation [60]. One Western equivalent to nonpossession trance could be nonpathologic dissociation (eg, psychologic absorption, daydreaming, hypnosis, or trance music and dance). Nonpossession trance could also represent a need to participate in dissociative processes intended to break away from irreconcilable conflicts through the creation of reality-altering solutions that are congruent with existing cultural constructions of reality. Probable Western equivalents would be maladaptive daydreaming [61] and the use of chemical dissociation through the ingestion of alcohol or cannabis [62]. In addition, nonpossession trance may provide a healthy, culturally sanctioned form of affect regulation not otherwise available to individuals but, in this case, provided by group experience.

Possession trance

Possession trance is defined as a single or episodic alteration in the state of consciousness characterized by the replacement of customary sense of personal identity with a new identity. This kind of trance is attributed to the influence of a spirit, power, deity, or other person [1]. Goodman [18] suggested that we might think of the entire phenomenon as representing a range of experience spanning from the socially sanctioned, construed, learned, and ritually controllable possession by revered deities at one end of the spectrum, to the unauthorized, unruly, and threatening occurrences of demonic possession at the other. Demonic possession syndromes are often time-limited, dramatic behaviors specific to a particular culture and are recognized as discrete by local informants and by medical observers. Similar to dissociative psychopathology, these unsolicited and socially nontolerated experiences cause considerable distress.

Possession trance and religion

For over a century, anthropologists have made observations and written reports on a diversity of cultures and societies that demonstrate a similar phenomenon of mind over mind, or spirit possession. Beliefs in the soul, spirits, and demons permeate Western and Eastern cultures and often are part of mainstream religion, frequently representing idioms of evil and sin. Developing countries are not the exclusive terrain of possession disorders and exorcism practices. Reports on these conditions were based on observations from countries in North America [63–65] and Latin America [66], the United Kingdom [67], Switzerland [68], Italy [69], France [70], Greece [71], Israel [30,72,73], Korea [74], and Russia [75]. A *Barna Research* poll showed that 54% of adult Americans believe that "a human being can be under the control or the influence of spiritual forces such as demons" [76]. Belief in demonic spirits is particularly common among conservative Christians, Roman Catholics, and Protestants, who believe in the inerrancy of the Bible. The phenomenon was recently the focus of academic interest in Rome when about 100 priests enrolled in an 8-week study of exorcism held at the prestigious Regina Apostolorum pontifical university [77].

The other major religions espouse similar conceptions. Islam refers to the world of the jinn (demons) as a potential source of possessing agents. The Qur'an and Sunnah indicate that jinn exist and that there is a purpose for their existence in this life, which is to worship Allah. The word *jinn* comes from an Arabic root meaning "hidden from sight." The ability to possess and take over the minds and bodies of other creatures is one of the powers attributed to the jinn.

In Judaism, possession trance is probably best understood within the context of Kabbalist polypsychic philosophy. The Kabbalist book, *The Teachings of the Zohar* [78], is a mainstay of Jewish sacred thought and describes the human psyche as composed of three main souls; it also elucidates the spiritual meaning of *gilgul*, the transmigration of souls. Many folkloristic possession tales inspired by Kabbalist tradition also contain the term *dybbuk*, a Hebrew word denoting a clinging, clutching, adhering agent for a sinner's transmigrating soul seeking correction [72].

Hinduism, one of the oldest religions of the world and the largest in India, promotes belief in reincarnation, the continuity of life from one birth to the next until the soul is realized and reaches nirvana [79]. Illness and misfortune are frequently regarded in India as the result of possession by a spirit, or *bhut bhada*. Benevolent possession by a deity is not considered a problem. When a demon or a harmful spirit is the possessing agent, treatment is sought, usually from a traditional healer [80]. Practitioners of the ancient Hindu system of medicine, the Ayurveda, often use their own possession states for diagnosis and confrontation with their patients' possessing spirits [81]. It was reported that 75% of psychiatric patients in India consulted religious healers about possession [82].

In China, Taiwan, and Korea, religious beliefs are mostly influenced by Confucianism, an obedience- and conformity-promoting faith, and by Taoism, a creed that embraces the principles of dual energies (yin and yang) and of a spirit world of immortal creatures that could intercede for devotees. Reports from rural areas in these parts of the world, where people cling to their religious convictions, describe possession agents representing spirits of deceased individuals, deities, animals, and devils, and describe possession as developing abruptly and manifested particularly among distressed women [83].

In Japan, most of the nation's many horticulturalist-, Shinto-, and Buddhist-derivate religions are said to attract individuals who have stress-related illness. Believers often consider illness as caused by *Dojo* possession: evil spirits, unhappy ghosts, or dangerous spirits of animals [18,84].

In the Pacific Islands of Polynesia, Melanesia, and Micronesia and among New Zealand's Maori, the prevailing faiths are associated with ancestor worship. Ancestor worship is based on the belief that the spirits of the dead continue to dwell in the natural world and have the power to influence the fate and fortune of the living. Ancestors are considered intermediaries between the supreme god (or the gods) and the people and can communicate with the living through dreams and by possession [85]. A recent study concluded that possession trance in the Pacific is widespread, predates contact with the Western civilization, and is now largely a female gender role [86].

Possession trance and dissociative disorders: culture-bound syndromes

Kluft [87] argued that in cultures that sanction indigenous possession states, multiple personality disorder (now known as dissociative identity disorder) would be uncommon. Ross [88] contended that pathologic multiplicity may develop more frequently in cultures such as the West, which is hostile to polypsychic views of the human experience. This argument may mean that culture provides a framework for reality perception and a blueprint for inner conflict and symptoms that are activated as a reaction to these conflicts. Martinez-Taboas [89] agreed that dissociation is a mechanism mediated by cultural expectations that influence the patient's perception, experience, expressions, and pattern of coping with stressors. This line of thought elucidates the potential for widely diverse expressions of dissociative mechanisms across the globe and regards dissociation as a constant factor in all human beings [90]. Although the present article addresses culture-bound syndromes of dissociation, to scrutinize only traditional cultures as potential shapers of dissociative expression would be incorrect. The symptoms of "Western" dissociative disorders have an intimate association with the existing cultural suggestions that envelop the individual who is constructing his or her emotional pain and fill it with "local content." A cultural perspective on Western dissociative disorders would contend that various attributes of these conditions are molded by cultural variables and organized in native semantic networks. Hacking [91] believes that multiple personality disorder/dissociative identity disorder is a recent and local phenomenon, stemming from nineteenth-century Western culture. A similar social constructionist view was presented by Spanos [5] who argued that whether enactments of multiple identities serve the purpose of promoting a religion or simply of getting care and attention for someone who feels they do not have enough, those enactments are guided by rules and expectations specific to the time and culture in which they are manifest, which are understood and given legitimacy by the authority figures involved (be they members of the clergy or psychotherapists) and the observing audience. I agree with Spanos that Western culture shapes many of the features of these conditions, but biologic and psychologic mechanisms are arguably mediated not primarily by local healers but by higher-level cultural idioms and meaning systems. Individualism, differentiation of the self, growth of the feminist movement, rising societal awareness, and concern over the issue of child abuse are powerful sociocognitive forces that have clearly been constitutive in Western dissociation. Regardless, similarities exist between Eastern and Western dissociative experience as serving an affect regulatory role.

Summary

Frequently, culture-bound dissociative syndromes convey not only an individual quandary but also principal societal tensions between the sexes, among age groups, or between the clergy and the laity. Because of their shared meaning, these occurrences often take place in well-defined situations, particularly when presented in collectivist cultures. In these milieus, such societal tensions, demonstrated by the "ailing" individual, can be played out and resolved. Clearly, these syndromes also have personal meaning and ameliorative functions for the characteristically socially weak protagonists, who can thereby regulate their circumstances in otherwise uncontrollable and generally depriving or oppressive conditions. This outcome can be achieved by invoking consensual, often sanctified community beliefs [92]. In more individualistic and modern societies, most oppressive structures operate within the family. Dissociation among Western individuals functions intrapsychically as an emotional analgesic and functions socially as a protector of the family institution. The common psychologic mechanism in dissociative conditions worldwide is self-hypnosis. Individuals may seek to induce ASC recreationally to enjoy metaphysical experiences. This conscious-altering process is exceedingly useful in the face of inescapable stress. Spontaneous self-hypnosis under duress has been established as a universal mechanism resulting in analgesia [93] and ASC [94]. The ameliorative function of dissociative conditions seems to stem from two recurring features, regardless of cultural context: (1) stress-induced self-hypnotic emotional and physical analgesia and (2) disguised and disowned cathartic expressions of forbidden feelings and behaviors.

This article highlights the great diversity of dissociative conditions globally and identifies probable commonalities in psychologic mechanisms and social functions. Future collaboration between anthropologists and mental health scholars is essential if we wish to advance cross-cultural investigation of dissociation. This sort of collaboration is essential for the refinement of the existing *Diagnostic and Statistical Manual of Mental Disorders/International Classification of Diseases* diagnostic criteria, which need to be made more relevant, more sensitive, and more specific to indigenous dissociation.

References

[1] American Psychiatric Association. Diagnostic and statistical manual for mental disorders. 4th edition, revised. Washington, DC: APA; 2000.
[2] Kluft RP. Multiple personality disorder. In: Tasman A, Goldfinger SM, editors. Annual review of psychiatry, vol. 10. Washington, DC: American Psychiatric Press; 1991. p. 161–88.
[3] Spiegel D, Cardeña E. Disintegrated experience: the dissociative disorders revisited. J Abnorm Psychol 1991;100:366–78.
[4] Piper A, Merskey H. The persistence of folly: a critical examination of dissociative identity disorder. Part I: the excesses of an improbable concept. Can J Psychiatry 2004;49:592–600.
[5] Spanos NP. Multiple identity enactments and multiple personality disorder: a sociocognitive perspective. Psychol Bull 1994;116(1):143–65.
[6] Horevitz R. Dissociation and multiple personality: conflicts and controversies. In: Lynn SJ, Rhue JW, editors. Dissociation: clinical and theoretical perspectives. New York: Guilford Press; 1995. p. 434–61.
[7] Bowers K. Dissociation in hypnosis and multiple personality disorder. Int J Clin Exp Hypn 1991;39(3):155–76.
[8] Frankel FH. Hypnotizability and dissociation. Am J Psychiatry 1990;147:823–9.
[9] Aldridge-Morris R. Multiple personality: an exercise in deception. Hillsdale (NJ): Erlbaum; 1989.
[10] Radwin JO. The multiple personality disorder: has this trendy alibi lost its way? Law Psychol Rev 1991;6:69–71.
[11] Devereux G. Normal and abnormal: the key problems of psychiatric anthropology. Some uses of anthropology: theoretical and applied. Washington, DC: Anthropological Society of Washington, 1956.
[12] Littlewood R. Pathologies of the West. Ithaca (NY): Cornell University Press; 2002.
[13] Yap PM. Classification of the culture-bound reactive syndromes. Aust N Z J Psychiatry 1967;1:172–9.
[14] Yap PM. Comparative psychiatry: a theoretical framework. Toronto: University of Toronto Press; 1974.
[15] Bourguignon E. Possession. San Francisco (CA): Chandler & Sharp; 1970.
[16] Bourguignon E, editor. Religion, altered states of consciousness, and social change. Columbus (OH): Ohio State University Press; 1973.
[17] Lewis-Fernandez R. The proposed DSM-IV trance and possession disorder category: potential benefits and risks. Transcultural Psychiatr Res Rev 1992;29:301–17.
[18] Goodman FD. How about demons? Possession and exorcism in the modern world. Bloomington (IN): Indiana University Press; 1988.
[19] Golub D. Cultural variations in multiple personality disorder. In: Cohen L, Berzoff J, Elin M, editors. Dissociative identity disorder. Northvale (NJ): Aronson; 1995. p. 285–326.
[20] Klienman A. Anthropolgy and psychiatry: the role of culture in cross-cultural research on illness. Br J Psychiatry 1987;151:447–54.
[21] Silverman J. Shamans and acute schizophrenia. American Anthropologist 1967;69:21–31.

[22] Weitzenhoffer AM. Hypnotism and altered states of consciousness. In: Sugerman AA, Tarter RE, editors. Expanding dimensions of consciousness. New York: Springer; 1978. p. 182–209.

[23] Hilgard ER, Hilgard JR, Macdonald H. Pain and dissociation in the cold pressor test: a study of hypnotic analgesia with "hidden reports" through automatic key pressing and automatic talking. J Abnorm Psychol 1975;84:280–9.

[24] Hannah JL. To dance is human. Austin (TX): University of Texas Press; 1979.

[25] Farr M. The role of dance/movement therapy in treating at-risk African American adolescents. Arts Psychother 1977;24(2):183–91.

[26] Hale-Benson JE. Black children: their roots, culture, and learning styles. Revised edition. Baltimore (MD): Johns Hopkins Press; 1986.

[27] Todson IL, Pasteur AB. Therapeutic dimensions of the Black aesthetic. J Non-White Concerns 1976;4(3):105–51.

[28] Kelly EF, Locke RG. Pre-literate societies. Parapsychol Rev 1982;13(3):1–7.

[29] Ramussen SJ. Reflections on Tamazai, a Tuareg idiom of suffering. Cult Med Psychiatry 1992;16(3):337–65.

[30] Somer E, Saadon M. Stambali: dissociative possession and trance in a Tunisian healing dance. Transcultural Psychiatry 2000;37(4):579–609.

[31] Jilek WG. Therapeutic use of altered states of consciousness in contemporary North American Indian dance ceremonials. In: Ward CA, editor. Altered states of consciousness and mental health. New York: Sage; 1989. p. 167–85.

[32] Fitzhenry J. Folk dancing as trance experience: some collected observations. Aust J Clin Exp Hypn 1985;13(2):134–8.

[33] Thong D. Psychiatry in Bali. Aust N Z J Psychiatry 1976;10(1):95–7.

[34] Becker-Blease KA. Dissociation states through age and electronic trace music. J Trauma Dissoc 2004;5(2):89–100.

[35] Francis LJ, Robbins M. Personality and glossolalia: a study among male evangelical clergy. Pastoral Psychol 2003;51(5):391–6.

[36] Douglas-Klotz N. Sufi approaches to transformational movement. Somatics 1984;5(1):44–52.

[37] Khan HI. The Sufi message, vol. 5. Metaphysics. Katwijk, Holland: Servire Publishers; 1962.

[38] Kennedy M. Participating in the life of Cairo: a letter on the Sufi dance. Catalyst 1985;16:21–3.

[39] Simons RC, Ervin FR, Prince RH. The psychobiology of trance I: training for Thaipusam. Transcultural Psychiatr Res Rev 1988;25(4):249–66.

[40] Amira J, Cornelius S. The music of Santeria, traditional rhythms of the Bata drums. Miami (FL): Crown Point; 1992.

[41] Akstein D. Terpsichoretrancetherapy: a new dimension in non-verbal psychotherapy. Presented at the International Congress for Psychosomatic Medicine and Hypnosis. Mainz, Germany, 1974.

[42] Stubbe H. Psychotherapy in Brazil. Z Psychosom Med Psychoanal 1980;26(1):79–93.

[43] Akstein D. Perspectivas Psicosociales de la aplicacion de la Terpsicoretranceterapia. Psychopathologie Africaine 1974;10:121–9.

[44] Prince R. Amok then and now. Transcultural Psychiatric Res Rev 1991;28:219–29.

[45] Kenny MG. Paradox lost: the latah problem revisited. J Nerv Ment Dis 1983;171(3):159–67.

[46] Ward CA. The cross-cultural study of altered states of consciousness and mental health. In: Ward CA, editor. Altered states of consciousness and mental health: a cross-cultural perspective. Newbury Park, CA: Sage; 1989. p. 125–44.

[47] Foulks EF. The transformation of "Arctic hysteria.". In: Simons RC, Hughes CC, editors. The culture-bound syndromes. Dordrech, Netherlands: Reidel; 1985. p. 307–24.

[48] Colson AC. Perceptions of abnormality in a Malay village. In: Wagner NN, Tan ES, editors. Psychological problems and treatment in Malaysia. Kuala Lumpur, Malaysia: University of Malaya Press; 1971. p. 85–103.

[49] Rubel A. The epidemiology of a folk illness. Ethnology 1964;5(3):268–83.

[50] Guarnaccia PJ, Canino G, Rubio-Stipec M, et al. The prevalence of *ataques de nervios* in the Puerto Rico disaster study. The role of culture in psychiatric epidemiology. J Nerv Ment Dis 1993;181:157–65.

[51] Escobar JI. Transcultural aspects of dissociative and somatoform disorders. Cultural Psychiatry 1995;18:555–69.

[52] Beng-Yeong N, Yiong-Huak C. Psychosocial stressors that precipitate dissociative trance disorder in Singapore. Aust N Z J Psychiatry 2004;38(6):426.

[53] Valla JP, Prince RH. Religious experiences as self-healing mechanisms. In: Ward CA, editor. Altered states of consciousness and mental health. New York: Sage; 1989. p. 149–66.

[54] El-Guindy H, Schmais C. The zar: an ancient dance of healing. Am J Dance Ther 1994;16(2): 107–20.

[55] El-Islam F. Culture-bound neurosis in Qatar women. Int J Soc Psychiatry 1974;11:167–8.

[56] Okasha AA. Cultural psychiatric study of el-zar cult in UAR. Br J Psychiatry 1966;112: 1217–21.

[57] Dwairy M, Van Sickle TD. Western psychotherapy in traditional Arabic societies. Clin Psychol Rev 1996;16(3):231–49.

[58] Saleh MA. Implications for counseling in the Arab world. Sch Psychol Int 1986;7:71–5.

[59] Geertz H. Latah in Java: a theoretical paradox. Indonesia 1968;5:93–104.

[60] Herskovits MJ. Life in a Haitian valley. Garden City (NY): Doubleday; 1971.

[61] Somer E. Maladaptive daydreaming: a qualitative inquiry. J Contemp Psychother 2002; 32(2):195–210.

[62] Somer E, Avni R. Dissociative phenomena among recovering heroin users and their relationship to duration of abstinence. J Soc Work Pract Addict 2003;3(1):25–38.

[63] Rosik CH, Rosik CH. Possession phenomena in North America: a case study with ethnographic, psychodynamic, religious and clinical implications. J Trauma Dissoc 2004;5: 49–76.

[64] Bull DL, Ellason JW, Ross CA. Exorcism revisited: positive outcomes with dissociative identity disorder. J Psychol Theol 1998;26:188–96.

[65] Buch M. Exorcism-seekers: clinical and personality correlates. Vancouver: University of British Columbia, Canada; 1995.

[66] Krippner S. Cross-cultural treatment perspectives on dissociative disorders. In: Rhue JW, Lynn SJ, editors. Dissociation: clinical and theoretical perspectives. New York: Guilford Press; 1994. p. 338–61.

[67] Hale AS, Pinninti NR. Exorcism-resistant ghost possession treated with clopenthixol. Br J Psychiatry 1994;165:386–8.

[68] Pfeifer S. Belief in demons and exorcism in psychiatric patients in Switzerland. Br J Med Psychol 1994;67:247–58.

[69] Ferracuti S, Sacco R, Lazzari R. Dissociative trance disorder: clinical and Rorschach findings in ten persons reporting demon possession and treated by exorcism. J Pers Assess 1996; 66:525–39.

[70] Achaintre A. Exorcisme et pratique medicale [Exorcism and medical practice]. Psychol Med (Paris) 1988;20:733–5.

[71] Vlachos IO, Beratis S, Hartocollis P. Magico-religious beliefs and psychosis. Psychopathology 1997;30:93–9.

[72] Somer E. Trance possession disorder in Judaism: sixteenth-century dybbuks in the Near East. J Trauma Dissoc 2004;5:131–46.

[73] Daie N, Witztum E, Mark M, et al. The belief in the transmigration of souls: psychotherapy of a Druze patient with severe anxiety reaction. Br J Med Psychol 1992;65:119–30.

[74] Yi KY. Shin-byung (divine illness) in a Korean woman. Cult Med Psychiatry 2000;24: 471–86.

[75] Worobec CD. Possessed: women, witches, and demons in imperial Russia. DeKalb (IL): Northern Illinois University Press; 2001.

[76] The Barna Group. Americans draw theological beliefs from diverse points of view. Barna Research Online, 2002-OCT-8. Available at: http://www.barna.org/FlexPage. aspx?Page=BarnaUpdate&BarnaUpdateID=122. Accessed March 18, 2005.

[77] Wilkinson T. Priests sign up for exorcism. Los Angeles Times. February 18, 2005.

[78] Tishbi Y. *Torat ha-Zohar* [The teachings of the *Zohar*]. Jerusalem, Israel: Mosad Bialik; 1982.

[79] Juthani NV. Psychiatric treatment of Hindus. Int Rev Psychiatry 2001;13(2):125–30.

[80] Castillo RJ. Spirit possession in South Asia, dissociation or hysteria? I. Theoretical background. Cult Med Psychiatry 1994;18(1):1–21.

[81] Gadit AA. Ethnopsychiatry—a review. J Pakistan Med Assoc 2003;53(10):1–6.

[82] Campion J, Bhugra D. Religious healing in South India. Presented at the World Association of Social Psychiatry Meeting. Hamburg, Germany, 1994.

[83] Gaw AC, Qin-zhang D, Levine RE, et al. The clinical characteristics of possession disorder among 20 Chinese patients in the Hebei province of China. Psychiatr Serv 1998;49:360–5.

[84] Davis W. Dojo: magic and exorcism in modern Japan. Stanford (CA): Stanford University Press; 1980.

[85] Frazer JG. The belief in immortality and the worship of the dead [three vols., 1913–24, reprinted]. New York: Macmillan; 1968.

[86] Dobin JD, Hezel FX. The distribution of spirit possession and trance on Micronesia. Pac Stud 1996;19(2):105–48.

[87] Kluft RP. Multiple personality disorders. In: Spiegel D, editor. Dissociative disorders: a clinical review. Baltimore (MD): Sidran Press; 1993. p. 17–44.

[88] Ross C. The dissociated executive self and the cultural dissociation barrier. Dissociation 1991;3:64–5.

[89] Martinez-Taboas A. Multiple personality disorder as seen from a social constructionist viewpoint. Dissociation 1991;4:129–33.

[90] Schumaker JF. The corruption of reality: a unified theory of religion. Amherst (NY): Prometheus; 1995.

[91] Hacking I. Multiple personality and the sciences of memory. Princeton (NJ): Princeton University Press; 1995.

[92] Lewis IM. Spirit possession and deprivation cults. Man 1966;1:307–29.

[93] Van der Kolk BA, Greenberg MS, Orr SP, et al. Endogenous opioids, stress induced analgesia, and posttraumatic stress disorder. Psychopharmacol Bull 1989;25(3):417–21.

[94] Cancio LC. Stress and trance in freefall parachuting: a pilot study. Am J Clin Hypn 1991; 33(4):225–34.

ELSEVIER
SAUNDERS

PSYCHIATRIC
CLINICS
OF NORTH AMERICA

Psychiatr Clin N Am 29 (2006) 227–244

The Scope of Dissociative Disorders: An International Perspective

Vedat Sar, MD

Clinical Psychotherapy Unit and Dissociative Disorders Program,
Medical Faculty of Istanbul, Istanbul University, 34390 Capa, Istanbul, Turkey

In contrast to the meaning that the unfortunate term "posttraumatic stress disorder" imposes, trauma is not identical with a noxious event [1]. It is a complex sociopsychologic process with subjective and objective components following traumatic experience that is embedded in past, present, and future. A comprehensive definition of psychic trauma is the loss of cohesion in internal world, in external reality, and between them; creating loss of psychic harmony in a given time point and across the life span. In that sense, trauma and dissociation are concepts that dissolve in each other [2]. An approach to trauma without understanding dissociation remains meaningless from both psychiatric and sociopsychologic point of views. Extracting dissociation from concepts and adaptations of everyday life or from general psychopathology empties its content and marginalizes it (ie, it is a disservice to both the traumatized person and the professional who wants to help them).

This issue includes a special article about culture-bound aspects of dissociation (see the article by Somer elsewhere in this issue). This article is concerned mainly with the documentation of the universality of dissociative disorders as presented by empirical studies conducted in various countries using standardized assessment instruments. The similarities between dissociative patients in various cultures are obvious [3,4]. Cultural differences between perceptions and conceptualizations of researchers and mental health professionals in psychiatry are higher than those in any other medical specialty. This seems to be the main reason why dissociative disorders have been considered by some authors as culture bound syndromes; somewhat paradoxically, either as a merely North American disorder or a premodern phenomenon seen in exotic cultures, primitive societies, or mystic-religious communities. Modern pioneers of the field initiated a rising wave of

---

E-mail address: vsar@istanbul.edu.tr

0193-953X/06/$ - see front matter © 2005 Elsevier Inc. All rights reserved.
doi:10.1016/j.psc.2005.10.007

dissociation studies in North America in the 1980s, to be slowed down in 1990s by the so-called "backlash" movement, which has been balanced by a steadily enlarging and emerging international research. Large-scale systematic studies on dissociative disorders in this initial period of international research flourished mainly in The Netherlands [3], Turkey [4], and Germany [5]. Case series also have been published from Switzerland [6] and Australia [7]. Case presentations and many other contributions continue to come from many countries throughout the world. This article does not claim to be an exhaustive one. Rather, to elucidate the way for future research, it tries to evaluate the key aspects of this mosaic of clinical and scientific endeavors.

Epidemiology of dissociation: a common psychiatric disorder

Most of the screening studies on dissociative disorders have been conducted in clinical settings (Table 1). Studies on dissociative disorders in Istanbul, Turkey, yielded prevalence slightly above 10% among psychiatric inpatients and outpatients [8–10]. Although still considerable, these rates were lower in The Netherlands [11], Germany [5], and Switzerland [6] among inpatients (between 4.3% and 8%). A Finnish study [12] reported higher rates for psychiatric outpatients (14%) and inpatients (21%). A study conducted among emergency admissions in Istanbul yielded the highest rate (35.7%) [13].

Two large-scale studies conducted in the general population of Sivas, Turkey, provided detailed information about the prevalence of all dissociative disorders in the community. The first one was conducted on a representative sample of 994 participants from both genders [14]. Although there was no difference in average Dissociative Experiences Scale (DES) scores between genders, there were two times more women than men among high scorers. The second study was conducted on a representative female sample of 648 participants in the same city using a structured diagnostic interview (ie, the Dissociative Disorders Interview Schedule) [15]. The overall prevalence of dissociative disorders was 18.3%. The largest group was Dissociative Disorder not Otherwise Specified (DDNOS) (8.3%). A total of 7.3% of the population reported having had dissociative amnesia at least once throughout their life. The prevalence of depersonalization disorder was 1.4%, whereas 1.1% of the population had Dissociative Identity Disorder (DID). Conditions based primarily on presence of distinct personality states (ie, DID and allied forms of DDNOS) together built up a prevalence of 5.2%. Only one proband (0.2%) had dissociative fugue as a solitary phenomenon; when present it was usually part of a more complex dissociative disorder (DID or DDNOS).

In The Netherlands, 378 subjects from a nonclinical population were screened using the Dissociation Questionnaire, a self-rating scale of European origin [16,17]. A total of 2.1% of the participants had a score above the

Table 1
Summary of dissociative disorder prevalence studies among psychiatric patients in four countries: Turkey, Switzerland, Germany, and The Netherlands

Study	% Inclusion rate	Number of subjects	Diagnostic instrument	Cutoff on dissociative experiences scale	% Rate of dissociative identity disorder	Rate of dissociative disorder	Dissociative experiences scale score		
							mean	SD	> %DES[b]
Psychiatric inpatients									
Tutkun et al [8]	63.6	166	DDIS	30	5.4[a]	10.2[a]	17.8	14.9	14.5
Modestin et al [6]	—	207	DDIS	20	0.4	5	13.7	13.5	12
Gast et al [5]	—	115	SCID-D	20	0.9	4.3	—	—	21.7
Friedl and Draijer [11]	50.4	122	SCID-D	25	2	8	20	18.1	29.5
Psychiatric outpatients									
Sar et al [9]	81.5	150	DDIS	30	2[a]	12[a]	15.3	14	15.3
Sar et al [10]	79.5	240	SCID-D	25	2.5	13.8	20	18.9	27.9
Psychiatric emergency unit									
Sar et al [13]	43.3	44	SCID-D	25	13.6	35.7	23.3	19.1	38.6

Abbreviations: DDIS, Dissociative Disorders Interview Schedule; DES, Dissociative Experiences Scale; SCID-D, Structured Clinical Interview for Dissociative Disorders.
[a] Clinically confirmed diagnosis.
[b] Percentage of patients with a Dissociative Experiences Scale score above cutoff point.

cutoff point (score of 2.5), and 0.5% had a score comparable with those of patients with dissociative disorders (scores of 3 or higher). Of the eight high scorers, seven were women. A total of 2.9% of the women and 0.7% men had scores above the 2.5 cutoff, a ratio of 4 to 1. In a large general psychiatric population in Germany [18], there were no significant gender differences in the distribution of high dissociators.

In Germany, a screening study was conducted on 51 male criminal offenders admitted to a medicolegal institution by the court so as to understand diminished or lack of responsibility for the offense because of psychiatric disorder, including a large group of persons with substance-use disorders [19]. Using the Structured Clinical Interview for Diagnostic and Statistical Manual (DSM)-IV Dissociative Disorders [20], a high prevalence of dissociative symptoms and disorders (23.5%), mostly DDNOS, were demonstrated. A total of 22.6% of the group had a DES score 20 or higher. In Turkey [21] 26.8% of 108 male prisoners in a regular correctional center had a DES score 20 or above. This rate was 18.5% for DES scores 30 or above. According to the Structured Clinical Interview for DSM-IV Dissociative Disorders, 15.7% of the subjects had a dissociative disorder, either DDNOS (N = 10) or dissociative amnesia (N = 7). Interestingly, only 2.8% of the prisoners fit the DSM-III-R borderline personality disorder criteria, whereas this rate was 28% for antisocial personality disorder and 66.4% for lifetime posttraumatic stress disorder diagnosis [21].

Overall, independent studies from various countries clearly demonstrate that dissociative disorders constitute a common mental health problem not only in clinical practice but also in the community. The lack of dissociative disorder sections in commonly used general psychiatric screening instruments has led to the omission of dissociative disorders in large-scale epidemiologic studies. Although studies using specific instruments have began to correct this perception, the inclusion of dissociative disorders in general psychiatric screening studies will help to gather detailed information about comorbidity issues (see the article by Sar and Ross elsewhere in this issue). Differences between rates obtained in various settings may be related to differences in treatment-seeking behavior and in mental health delivery systems. In particular, the relatively high prevalence of DDNOS both in clinical settings and in the community points to the necessity for a thorough revision in the DSM-IV dissociative disorders section.

Somatoform aspect of dissociative disorders: conversion disorder

There has been a common belief that somatization is a phenomenon seen among people with low socioeconomic level and in less industrialized countries. Several studies on conversion disorder in The Netherlands, Turkey, and Germany, however, challenged this notion. Moreover, there are great similarities in symptom patterns between Turkish and Dutch samples (ie, only pseudoseizure was more frequent among Turkish dissociative patients). Pseudoseizure has been known as the most prevalent conversion symptom in Turkey [22,23].

Conversion disorder is extremely common in Turkey. All Turkish psychiatrists are faced virtually with hundreds, if not thousands, of conversion disorder patients throughout their careers. In a screening study conducted in a primary health care center in semirural area near Ankara, Turkey, the prevalence of conversion symptoms (ie, somatoform dissociation) in the preceding month was 27.2%, and the lifetime rate increased to 48.2% [24]. This phenomenon is exactly in accordance with the high prevalence rates obtained for dissociative disorders in Turkey. A 2-year follow-up study in Sivas, Turkey, demonstrated that 47.4% of patients diagnosed as having conversion disorder previously had a DSM-IV dissociative disorder on the first axis (ie, an overt psychoform dissociative condition) [25]. This figure was 30.5% in a screening study conducted among inpatients with conversion disorder in Elazig, Turkey [26]. The rates obtained for conversion disorder serve as direct indicator of the prevalence of dissociative disorders as a common psychiatric disorder.

Besides the large overlap with dissociative disorders, patients with conversion disorder have overall psychiatric symptom scores close to those of general psychiatric patients, suggesting high general psychiatric comorbidity [27,28]. In a primary health care center near Ankara, Turkey, conversion symptoms were more frequently observed among subjects who had an International Classification of Diseases (ICD)-10 diagnosis [24]. Depression, generalized anxiety disorder, and neurasthenia were the most prevalent psychiatric disorders among them. Dissociative disorder comorbidity, however, is a significant predictor of this pattern (ie, higher general psychiatric comorbidity including somatization disorder, dysthymic disorder, major depression, and borderline personality disorder, with self-destructive behavior and suicide attempts) [25]. There was high comorbidity between dissociative disorder and borderline personality disorder in this spectrum, whereas generalized anxiety disorder was the sole category distributed homogenously between dissociative and nondissociative groups.

Studies in The Netherlands and Turkey documented that patients with conversion disorder reported high levels of childhood trauma [25,29]; moreover, two Turkish studies documented that conversion disorder patients with a dissociative disorder report childhood trauma more frequently than those without [25,26]. In contrast, a Dutch study on patients with conversion disorder or chronic pelvic pain did not demonstrate a relationship between childhood trauma and dissociation; only somatoform dissociation was related to physical abuse in childhood. After controlling for the overall level of psychopathology, the authors recommended that clinicians be more alert to recent potentially traumatizing experiences or comorbid psychiatric disorders [30]. Another Dutch study did not find higher levels of hypnotizability among patients with conversion disorder compared with normal controls [31]. Although the patients had frequent childhood trauma histories and elevated dissociation scores, after controlling the effect of overall psychopathology, the authors concluded that the role of childhood trauma and dissociation in conversion disorder is not clear either. They underline that psychoform dissociation scales might not be able to assess dissociation in conversion disorder, but a measure specific for somatoform dissociation might demonstrate this relationship better [32]. A study in patients with chronic headache and low back pain in Turkey supported this observation (ie, there was no relationship between childhood trauma and DES scores; however, patients with a childhood history of neglect had higher somatoform dissociation scores) [33]. See the article by Lyons-Ruth elsewhere in this issue regarding relational versus physical or sexual trauma in the etiology of dissociative disorders.

The large overlap with psychoform dissociative disorders and the relationship between childhood trauma and somatoform symptoms support Janet's notion that conversion disorder is the somatoform aspect of dissociation [34,35]. A Dutch group [36] hypothesized that there is a similarity between evolutionary animal defensive responses to variable predatory imminence and injury and certain somatoform dissociative symptoms of trauma-reporting patients who have dissociative disorder (eg, freezing and anesthesia-analgesia). Other pathways facilitating somatoform type of dissociation and choice of a particular symptom (eg, pseudoseizure) need to be explored. There is growing interest in this issue among clinicians and researchers in neurology (see the article by Bowman elsewhere in this issue).

Borderlands of dissociative disorders: from psychosis to obsessions

Dissociative disorders can easily be differentiated from schizophrenic disorder using standardized assessment instruments [37]. An acute psychotic disorder, "hysterical psychosis," however, has a special place in this context. It has been well known in Turkish mainstream psychiatry that hysterical psychosis has a dissociative nature and is qualitatively different from schizophrenic disorder [38]. This condition has been considered as a "pseudopsychotic dissociation," which does not constitute an indication for neuroleptic drug treatment [38]. It should be held separate from other psychotic disorders and should rather be classified among dissociative disorders. Short-term hospitalization, supportive psychotherapy, and especially separation from a distressing family environment have been the most useful measures for the management of the disorder. According to a retrospective investigation of a large series of consecutive patients hospitalized in a Turkish university psychiatry clinic between 1970 and 1980 and diagnosed as some form of "hysteria," who constituted 6% of the whole inpatient population in a 10-year period at this institution, 7.8% were diagnosed as hysterical psychosis [39]. Fully in accordance with these observations, after evaluation of an Israeli case, Van der Hart and coworkers [40] emphasized that dissociative psychosis may last even longer than a few weeks and the main characteristic of this condition is not the acute course but its dissociative nature.

Observations on dissociative psychosis are not limited to certain cultures [41]. Besides the concept of trauma-induced psychosis [40], dissociative psychosis can also be linked to the psychogenic or reactive psychosis concepts of European psychiatry [42,43]. Besides being a discernable diagnosis, dissociative psychosis may happen in patients with dissociative identity disorder as a result of decompensation after an acute stressful life event. This may manifest itself as a struggle for control and influence between alter identities carrying frightening, fearful, aggressive, or delusional features, some of whom may had been dormant for a long time [44]. Consequently, hysterical psychosis, for which I propose a more parsimonious name (dissociative psychosis), has been the diagnostic starting point that led to the recognition of dissociative identity disorder in Turkey [44,45].

A more difficult conceptual problem exists between dissociative disorders and borderline personality disorder. Obviously, the borderline personality disorder criteria identify a group of patients with certain features. Although highly sensitive, they are not very specific. Hudziak and coworkers [46] found no cases of pure borderline personality disorder (ie, borderline personality disorder without comorbidity). It is not known if these other disorders define these patients more appropriately with regard to choice of and response to treatment, natural history, outcome, and family illness patterns. In a recent study in Turkey [10], 64% of the outpatients with DSM-III-R borderline personality disorder had a DSM-IV dissociative disorder in the first axis (see the article by Classen and coworkers elsewhere in this issue). This figure is 72.5% for college students with DSM-IV borderline personality disorder, and 69.2% for women with DSM-III-R borderline personality disorder in the general population (Sar and coworkers, unpublished data) with both diagnoses having the highest scores of childhood trauma [10]. A total of 8.5% of college students fit the DSM-IV borderline personality disorder criteria (Sar and coworkers, unpublished data). This rate is too high to be covered by a personality disorder category and points to a conceptual problem. It could be that borderline features develop in response to living with the core symptoms related to dissociative adaptations to traumatic experience.

Somewhat paradoxically, many dissociative patients have comorbid obsessive-compulsive disorder (OCD). In a German study investigating the relationship between dissociation and OCD on a symptomologic level, checking, symmetry, and ordering were significantly related to dissociative symptomatology among OCD patients. A lack of association was found in washing and cleaning, counting and touching, and aggressive impulses and fantasies [47]. In a study from South Africa, 15.8% of patients with OCD and 18.8% of patients with trichotillomania had DES scores of 30 or above [48]. In the OCD group, high dissociators were significantly younger than low dissociators, and significantly more high dissociators than low dissociators reported a lifetime history of tics, Tourette's syndrome, bulimia nervosa, and borderline personality disorder. In the trichotillomania group, significantly more high dissociators than low dissociators reported lifetime kleptomania and depersonalization disorder. Significant positive correlations were found between DES scores and emotional, sexual, and physical abuse and physical neglect scores in both diagnostic groups. Overall, the study yielded a comorbidity profile with increased incidence of impulse dyscontrol disorders in the dissociative groups in both disorders. Dissociative processes are ubiquitous in a number of psychiatric disorders across a number of cultures.

The study on OCD and trichotillomania [47] demonstrated a further link between childhood trauma and dissociative experiences. Moreover, in the OCD group, investigation of genetic polymorphisms involved in monoamine function revealed no significant differences between high and low dissociator groups [47]. These findings are against the validity of a genetic hypothesis in the origins of dissociative symptomatology. In a similar manner, a German study of clinical and nonclinical populations, for both genders, showed that the character traits of self-transcendence and self-directedness were significant and independent predictors of dissociation [49]. The authors propose that these results support the hypothesis that dissociative symptoms are caused by environmental factors and point against a genetic predisposition in the development of dissociative symptoms.

The studies on these gray areas provide hints for many new insights in psychiatry. First, dissociation is not an issue limited to dissociative disorders; like anxiety and depression, it has an important place in general psychopathology across many diagnostic categories. Furthermore, although anxiety and depression may be phenomena representing final common pathways, dissociation may contribute to the pathophysiology of many psychiatric disorders including nonschizophrenic psychotic phenomena [50]. This seems to be true across many cultures.

Brain imaging in dissociative disorders: more questions than answers?

Although limited in number, studies from The Netherlands, Turkey, and Germany demonstrated preliminary data on the dissociative disorders that encouraged further research. Two perspectives have been pursued: comparison of dissociative disorders, as a diagnostic category, with a control population, or attempts to demonstrate that dissociative mechanisms, per se, focus on differences between distinct mental states.

Sar and coworkers [51] did not find any difference between brain perfusion assessment in alter and host personality states of five patients with DID, in repeated single-photon emission CT evaluations. In comparison with a nondissociative, nondepressive, and nontraumatized control group, however, 15 patients with DID had diminished perfusion bilaterally in orbitofrontal regions, and increased perfusion in the left (dominant) lateral temporal region. Besides supporting an orbitofrontal hypothesis of dissociative disorder [52], this study was at least able to demonstrate a significant abnormality in brain perfusion of these patients. Because data obtained from control groups with other psychiatric disorders were not provided, specificity of these findings for dissociative disorders has not yet been proved (eg, contribution of depression is not known).

Reinders and coworkers [53] investigated 11 women with DID using a symptom provocation paradigm and positron emission tomography. They concluded that different regional blood flow patterns exist for different senses of self. They demonstrated specific changes in localized brain activity consistent with their subject's ability to generate at least two distinct mental states of self-awareness, each with its own access to autobiographic trauma-related memory. The medial prefrontal cortex and the posterior associative cortices seemed to have an integral role in conscious experience.

In a Turkish study based on single-photon emission CT technology, four of five patients with conversion disorder (astasia-abasia) had left temporal, and one patient had left parietal, perfusion defects [54]. A further study on two patients with conversion disorder (having severe gait disturbance) yielded near-total absence of somatosensory-evoked potential responses on the scalp during the symptomatic period, which normalized after recovery [55]. The authors hypothesized that this is likely to be caused by the inhibition of afferent signals at the level of thalamus rather than primary somatosensory areas. The thalamus, as the main relay of afferents to the cortex, modulates sensory and motor signals, and it may control the selective engagement of cortical areas involved in motor and cognitive function [56].

The findings of these preliminary studies point out the need for additional controlled studies. The relationship and possible differences between dissociative, depressive, and anxiety disorders should be clarified using appropriate study designs (eg, nondissociative control groups). Beside trait measures, use of state scales is also important. Because high comorbidity is a rule rather than exception in these diagnostic groups and among patients with dissociative disorder in particular, the effect of overall severity of the psychiatric condition should be taken into consideration.

Amnesia, alexithymia, and depersonalization: controversial aspects

Amnesia was added to the diagnostic criteria of dissociative identity disorder in the DMS-IV. Huntjens and coworkers [57] found, in contrast to patient's reports, evidence of intact memory functioning in dissociative identity disorder. In a further study [58], although dissociative patients showed a slower response pattern, simulators were able to mimic patient pattern. The authors propose that simulation in implicit memory tasks is possible. This may need to be taken into consideration in future study designs. An experimental study in The Netherlands on high and low dissociators selected from normal population indicated a relation between dissociation and memory disturbances that seemed to be confined to the subjective experience of memory [59]. A functional MRI study on healthy low and high dissociators yielded results compatible with the conceptualization of nonpathologic dissociation as an information-processing style characterized by distinct attentional and mnemonic abilities (ie, increased verbal working memory) [60].

Dorahy and coworkers [61] studied the relationship between increased arousal, inhibitory functioning, dissociation, and information processing. Participants with dissociative identity disorder displayed a greater degree of self-reported anxiety and reduced inhibition in the negative context but not in the neutral context. The degree of negative priming for the depressed and the general population samples remained stable across contexts as did their anxiety levels. In a subsequent study, patients with dissociative identity disorder displayed effective cognitive inhibition in the neutral but not the anxious content [62]. Because the generalized anxiety disorder sample displayed the opposite findings, this reduced functioning may not be directly accounted for by anxiety. The authors propose that reduced inhibition in dissociative identity disorder may represent an adaptive functional reorganization of cognitive operations in contexts perceived as threatening. These observations also may have implications for psychotherapy of dissociative disorders.

Markowitsch [63] reported that similarities between organic and psychogenic (dissociative) forms of retrograde amnesia do exist. He hypothesizes that psychogenic and organic amnesia may be caused by a desynchronization (or blockade) of the trigger mechanisms or pathways. Recovering from retrograde amnesia is consequently viewed as a reinstatement of synchrony, or as a deblocked gating mechanism. This led him to define the "mnestic block syndrome" [64,65], which is considered to be related to an altered brain metabolism that may include changes in various transmitter and hormonal systems (γ-aminobutyric acid agonists, glucocorticoids, acetylcholine). Whether depression contributes to this syndrome is uncertain, but may be a possibility.

Another well-investigated but still controversial theme has been alexithymia. In a nonclinical young population in Switzerland [66], both personality characteristics, such as alexithymia and neuroticism, and to a modest degree environmental factors in terms of the lack of parental care, contributed to the dissociation variance. A Turkish study [67] reported, however, after multivariate analysis, that alexithymia was not related to dissociation among psychiatric outpatients. This study suggested that dissociation is fundamentally a different construct from alexithymia, which was closely related to state and trait anxiety.

Depersonalization is a major concept of traditional clinical psychopathology [68]. Like anxiety, depersonalization may be part of any psychiatric disorder including schizophrenia. It can also constitute a psychiatric disorder on its own: depersonalization disorder. This overall presence has delayed the recognition of depersonalization both as a central mechanism in dissociation and as a diagnostic category among other dissociative disorders.

There is an interest in depersonalization among researchers in the United Kingdom. A study in London demonstrated that whereas depersonalization disorder can be distinguished from other psychiatric disorders, symptoms of primary and secondary depersonalization overlap largely, and anxiety and especially depression were correlated with depersonalization symptoms [69]. A further study conducted on a large depersonalization disorder series concluded that links with anxiety and depression seem to be stronger than dissociation. They propose that depersonalization disorder should be classified under mood or anxiety disorders [70]. Trauma (including physical or sexual abuse) was recorded as a contributing factor in only 14% of the cases in this study. Interestingly, the authors were able to separate an early onset group (5–16 years) who seemed to have a more severe disorder in that they were more likely to report higher depersonalization disorder symptomatology and greater levels of anxiety and depression. The authors state that "they also endorsed a question regarding hallucinations of voices, however it is reassuring that in most cases several years had passed without any suggestion of a psychotic illness developing." Just under half of all participants suffered from tinnitus or migraine. Unfortunately, the authors did not consider these issues as clinically significant. They are, in fact, phenomena highly suspect for complex dissociative disorders when occurring in the context of depersonalization. In a subgroup of patients diagnosed as having DDNOS in Turkey, there were many cases who reported both depersonalization symptoms and dissociative amnesia without cues of identity confusion or alteration [25]. Interestingly, most of these patients reported amnesia for childhood events in addition to memory gaps in daily life. This may point to an intermediate stage in processing of developmental trauma. These studies illustrate the care that must be taken to discern thoughtfully the extent to which dissociative experiences occur in different clinical populations or risk research that does not accurately represent a clinical population. The same problem exists across cultures, and in some settings may be even more challenging because of a preponderance of particular variations in presentation of patients (eg, the extent of conversion disorders in Turkey).

Families, adolescents, and children

In contrast to previous reports about high transgenerational incidence of dissociative disorders in North America [71,72], a screening study conducted on first-degree relatives of dissociative patients in Istanbul led to zero (0%) prevalence [73]. This observation led to definition of a specific dysfunctional family type: apparently normal (dissociative) family. Although these parents were traumatized more frequently than controls, their dissociative psychopathology remained in subclinical level. These observations also led the authors to consider that despite their ordinary outside appearance, certain dysfunctional family types might have importance in the development of dissociative disorders, and childhood traumata other than sexual or physical abuse also may have severe impact.

A Dutch study demonstrated that besides childhood sexual and physical abuse, maternal dysfunction is related to the level of dissociation, whereas dissociation also may be related to neglect [74]. Higher prevalence for sexual or physical abuse in patients with conversion disorder was demonstrated, whereas dissociation severity was correlated with parental dysfunction by the mother but not by the father [29]. A dual-personality type of dissociative disorder has been reported in Japan [75]. This endemic condition called "hikikomori" (social withdrawal) originated most commonly among young offspring of middle and upper class families with pseudomutual relationships. Close family relations are also supported culturally in the Middle East (eg, in Israel [76] and Turkey). Many family patterns noted in North American research on families of schizophrenic patients a few decades ago may have some importance in inquiring about families of dissociative subjects in various cultures (eg, pseudomutuality [77], marital schism [78], schizophrenogenic mother [79], and double-bind [80]).

Pasquini and coworkers [81] concluded that not only are interfamilial childhood abuses inflicted on the patient a risk factor, but major losses or other severe life events suffered by the mother within 2 years of a patient's birth are risk factors for the development of dissociative disorders. A possible explanation of these findings was that disorganized or insecure attachment may increase susceptibility to traumatic experiences and propensity to dissociation in adult life (ie, disorganized attachment behavior in the infant is linked to losses and other severely distressing events in the life of the caregiver) [82]. Ozturk [83] documented that among girls, siblings in the first rank of sibling order tend to develop conversion disorder perhaps because these children occupy a special position in the family system [84]. This role is characterized by carrying adult responsibilities in an early age (eg, caring for siblings) without showing any opposition and continuing to do so in further life (complacent overadjustment) [38]. These findings were replicated in a large series of inpatients diagnosed as having hysteria in the 1970s [39].

Besides nosologic issues, family studies are important for elucidation and treatment of dissociative disorders among children and adolescents. Case studies and series of dissociative children and adolescents have been published in Turkey [85–88]. A screening among high school students revealed the relationship between childhood trauma, dissociation, suicide, and self-mutilation in this age group; there was no gender difference on average DES scores [89]. In a study on a normative sample in Sweden, 8.8% of the adolescents reported scores above the cutoff point of 2.5 on the Dissociation Questionnaire, with a female to male ratio of 2.6:1 [90].

Dissociation pathway to substance dependency: chance for early intervention?

A Finnish study yielded a substance abuse history in 50% of dissociative patients [12]. These rates remained lower in Turkey (ie, 29.4% among dissociative inpatients and 22.2% among dissociative outpatients) [8,9]. It is possible, however, that dissociative patients who have substance abuse histories are usually admitted to drug dependency treatment units because of the severity and priority of treating their substance abuse. Nevertheless, in a large group of treatment-seeking inpatients with drug or alcohol abuse in Istanbul, the prevalence of dissociative disorders was 17.2% [91]. A total of 67.6% of the dissociative group reported that their dissociative experiences started before onset of substance use (ie, the interval was 3.6 years in average with a range of 1–11 years). These patients were younger, had shorter remission durations, and tended to use drugs rather than alcohol, whereas the number of substances used was correlated with the severity of current dissociative disorder. Female gender, childhood emotional abuse, and suicide attempts predicted a dissociative disorder diagnosis among them. The prevalence of dissociative disorders increased to 26% among inpatients with drug abuse (Tamar-Gurol and coworkers, unpublished data). It is noteworthy, that significantly more substance-dependent inpatients with dissociative disorder ceased treatment program prematurely [91]. These findings are alarming, because they demonstrate the importance of the recognition of dissociative disorders for prevention and successful treatment of substance dependency among adolescents and young adults. Gender differences were prominent among alcohol-dependent inpatients in particular. The small female group tended to have a clear-cut dissociative disorder, whereas a large part of the male patients seemed to provoke dissociation by using alcohol [92]. The Turkish experience suggests that screening for dissociative disorders in substance abuse treatment settings should be routine.

Dissociated identities in an age of globalism: what psychiatry has to tell

This attempt to paste together the mosaic of international research has provided a unique view about the scope of dissociation as perceived by scientists from different cultures. Based on local factors, such as technologic or financial opportunities, acknowledgment of this work by the clinical psychiatry establishment, and characteristics of the mental (and general) health care delivery system, the interested researcher may be able to attend to different aspects of this broad area of psychology and psychopathology. What is clear is that dissociative processes are ubiquitous across cultures, are part of the picture of many psychiatric syndromes, and are a discernable and useful diagnostic category that provides a window of hope for patients when it is recognized.

Remarkably, the final answer of this question is not yet clear: what is dissociation? Although dissociation may affect several mental faculties, such as consciousness, memory, the perception of self and other, perception of the environment, mood, behavior, and both motor and sensorial abilities, a supraordinate definition of dissociation is elusive (see the articles by Dell and Way elsewhere in this issue). What is the core of this human condition, which is characterized by the loss of internal and external harmony? What is the origin of excruciating feelings of emptiness, boredom, and loneliness? Why is there such preoccupation with death, suicide, and self-destructiveness that resist known biologic treatment tools? Besides diverse effects of local cultures, can one speak about dissociogenic effects of society on the individuum in this Zeitgeist of consumerism and globalism [93]?

Dissociative disorders are categorically modern carriers of two basic concepts in clinical psychopathology: depersonalization and identity [94]. Once popular, the concept of identity has disappeared from psychiatry; the identity disorder category of the DSM-III does not exist anymore. For identity confusion, there is no niche remaining other than dissociative disorders, except borderline personality disorder, which extends the issue to that of a long-term personality disorder. In an allegedly atheoretical age of psychiatric nosology and classification, the impaired contact of psychiatry with general clinical psychopathology [95] has blurred the importance of these concepts in clinical practice. Even in a period of growing recognition of psychic trauma, however, hysteria does not tend to disappear from psychiatric clinics and from medicine in general; these patients are everywhere if one just looks. Neither do they get usually appropriate treatment; they remain one of psychiatry's most hopeful [96] but still poorly treated population. Although the clinical path is still filled with pitfalls, thanks to the current unprecedented opportunities for worldwide communication, it is hoped that an international scientific perspective on the dissociative disorders and dissociation will contain and correct aberrations caused by local controversies.

References

[1] Fischer G, Riedesser P. Lehrbuch der psychotraumatologie [Textbook of Psychotraumathology]. München: Ernst Reinhardt Verlag; 1999.
[2] Sar V, Ozturk E. What is trauma and dissociation? Journal of Trauma Practice, in press.
[3] Boon S, Draijer N. Multiple personality disorder in the Netherlands: a clinical investigation of 71 patients. Am J Psychiatry 1993;150:489–94.
[4] Sar V, Yargic LI, Tutkun H. Structured interview data on 35 cases of dissociative identity disorder in Turkey. Am J Psychiatry 1996;153:1329–33.

[5] Gast U, Rodewald F, Nickel V, et al. Prevalence of dissociative disorders among psychiatric inpatients in a German university clinic. J Nerv Ment Dis 2001;189:249–57.

[6] Modestin J, Ebner G, Junghan M, et al. Dissociative experiences and dissociative disorders in acute psychiatric inpatients. Compr Psychiatry 1996;37:355–61.

[7] Middleton W, Butler J. Dissociative identity disorder: an Australian series. Aust N Z J Psychiatry 1998;32:794–804.

[8] Tutkun H, Sar V, Yargic LI, et al. Frequency of dissociative disorders among psychiatric inpatients in a Turkish university clinic. Am J Psychiatry 1998;155:800–5.

[9] Sar V, Tutkun H, Alyanak B, et al. Frequency of dissociative disorders among psychiatric outpatients in Turkey. Compr Psychiatry 2000;41:216–22.

[10] Sar V, Kundakci T, Kiziltan E, et al. Axis I dissociative disorder comorbidity of borderline personality disorder among psychiatric outpatients. J Trauma Dissociation 2003;4:119–36.

[11] Friedl MC, Draijer N. Dissociative disorders in Dutch psychiatric inpatients. Am J Psychiatry 2000;157:1012–3.

[12] Lipsanen T, Korkeila J, Peltola P, et al. Dissociative disorders among psychiatric patients: comparison with a nonclinical sample. Eur Psychiatry 2004;19:53–5.

[13] Sar V, Koyuncu A, Öztürk E, et al. Prevalence of dissociative disorders among emergency psychiatric admissions. Presented at the Annual Conference of the International Society for the Study of Dissociation. Chicago, IL; November 2–4, 2003.

[14] Akyüz G, Dogan O, Sar V, et al. Frequency of dissociative identity disorder in the general population in Turkey. Compr Psychiatry 1999;40:151–9.

[15] Sar V, Akyüz G, Kundakci T, et al. Prevalence of trauma-related disorders in Turkey: an epidemiological study. In: Proceedings of the 14th Annual Meeting of the International Society for Traumatic Stress Studies. Washington: International Society for Traumatic Stress Studies. November 20–22, 1998. p. 90.

[16] Vanderlinden J, Van Dyck R, Vandereycken W, et al. Dissociation and traumatic experiences in the general population of the Netherlands. Hosp Community Psychiatry 1993;14:786–8.

[17] Vanderlinden J, Van Dyck R, Vandereycken W, et al. The Dissociation Questionnaire (DIS-Q). Development and characteristics of a new self-reporting questionnaire. Clin Psychol Psychother 1993;1:21–7.

[18] Spitzer C, Klauer T, Grabe HJ, et al. Gender differences in dissociation: a dimensional approach. Psychopathology 2003;36:65–70.

[19] Spitzer C, Liss H, Dudeck M, et al. Dissociative experiences and disorders in forensic inpatients. Int J Law Psychiatry 2003;26:281–8.

[20] Steinberg M. Structured Clinical Interview for DSM-IV Dissociative Disorders- Revised (SCID-D-R). Washington: American Psychiatric Press; 1994.

[21] Sar V, Akyuz G. Trauma and dissociation among prisoners. In: Proceedings of the 20th Annual Conference of the International Society for the Study of Dissociation. Baltimore: International Society for the Study of Dissociation. 2002.

[22] Sar I, Sar V. Konversiyon bozukluğunda belirti dağılımı [Symptom frequencies in conversion disorder]. Journal of Uludag University Faculty of Medicine 1990;17:67–74.

[23] Sar V, Kundakci T, Kiziltan E, et al. Differentiating dissociative disorders from other diagnostic groups through somatoform dissociation in Turkey. J Trauma Dissociation 2000;1:67–80.

[24] Sagduyu A, Rezaki M, Kaplan I, et al. Saglik ocagina basvuran hastalarda dissosiyatif (konversiyon) belirtiler [Prevalence of conversion symptoms in a primary health care center]. Turk J Psychiatry 1997;8:161–9.

[25] Sar V, Akyüz G, Kundakci T, et al. Childhood trauma, dissociation and psychiatric comorbidity in patients with conversion disorder. Am J Psychiatry 2004;161:2271–6.

[26] Tezcan E, Atmaca M, Kuloglu M, et al. Dissociative disorders in Turkish inpatients with conversion disorder. Compr Psychiatry 2003;44:324–30.

[27] Spitzer C, Freyberger HJ, Kessler C, et al. Psychiatrische komorbiditaet dissoziativer störungen in der neurologie [Psychiatric comorbidity of dissociative disorders in a neurological clinic]. Nervenarzt 1994;65:680–8.

242 SAR

[28] Spitzer C, Spelsberg B, Grabe HJ, et al. Dissociative experiences and psychopathology in conversion disorders. J Psychosom Res 1999;46:291–4.
[29] Roelofs K, Keijsers GPJ, Hoogduin KA, et al. Childhood abuse in patients with conversion disorder. Am J Psychiatry 2002;159:1908–13.
[30] Spinhoven P, Roelofs K, Moene F, et al. Trauma and dissociation in conversion disorder and chronic pelvic pain. Int J Psychiatry Med 2004;34:305–18.
[31] Moene FC, Spinhoven P, Hoogduin KA, et al. Hypnotizability, dissociation, and trauma in patients with a conversion disorder: an exploratory study. Clin Psychol Psychother 2001;8: 400–10.
[32] Nijenhuis ERS, Spinhoven P, Van Dyck R, et al. The development and psychometric characteristics of the Somatoform Dissociation Questionnaire (SDQ-20). J Nerv Ment Dis 1996; 184:688–94.
[33] Yucel B, Ozyalcin S, Sertel HO, et al. Childhood traumatic events and dissociative experiences in patients with chronic headache and low back pain. Clin J Pain 2002;18:394–401.
[34] Nijenhuis ERS, Van der Hart O. Somatoform dissociative phenomena: a Janetian perspective. In: Goodwin JM, Attias R, editors. Splintered reflections: images of the body in trauma. New York: Basic Books; 1999. p. 89–127.
[35] Nijenhuis ERS, Spinhoven P, Vanderlinden J, et al. Somatoform dissociative symptoms as related to animal defensive reactions to predatory threat and injury. J Abnorm Psychol 1998; 107:63–73.
[36] Nijenhuis ERS, Spinhoven P, Van Dyck R, et al. Degree of somatoform and psychological dissociation in dissociative disorder is correlated with reported trauma. J Trauma Stress 1998;11:711–30.
[37] Yargic LI, Sar V, Tutkun H, Alyanak B. Comparison of dissociative identity disorder with other diagnostic groups using a structured interview in Turkey. Compr Psychiatry 1998;39:345–51.
[38] Öztürk OM, Gögüs A. Agir regressif belirtiler gösteren histerik psikozlar [Hysterical psychoses presenting with severe regressive symptoms]. In: Proceedings of the 9th National Conference of Psychiatry and Neurology. Ankara, Turkey: Meteksan; 1973. p. 155–64.
[39] Sar I. 1970–1980 yılları arasında Hacettepe Universitesi Psikiyatri Klinigine yatarak tedavi gören hastalardan "histeri" tanısı alanların değerlendirilmesi [A retrospective evaluation of inpatients diagnosed as "hysteria" in Hacettepe University Psychiatric Clinic between 1970–1980] [doctoral dissertation]. Ankara, Turkey: Hacettepe University; 1983.
[40] Van der Hart O, Witztum E, Friedman B. From hysterical psychosis to reactive dissociative psychosis. J Trauma Stress 1992;6:43–64.
[41] Modestin J, Bachman KM. Is the diagnosis of the hysterical psychosis justified? Clinical study of hysterical psychosis, reactive/psychogenic psychosis, and schizophrenia. Compr Psychiatry 1992;33:17–24.
[42] Strömgren E. Psychogenic psychoses. In: Hirsch SR, Shepherd M, editors. Themes and variations in European Psychiatry. Bristol: Wright; 1974. p. 97–120.
[43] Strömgren E. The development of the concept of reactive psychoses. Psychopathology 1986; 20:62–7.
[44] Tutkun H, Yargic LI, Sar V. Dissociative identity disorder presenting as hysterical psychosis. Dissociation 1996;9:241–9.
[45] Sar V, Tutkun H. The treatment of dissociative identity disorder in Turkey: a case presentation. Dissociation 1997;10:146–52.
[46] Hudziak JJ, Boffeli TJ, Kriesman JJ, et al. Clinical study of the relation of borderline personality disorder to Briquet's syndrome (hysteria), somatization disorder, antisocial personality disorder, and substance abuse disorders. Am J Psychiatry 1996;153:1598–606.
[47] Grabe HJ, Goldschmidt F, Lehmkuhl L, et al. Dissociative symptoms in obsessive-compulsive dimensions. Psychopathology 1999;32:319–24.
[48] Lochner C, Seedat S, Hemmings SMJ, et al. Dissociative experiences in obsessive-compulsive disorder and trichotillomania: clinical and genetic findings. Compr Psychiatry 2004;45: 384–91.

[49] Grabe HJ, Spitzer C, Freyberger HJ. Relationship of dissociation to temperament and character in men and women. Am J Psychiatry 1999;156:1811–3.

[50] Sar V. Do we really know what schizophrenia is? J Trauma Dissociation, in press.

[51] Sar V, Unal SN, Kiziltan E, et al. HMPAO SPECT study of cerebral perfusion in dissociative identity disorder. J Trauma Dissociation 2001;2:5–25.

[52] Forrest K. Toward an etiology of dissociative identity disorder: a neurodevelopmental approach. Conscious Cogn 2001;10:259–63.

[53] Reinders AATS, Nijenhuis ERS, Paans AMJ, et al. One brain, two selves. Neuroimage 2003; 20:2119–25.

[54] Yazici KM, Kostakoglu L. Cerebral blood flow changes in patients with conversion disorder. Psychiatry Res 1998;83:163–8.

[55] Yazici KM, Demirci M, Demir B, et al. Abnormal somatosensory evoked potentials in two patients with conversion disorder. Psychiatry Clin Neurosci 2004;58:222–5.

[56] Vuilleumier P, Chicherio C, Assal F, et al. Functional neuroanatomical correlates of hysterical sensorimotor loss. Brain 2001;124:1077–90.

[57] Huntjens RJC, Peters ML, Postma A, et al. Transfer of newly acquired stimulus valence between identities in dissociative identity disorder. Behav Res Ther 2005;43:243–55.

[58] Huntjens RJC, Postma A, Woertman L, et al. Procedural memory in dissociative identity disorder: when can inter-identity amnesia truely established? Conscious Cogn 2005;14: 377–89.

[59] Kindt M, Van den Hout M, Buck N. Dissociation related to subjective memory fragmentation and intrusions but not to objective memory disturbances. J Behav Ther Exp Psychiatry 2005;36:43–59.

[60] Veltman DJ, deRuiter MB, Rombouts SA, et al. Neurophysiological correlates of increased verbal working memory in high dissociative participants: a functional MRI study. Psychol Med 2005;35:175–85.

[61] Dorahy MJ, Middleton W, Irwin HJ. The effect of emotional context on cognitive inhibition and attentional processing in dissociative identity disorder. Behav Res Ther 2005;43:555–68.

[62] Dorahy MJ, McCusker CG, Loewenstein JL, et al. Cognitive inhibition and interference in dissociative identity disorder: the effects of anxiety on specific executive functions. Behav Res Ther, in press.

[63] Markowitsch HJ. Retrograde amnesia: similarities between organic and psychogenic forms. Neurol Psychiatry Brain Res 1996;4:1–8.

[64] Markowitsch HJ. Functional neuroimaging correlates of functional amnesia. Memory 1999; 7:561–83.

[65] Markowitsch HJ, Kessler J, Russ MO, et al. Mnestic block syndrome. Cortex 1999;35: 219–30.

[66] Modestin J, Lötscher K, Erni T. Dissociative experiences and their correlates in young nonpatients. Psychol Psychother 2002;75:53–64.

[67] Tutkun H, Savas HA, Zoroglu SS, et al. Relationship between alexithymia, dissociation and anxiety in psychiatric outpatients from Turkey. Isr J Psychiatry Relat Sci 2004;41:118–24.

[68] Jaspers K. Allgemeine psychopathologie [General psychopathology]. Berlin: Springer Verlag; 1913.

[69] Lambert MV, Senior C, Fewtrell WD, et al. Primary and secondary depersonalization disorder: a psychometric study. J Affect Dis 2001;63:249–56.

[70] Baker D, Hunter E, Lawrence E, et al. Depersonalisation disorder: clinical features of 204 cases. Br J Psychiatry 2003;182:428–33.

[71] Kluft RP. Multiple personality in childhood. Psychiatr Clin North Am 1984;7:121–34.

[72] Braun BG. The transgenerational incidence of dissociation and multiple personality disorder: a preliminary report. In: Kluft R, editor. Childhood antecedents of multiple personality. Washington: American Psychiatric Press; 1985. p. 127–50.

[73] Ozturk E, Sar V. Apparently normal family: a contemporary agent of transgenerational trauma and dissociation. Journal of Trauma Practice, in press.

[74] Draijer N, Langeland W. Childhood trauma and perceived parental dysfunction in the etiology of dissociative symptoms in psychiatric patients. Am J Psychiatry 1999;156:379–85.
[75] Hattori Y. A case study of 35 hikikomori clients: social withdrawal of young people in Japan. Journal of Trauma Practice, in press.
[76] Somer E. Advances in dissociation research and practice in Israel. Journal of Trauma Practice, in press.
[77] Wynne LC, Ryckoff IM, Day J, et al. Pseudomutuality in the family relations of schizophrenics. Psychiatry 1958;21:204–19.
[78] Lidz T, Fleck S, Cornelison AR. Schizophrenia and the family. New York: International Universities Press; 1965.
[79] Fromm-Reichmann F. Principles of intensive psychotherapy. Chicago: University of Chicago Press; 1950.
[80] Bateson G, Jackson DD, Haley J, et al. Toward a theory of schizophrenia. Behav Sci 1956;1: 251–64.
[81] Pasquini P, Liotti G, Mazzotti E, et al. Risk factors in the early family life of patients suffering from dissociative disorders. Acta Psychiatr Scand 2002;105:110–6.
[82] Main M, Morgan H. Disorganization and disorientation in infant strange situation behavior: phenotypic resemblance to dissociative states. In: Michelson LK, Ray WJ, editors. Handbook of dissociation: theoretical, empirical, and clinical perspectives. New York: Plenum Press; 1996. p. 107–38.
[83] Ozturk M. Histeri belirtileri gösteren çocukların aile içindeki özel yeri [The special position of the children with hysteria symptoms in the family]. Turk J Pediatr 1976;19:93–107.
[84] Sar I, Sar V. Histerik hastanın kardes dizisindeki yeri [Early birth order in hysteria]. Medical Bulletin of the Sisli Children's Hospitalospital 1991;25:114–22.
[85] Sar V, Öztürk E, Kundakci T. Psychotherapy of an adolescent with dissociative identity disorder: change in Rorschach patterns. J Trauma Dissociation 2002;3:81–95.
[86] Zoroglu SS, Sar V, Tuzun U, et al. Reliability and validity of the Turkish version of the Adolescent Dissociative Experiences Scale. Psychiatry Clin Neurosci 2002;56:551–6.
[87] Zoroglu SS, Tüzün Ü, Öztürk M, et al. Reliability and validity of the Turkish version of the Child Dissociation Checklist. J Trauma Dissociation 2002;3:37–49.
[88] Zoroglu SS, Yargic LI, Tutkun H, et al. Dissociative identity disorder in childhood: five Turkish cases. Dissociation 1996;9:250–5.
[89] Zoroglu SS, Tüzün Ü, Sar V, et al. Suicide attempt and self-mutilation among Turkish highschool students in relation with abuse, neglect and dissociation. Psychiatry Clin Neurosci 2003;57:119–26.
[90] Svedin CG, Nilsson D, Lindell C. Traumatic experiences and dissociative symptoms among Swedish adolescents. A pilot study using DIS-Q-Sweden. Nord J Psychiatry 2004;58:349–55.
[91] Karadag F, Sar V, Tamar-Gürol D, et al. Dissociative disorders among inpatients with drug or alcohol dependency. J Clin Psychiatry 2005;66:1247–53.
[92] Evren C, Sar V, Karadag F, et al. Dissociative disorders among alcohol-dependent inpatients. Psychiatry Res, in press.
[93] Sar V, Ozturk E. A new core psychological structure in understanding dissociation: the sociological self. Newsletter of the International Society for the Study of Dissociation 2003;21: 4–5.
[94] Erikson EH. Identity, youth and crisis. New York: Norton; 1968.
[95] Jaspers K. Klinische psychopathologie [Clinical psychopathology]. Berlin: Springer Verlag; 1913.
[96] Kandel ER. Biology and the future of psychoanalysis: a new intellectual framework for psychiatry revisited. Am J Psychiatry 1999;156:505–24.

ELSEVIER
SAUNDERS

PSYCHIATRIC
CLINICS
OF NORTH AMERICA

Psychiatr Clin N Am 29 (2006) 245–262

Therapeutic Interventions in the Treatment of Dissociative Disorders

Joan A. Turkus, MD*, Jennifer Aloe Kahler, PsyD

The CENTER: Posttraumatic Disorders Program, The Psychiatric Institute of Washington, D.C., 4228 Wisconsin Avenue, NW, Washington, DC 20016, USA

Many clinicians who treat patients who have dissociative disorders are often puzzled about how to approach this difficult population. According to the *Diagnostic and Statistical Manual for Mental Disorders, Fourth Edition,* the essential features of dissociation are a disruption of the normal integrative functions of consciousness, memory, identity, and perception of the environment [1]. These patients often present with challenging symptomatology that even a seasoned clinician can find overwhelming. However, ego-strengthening skills and principles are available that should be taught and emphasized early in therapy to help stabilize the patient and allow the treatment to progress. The resulting skills and ego strength create a psychologic foundation for processing trauma. They need to be maintained and reworked to sustain overall function.

Based on years of experience working with this population, we have learned that we must be flexible in our approach to these patients and must apply these techniques within an overall psychodynamic framework. Approaching these patients from a psychodynamic perspective is crucial for recognizing the devastating effects that past trauma has had on their lives and their current states of dysfunction. Applying skill-building interventions in the beginning stages of treatment is also useful to ameliorate the disabling dissociative symptoms and to help patients cope with painful affect and recollections of traumatic experience. It is simply not enough to work through past trauma without also teaching skills to manage the acute symptoms that the patient may be experiencing. In fact, if a patient is not able to remain "in the present" long enough to maintain daily function and process past trauma, the therapy will not be fruitful. Therefore, the patient must be taught symptom management and coping skills before he or

* Corresponding author. 200 Little Falls Street, Suite 205, Falls Church, VA 22046.
E-mail address: joan.turkus@verizon.net (J.A. Turkus).

0193-953X/06/$ - see front matter © 2005 Elsevier Inc. All rights reserved.
doi:10.1016/j.psc.2005.10.015

she progresses further into the treatment. Clinicians who undertake this work should seek continuing education in posttraumatic and dissociative disorders. In addition, the clinician should pursue additional training in cognitive-behavioral therapy and clinical hypnosis.

We have outlined 10 key skills and techniques that are helpful in the beginning stages of treatment for patients who have dissociative disorders. These skills are discussed in the sequence we suggest they be applied during treatment.

Psychoeducation

Education is an invaluable tool for treating dissociative disorders. It helps to undo the stigmatization and shame associated with being ill. We have heard the words *insane, crazy,* and *freak* many times from patients who are traumatized. In fact, patients on our trauma unit have requested that we change the group name to *psycheducation,* to eliminate any implication of *psycho.* Education shifts the focus from "What's wrong with you?" to understanding the patients' experiences as normal human responses to trauma and how it disrupts one's life. Education appeals to intellectual strengths, and the practice of coping skills improves function and resilience. Psychoeducation can be accomplished in focused skill-building groups, which also have the advantage of increasing interpersonal connection [2]. If groups are not available, the material can be integrated judiciously into individual psychotherapy.

Several workbooks and self-help books are available. Browsing in the self-help section of a bookstore is an education in itself; the clinician should remember that this is what patients do. This article's reference list includes books we have found particularly useful in practice [3–6]. Basic information on posttraumatic stress disorder and dissociation is helpful. We often start with the "Expert Consensus Treatment Guidelines for Posttraumatic Stress Disorder: A Guide For Patients and Families" [7]. Therapists must review carefully any material or books recommended to patients, and encourage patients to read and question with intellectual curiosity and discuss what fits and what does not. Many patients are prolific readers in the field of trauma and dissociation (and keep up with the latest talk shows). Some of them may have read more books and articles, searched the Internet, or seen more television shows and films on the subject than many therapists. Therefore, clinicians are encouraged to discuss this material and offer wise suggestions about what may not be appropriate for patients because of the risk for overstimulation and confusion.

Research in the neurobiology of trauma has advanced in the past decade. Increasing literature on the effects of stress on children is also available [8]. Therapists may find it useful to normalize physiologic reactions to traumatic stress, such as "freezing," as a response guided by the limbic system. This explanation allows the patient to stop blaming themselves for passively submitting to victimization. Psychoeducation, as interpretation, can transform a worried patient's "weird, crazy experience" into a lesson about normal human biology (eg, the psychophysiologic consequences of sleep deprivation or hypoglycemia). Therapists can also simplify neuroscience and educate patients about the plasticity of the brain, ongoing neurogenesis, and the development of new neural nets to instill hope of trauma resolution and recovery [9].

One strategy to stimulate patient interest in learning is to compare survival behaviors with recovery skills. Examples include the survival response of secrecy in contrast with the recovery skill of discretion or privacy, or the survival mode of dissociation in contrast with grounding and the paced reassociation of the recovery process. Cognitive-behavioral interventions in psychotherapy include, but are not limited to, the topics of: (1) self-nurturing, self-soothing strategies, (2) boundaries and relationships, (3) self-injurious behaviors, (4) understanding substance abuse within a trauma history [10], (5) affect management, (6) grief and loss, (7) organization and problem-solving, (8) responsible assertion, (9) safety planning, and (10) maintaining social support and connection. Psychotherapists must not only teach these to the patient but also encourage the patient to practice these interventions on a regular basis and review them in psychotherapy periodically. Skill building is always a work in progress; patients' self-reports should be discussed and revisions made as part of the ongoing process. Skills are gained over time and through diligence; however, it is well worth the effort for the "teacher" and the "student." Successes in these areas, even small steps, create a cumulative resource for inspiration and hope, and a credible database for evidence of progress and recovery.

Pacing and containment

Pacing and containment are critical in building a foundation and framework for therapy. One of the essential goals of therapy with patients who have dissociative disorders is to maintain function while doing the work. This task is not easy because of the propensity for flooding of painful material and the intensity of the accompanying affect, against which the dissociation has been a lifelong defense. In the process of psychotherapy, the therapist encourages dissociative barriers to become more permeable and finally to collapse. The patient must learn the ego defense of suppression. Suppression is the conscious postponement of dealing with difficult material until an opportune time so that one may go on with ordinary life activities. In dissociative identity disorder (DID), the parts of self have to communicate and cooperate to accomplish this task.

Patients are often resistant to practicing the skills of pacing and containment. The concepts are not familiar to patients who dissociate and alternate between flooding of intense affect and numbing or avoidance. Patients sometimes express a magical wish that therapy will "get it all out quickly" and make them well. Misunderstandings about containment are common, such as angrily interpreting it as the therapist's directive "to forget it and get over it." Patients may have encountered similar messages from family members in denial or from nonsupportive friends. The denial of trauma may also have been framed in a religious directive, such as "just pray about it." Therapists may find it helpful to reframe pacing and containment as skills to be used in adult life and not just tools for psychotherapy.

Pacing is a task shared by the therapist and patient. The therapy must be planned and paced as much as possible—broadly over time and in individual sessions. Having a working understanding of stage-oriented treatment is the ground for the therapeutic process [11–13]. The first stage of therapy is the establishment of safety and stabilization and the building of the therapeutic alliance. The second is of trauma processing; the integration of traumatic recollections and intense affect. The third is postintegrative self and relational development. Skill building is clearly the focus in the first stage of therapy. This task may have to be reworked during the trauma processing stage, which is often destabilizing despite the best efforts of the therapist and patient. Individual sessions should have a beginning, middle, and end, with time dedicated for wrap-up toward the end of each session. Therapists may find it useful to announce that there are 10 minutes left in the session and use that time to recap the session and be certain that the patient is "grounded" in the present. Grounding is explored later as a separate topic.

Containment skills can be taught through psychoeducation and imagery. Therapists must start by normalizing feelings ("gut feelings") as an integral part of a human being. Affect modulation involves the identification of feelings, followed by the contextual relationship, and then modulation. Patients often feel "bad" or "in pain," but are unable to discriminate sadness, guilt, shame, or anger. Learning to identify a specific feeling and give it context is the beginning of control and understanding. In patients who have dissociative disorders, complex, mixed feelings, such as love and anger, are usually dissociated. Teaching patients that ambivalence is normal and understandable, particularly viewed through the lens of a trauma history, promotes growth and maturity as whole persons. Instruction on how to modulate affect may be as simple as "sitting with the feeling" and waiting for the normal fading of the feeling and the physical sensations. Allowing oneself to cry as a release for sadness and grief is a normal experience to be reclaimed.

Modulation also involves teaching self-soothing, mindfulness, or distracting strategies [14]. Patients who have dissociative disorders and were raised in dysfunctional families are unfamiliar with the benefits of common activities such as taking a walk, having a cup of tea, breathing deeply, or relaxing to soothing music. The therapist and patient can collaboratively create a list of strategies to keep at hand for difficult moments or days. Keeping such a list on an index card in a wallet or purse may be helpful as an orienting strategy.

Containment imagery may involve various techniques. The clinical hypnosis literature offers many suggestions [15,16]. These include counting down or dialing down dysphoric feelings, or releasing painful affect to the universe or earth in a slow, controlled, and tolerable way. Traumatic recollections and painful affect may be contained in imaginary physical objects, such as videotapes to be viewed later or a locked trunk or box to be opened with care in a therapy session. The imagery can be as creative as the therapist and patient make it, but should fit the patient's personality and internal world. Negative or persecutory images, such as incarceration of an offending thought, feeling, or parts of self in an "internal jail," or being punished for an act, should not be used. These images reenact and reinforce traumatic experience.

Grounding skills

Dissociative processes adaptively modulate the intolerable anxiety and stress resulting from trauma at the same time that these processes exact the price of destroying the context and meaning of experience. For example, many patients who are dissociative speak of memory gaps and time loss that are too large to be accounted for by normal forgetting. They may experience the physical sense of floating or feeling outside the body (depersonalization) when they experience stress, anxiety, or fear. A common struggle when working in therapy with a patient who is dissociative is that the patient continues to experience these symptoms from past events, although the present situation no longer poses danger or ongoing trauma. Of course, the therapist must always determine whether a patient is still in an abusive or dangerous relationship or life circumstance. Therapists often speak of having an intense session with a patient, only to have that patient later forget that the session even took place. At other times, the patient may present for therapy in a highly distraught state, unable to recall what precipitated the crisis. A basic and central skill-set for the alleviation of symptoms of dissociative disorders is *grounding*. Grounding is the process of being psychologically present. It is helpful in "facilitat[ing] clear reality contact... reduc[ing] posttraumatic experiences... and reduc[ing] dissociative experiences (i.e., spontaneous trance, depersonalization, time loss, and uncontrolled switching)" [6]. Grounding skills are beneficial in the treatment of not only dissociation but also posttraumatic stress disorder, which is a common comorbid diagnosis. Grounding skills can be divided into two areas: sensory awareness and cognitive awareness.

Sensory awareness grounding skills encourage patients focus in the present by using all five senses in awareness of their body position. Asking the patient to identify an object in the clinician's office to serve as a visual reminder of physical surroundings during the session can also be helpful. This object can also serve as a constant and familiar item for the patient. Patients often find it helpful to hold a stress ball, small stone, or other palm-sized object to enhance their sense of touch. The object can easily be transported to and from sessions and used between sessions to facilitate the reduction of symptoms. Patients may use a favorite lotion or perfume to enhance the sense of smell. Focusing on the sound of a watch or clock ticking, or even asking the patient to focus on the therapist's voice, is valuable for grounding. And finally, encouraging the patient to carry gum, mints, or hard candy can be useful for enhancing the sense of taste.

Cognitive awareness grounding skills involve orienting the patient to name, day, date, age, and location. Patients who have severe trauma histories may often be confused about the safety of the therapist's office, worrying that a perpetrator may be in the hall or just outside the door. Patients who have DID may present in a self-state that believes they are decades younger or older than their present age. The patient may even be confused about the identity of the therapist and require a reminder and reorientation to the therapist's role and name. Therapists must practice cognitive awareness in session so that the patient's dissociative symptoms in day-to-day life decrease.

Therapists must maintain appropriate boundaries when using grounding skills with a patient. Certainly sitting with a patient who is suddenly wracked with posttraumatic symptoms can create intense countertransference, especially when the therapist wishes to comfort or even hold the patient. However, this situation can be very confusing for a patient. It also creates a potential ethical or legal dilemma if the patient confuses the clinician's physical attempts to soothe with elements of past abuse. Therapists must appreciate that some of their innocuous actual behaviors may feel threatening to the patient, and it may be useful to inquire if that is the case.

Encouraging the patient to rely solely on the therapist for grounding tends to backfire. For example, in our experience, when a patient has become conditioned to listening to a tape of the therapist's voice as the sole means of facilitating connection to the present, the patient does not have the opportunity to learn to do the work independently. This reliance, in turn, prevents the patient from moving forward in treatment and creates an unhealthy dependency on the therapist.

"Talking through" in dissociative identity disorder

One of the hallmarks of a patient's experience in the early stages of treatment for DID is what may be termed *internal conflict*. A patient who has DID often reports that many internal self-states are working against one another in a failed attempt to meet each one's needs. An internal struggle for power and control is often experienced. Such conflicts lead to a general state of chaotic dysfunction and to repeated crises involving the patient's safety. "Talking through" or talking to the personality system as a whole is an effective and useful technique in working with a patient who has DID [16–18]. The therapist must encourage all self-aspects, known and unknown, to become part of the treatment process.

This process can be accomplished by asking, in a directive manner, that all self-aspects focus on the therapist. One approach is to state:

> This is Dr. _____. I need all parts inside to listen to me now. You can listen through the ears or look through the eyes. We have a serious problem in front of us that must be addressed. There is a great deal of conflict inside that is wise not to continue. I am sure that even those inside who do not wish to cooperate at this time would agree that this conflict is problematic. No one is getting his or her needs met. As much as you may not like this, working together is essential to help all of you function. We must all find a way to work together. I am willing to help with this process if you are willing to listen.

The use of the objectified "the eyes" and "the ears" is intentional. Many patients who have DID experience depersonalization and do not feel connected to their own bodies. Using these objectified body references early in treatment can bypass internal resistance to "listening-in" and cooperating. The therapist also must not assume that each self-state is willing to assist with the treatment process. This potential obstacle should be recognized up-front by acknowledging the conflict and requesting that each self-state "listen-in" to the treatment process. The therapist must make this request throughout the therapy process, in every session. The end-result of this technique will be an increased coconsciousness and awareness of one's own internal processes.

"Talking through" is useful in making safety contracts, establishing general principles or boundaries, informing the patient about events affecting the therapy (eg, vacations), and working with the patient in times of crisis [17]. A further benefit of addressing all self-states is an increase in coconsciousness. Coconsciousness is the internal awareness of the existence and experiences of other self-aspects. The reduction of dissociative symptoms must encourage all self-aspects to "listen in" and become part of the treatment process. Therapists will also find that more of the therapy material is absorbed by the patient and that treatment progresses at a steadier pace with this technique. The patient will eventually experience fewer episodes of time loss, fewer behaviors outside of awareness, and an improvement in general functioning.

"Internal meetings" in dissociative identity disorder

In our experience, it is counterproductive and ineffective for the therapist to ignore the patient's experience of self-states. In addition, the internal conflict described in the earlier section on "Talking Through" is a chief complaint among most patients who have DID. Many patients in the early stages of treatment for DID report that they cannot achieve internal cooperation and communication; they feel helpless to know where to begin the process of working with internal self-states. In addition, "in many cases the patient finds the idea of alter selves so frightening that communication only succeeds when it is first distanced ... through the therapist ..." [17]. This task seems daunting to many therapists when faced with a very challenging dissociative patient.

We commonly teach patients a skill called *internal meetings*. This technique is a modified version of the "Dissociative Table Technique" [19]. The Dissociative Table Technique offers an intervention that allows clients to recognize internal ego states and to structure and control switching and internal communication. It is an adjunctive strategy to psychotherapy and has proven successful in establishing internal cooperation and integration of the various ego states. We have found internal meetings to be effective in reducing internal conflict and resolving safety issues. Often this skill serves to more quickly identify the suicidal or most hopeless self-aspect. Thus, internal meetings become useful in planning for safety. Clinicians must assess the appropriateness of this intervention on a case-by-case basis. The patient who is too agitated or unable to agree with the guidelines (discussed later) may not be ready for this skill. A patient who is acutely suicidal might be hospitalized before using this technique. As always, risk should be assessed carefully before proceeding with a new technique or special intervention.

We find that the more organized a patient's internal meetings are initially, the more successful the outcome. We first explain to the patient that internal meetings are useful for problem-solving and decreasing internal conflict. The patient is assigned a topic for the meeting. For example, if a patient has little awareness of one's internal system, the first topic may simply be "introductions"—that is, asking each self-state to "introduce" oneself and reveal age (if known), likes/dislikes, needs/wants, and internal role or "job" (if known). A second topic might be, "What does each part need to begin working on together?" As patients become adept at internal meetings, they will begin to conduct them daily and self-initiate the activity. Internal meetings will become an integral part of the treatment process and the patient's daily increasing awareness of internal experiences.

We instruct patients to set clear guidelines for self-states who participate in the meetings. For example, patients are instructed to avoid graphic language, name-calling, or threats between self-states. An agreement must be made that self-states stay safe before, during, and after the meetings. Suggesting that only one self-state speak at a time so that each part has a chance to participate may also be helpful.

Patients often find it useful for some self-states attending the internal meeting to have roles or jobs. For example, we often request one self-state be the secretary. This role involves recording verbatim in a journal what is discussed in the internal meeting. The journal record provides rich material for therapy sessions. Second, a self-state is often asked to become the timekeeper. In this role, a self-state helps monitor the length of the internal meeting, which we suggest is kept to 30 minutes. Some patients also find it helpful to have a moderator who ensures that decorum is kept and each self-state participates. Other roles can be developed as the patient wishes.

Another important aspect of this skill is the use of an internal meeting space. This concept helps the patient become more organized and focused when using the skill. Fraser [19] suggests using the image of a table in a safe room, with chairs for the ego states. This image can be useful, although we further agree with Fraser that some clients may not wish to use such a closed-in setting. Some may choose a scene such as sitting on a beach or in a field on blankets, or another less restrictive outdoor setting.

It may be helpful for the patient to begin conducting internal meetings in the presence of the therapist, then practice having them on their own. As the treatment progresses, the therapist can often direct a patient to have an internal meeting if a safety crisis occurs. The patient can "check inside" to determine the cause of the crisis and even problem-solve a solution. Furthermore, this skill often leads to increased internal communication and eventually coconsciousness. It is remarkable to see the shift in internal awareness that patients experience as they become more aware of their internal system, including previously dissociated feelings, thoughts, and experiences. Overall, the internal meeting is a remarkable tool to promote change.

Traumatic reenactment

Traumatic reenactment, external and internal, is a common and frustrating experience for patients who have dissociative disorders. There are several psychologic and biologic theories to explain this revictimization, including repetition compulsion [20]; introjection of aggressive part-objects [21]; identification with the aggressor [22]; learned behavior; freezing and submission limbic states; and the neurobiology of disorganized attachment [9,23]. Significant research validates that a history of child trauma is a strong predictor of adult revictimization, particularly in the area of sexual abuse [24]. Patients who have dissociative disorders often report a history of childhood abuse or neglect, which may be polyabuse that includes physical, sexual, and emotional abuse. Dissociation creates a vulnerability to revictimization in the tendency to regress to a passive child-like state in a dangerous circumstance. These patients, despite their hypervigilance, may place themselves in risky situations as part of the pull toward reenactment, indifference to consequences, or acting out of a wish to self-punish or die.

One of the best and simplest models for understanding traumatic reenactment comes from the alcoholism literature, the Karpman Drama Triangle [25]. Karpman envisioned a family system triangle of shifting roles, including a persecutor, victim, and rescuer. A trauma triangle (Fig. 1) would also include the role of "nonrescuer" or "bystander" that our patients commonly describe.

These roles are not only repeated in patients' lives, but also in the internal world of DID. The self-aspects often represent these roles with persecutory

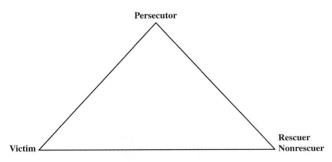

Fig. 1. Karpman Drama Triangle.

parts of self, victimized child parts, and helping parts [26]. These parts play out the drama of internal sadomasochism. Externally, patients who have dissociative disorders not only are subject to revictimization but also often exhaust themselves with rescuing and caretaking. For the most part, these patients tend to act out toward self rather than others; acting out toward others is an issue to be aware of and neutrally question. The Karpman Drama Triangle also models insights into transference and countertransference concerns.

Of particular concern in the treatment of DID is dealing with a patient's persecutory self-aspect, who may be threatening, hostile and especially uncooperative in helping to attain safety. Therapeutically, the therapist must stay calm and accept this aspect as part of the whole (the dissociative system often rejects and wants to rid itself of this aggressive part). The therapist's acceptance models the importance of working with this part's needs and the courage to deal with aggression as a problem, rather than remaining shame-bound or avoidant. Talking safely with a persecutory part of self can usually be done either directly or through other parts. Guidelines may need to be established about not hurting self, the therapist, or objects in the room; these guidelines can be reassuring to the patient and therapist.

Several techniques are useful when communication is achieved with a persecutory part of self. One technique is for the therapist to be empathic and gently confrontive about "this part also having been hurt," yet trying to be a protector, even when that part strongly identifies with an abuser. The protector part often uses strategies to regulate affect that caused dissociation at the hands of an abuser, but does so with a price. The existential loneliness and inner conflicts of this part may be pointed out. In addition, working with the whole system of dissociative aspects to help this part make a name or role change will usually be helpful (eg, going from "killer" to "Kerry"). This part may now be encouraged to alert the therapist when the work is going too fast, or to move from creating lack of safety to monitoring safety. It is not unusual for a persecutory self-aspect to turn out to be a child part, which is actually frightened underneath the aggressive presentation.

Safety planning

The specter of suicide is often present in the early treatment of patients who are severely traumatized [13]. In clinical experience, these patients have a high incidence of parasuicidal behaviors, suicide attempts, and completed suicides. Furthermore, many patients who have histories of childhood abuse exhibit self-harming behaviors, such as cutting, burning, intentional starvation, and placing oneself in dangerous situations. Patients who have DID often self-injure or attempt suicide outside of their awareness when another self-aspect has taken over functioning of the internal system. An internally collaborative safety plan is vital in the treatment process to manage safety crises and maintain safety.

Establishing a written safety plan with the patient that outlines actions the patient should take if in crisis can be very useful early in the treatment process when the therapist is developing a rapport with the patient. The basic tenet of such a plan is an agreement between patient and therapist that if the patient has attempted to manage the crisis independently using skills such as relaxation, grounding, containment, or journaling, that the patient will then contact the therapist before acting on any self-harming impulses and wait for the therapist to call back so that impulses can be discussed. This last instruction is important and must be specific because some patients may use concrete thinking to give themselves permission to self harm, such as "Well, I called you before I cut myself. Wasn't that our agreement?" The basics of a written safety agreement are, "I will not hurt myself or kill myself, nor anyone else, external or internal, accidentally or on purpose, at any time" [17].

A useful model for assisting the patient in determining which steps should be taken before contacting the therapist is the "Triangle of Choices for Safety" (Fig. 2) [27]. This model is based on the premise that patients have choices in the maintenance of their safety. As patients go through the predetermined choices and steps of the triangle, and if the options in each step are used and do not alleviate symptoms, then they progress to the next step. The choices become fewer and fewer as the interventions are not successful. Finally, as patients reach step 4, they should contact the therapist. If the intervention is not successful, they have a previously established commitment to use step 5; usually some form of hospitalization or a visit to the local emergency department.

The Triangle of Choices for Safety can be a useful approach to encouraging the patient to first try to use skills independently instead of immediately turning to the therapist for support. This method may serve to also minimize therapist burnout when a patient struggles frequently with safety issues.

The approach to patients diagnosed with DID is similar to that for those who have dissociative disorder not otherwise specified (DDNOS). However, significant variations may exist in the extent to which a person who has DDNOS has fully separate self-aspects, and this may require the therapist to tailor a cohesive internal safety commitment with all self-aspects.

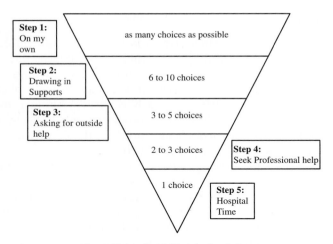

Fig. 2. Triangle of Choices for Safety.

Behavioral contracts between therapist and patient to set limits on unhealthy behavior and promote adaptive behavior are time-proven interventions in the treatment of DID [16–18,28]. This process may not come easily. A signed safety contract may not prevent suicide, regardless of such a promise, and thoughtful clinical judgment is always required when a patient is at high risk for self-harming behavior. Often, many self-states continue to believe that experiencing feelings is intolerable, and therefore must self-injure or turn to suicide if strong, painful feelings surface. Misguided protective self-aspects may believe that punishing other self-aspects is necessary to maintain secrets of past trauma. These trauma-distorted thoughts are challenged frequently in session.

One helpful tactic is to encourage the patient to use internal meetings to discuss the topic of safety with all self-aspects. Helpful beginning topics may be, "What does each part need to commit to safety?" or, "What needs to change in order for all parts to begin to work together towards safety?" Patients might also be encouraged to create an internal safety committee, wherein several self-aspects work together to monitor and maintain the safety commitment. If an impending crisis is sensed, the committee will bring it to the attention of the therapist for intervention. A written safety commitment that is widely used by clinicians states:

> I, _____ and all parts of my mind, known and unknown, agree to not intentionally or by accident hurt ourselves. If I am feeling unsafe, I will use _____ to stay safe. If those interventions do not help, I will contact my therapist, wait for help, and accept the help that is offered.

Many variations on this safety commitment exist. The safety plan will often need to be reworked as the treatment progresses. The therapist should check in frequently with the patient about any safety issues or concerns. The general principle is for patients to use intervention skills and not act on thoughts or plans, but wait until they speak with the therapist to discuss safety issues rather than acting on them.

Healing place

Clinical practice in the field of trauma and dissociation is replete with the creation of "safe place" imagery to manage fear and anxiety [16]. However, two issues arise with the concept of a safe place. First, many patients state that *safe* is a triggering word because they were never safe in the past. It is also not unusual for the word *safe* to have been used seductively in an abuse scenario. The patient may not be safe in the present, either. Second, therapists should emphasize the importance of normal vigilance in the world and not getting lost in internal imagery. "Healing place" is a more viable concept, because *healing* is an active and creative concept that connotes the power of process and hope.

The installation of a healing place is a valuable therapeutic intervention. Patients' willingness to use it is an indication that they are motivated and committed to the process of psychotherapy. The imagery itself has many variations and must be tailored to the individual patient. The therapist must not impose imagery, which may unwittingly trigger a recollection of abuse, but should first elicit suggestions or ideas from the patient. The therapist should include positive language in presenting the concept, such as "tapping into one's internal strengths and resources." The therapist and patient should spend some time in discussion, so that the work is collaborative and fruitful; it should not be a "cookbook" intervention, but limited only by imagination and good judgment (eg, should not include traumatizing imagery).

Many images can be used for a healing place. For example, the healing place may be focused on comforting frightened child aspects in DID and so includes a nursery full of toys, pillows, and a rocking chair for an "older" self-aspect to care for the "younger ones." This act is, of course, self-nurturing and self-parenting. It may be a place of healing and deep relaxation to calm psychologic and physiologic distress. It may be a place in nature in which to wonder and play and take in the beauty. Or, it may be a place of perspective and wisdom in which to ponder the past, gain insight, and weather the storms of life while healing continues. The therapist may ask the patient to include a symbol of hope. For many patients, a healing place connects with spirituality.

The installation and practice of a healing place should always include external safety and protected time to relax and heal. A generic script might be:

> This is a time for you to take for yourself, to facilitate the process of deep healing within. It is a time of invitation for all aspects of self, all parts of

your mind and your inner spirit to create this healing place. Focus inward and visualize this healing place just as you have talked about it. Fill the space with all the comforting and beautiful things that you wish to be there. Use your favorite colors. Experience it with all your senses, look around, touch things, breathe in the smells, hear the sounds, and move through all of the space. Spend as much time as you need to creatively fill the space and experience it fully. Know that you can return here at any time in which you are physically safe in the world and will not be interrupted. This place is only a thought away. It is your place of healing for all of your mind, body, and spirit. It is your creation.

The actual script would include details that have already been discussed and positive language. After installation of a healing place, the therapist should invite the patient to describe and share the experience for affirmation and reinforcement or to discuss any problems encountered. The place may need to be modified if there is intrusion of resistance or traumatic material. Not infrequently, a persecutory self-aspect in DID may want to prevent the creation of or threaten to destroy the healing place. That self-aspect then must first be won over in the spirit of cooperation, or at least noninterference. If that can be accomplished, then all self-aspects will gradually use the space. Overall, healing place imagery is ego-strengthening and self-soothing. In calming the mind and body, it also helps to undo the agitation and damaging physiologic effects of trauma [29].

Journaling and artwork

In our inpatient program, we regularly provide patients with journals and encourage them to use these throughout the hospitalization and continue the practice in outpatient therapy. We ask the patient to bring the journal to therapy sessions and discuss material that has been written. We always discuss the importance of protecting the journal and assure the patient that what is written is confidential. Some patients, however, balk at this request; usually it is not because of a fear of sharing the journal with the therapist, but instead of writing about personal thoughts and feelings and a fear that others may read the material. Usually this is a well-founded fear resulting from childhood trauma in which privacy and boundaries did not exist. In addition, a patient who has DID may be reluctant to use the journal because of "the experience of losing time or becoming profoundly depersonalized during the writing sessions, and sometimes finding strange, obscene, threatening or frightening messages in the journal" [17]. For patients who have been newly diagnosed with DID, this may be the first time they learn of other self-aspects. A helpful intervention to encourage the use of the journal by all self-aspects is to suggest folding the written page in the journal in half, indicating that the page should not be read until a therapy session. This strategy is particularly useful in the beginning stages of internal communication. For the therapist, journaling may prove to be very useful clinical material that aids in the diagnosis of DID, particularly if self-aspects identify themselves through a change in handwriting or the style of language (eg, grade school grammar versus college level).

It can be very organizing for a patient to be given the task of journaling between therapy sessions. We might suggest questions for the patient to contemplate and write about between sessions, usually stemming from topics discussed in the previous therapy session. We usually write the question or assignment directly in the journal so they can't claim to have forgotten the assignment and to emphasize the connection and collaboration with the therapist. (Some patients prefer that their therapist not write in their book. Asking permission is important.) This reminder keeps the patient on task. The use of an adjunctive workbook may also be valuable [30]. We also often encourage patients to take notes at the end of the therapy session (or during, if necessary). This practice is particularly useful when a patient is highly dissociative and loses time during the day.

Another expressive therapy that has proven to be useful in the treatment of dissociative disorders is art therapy. Finding an art therapist skilled in working with trauma and dissociation is often difficult. However, therapists may find it useful to adopt some basic artwork as part of the therapy work, being careful to keep it simple and contained. Therapists should keep in mind that artwork can be uncovering and destabilizing, so structured exercises are the best approach. *Managing Traumatic Stress Through Art* [31], a workbook written by informed art therapists, can be used as a guide. This workbook contains several carefully structured art projects with reproducible work sheets. The projects must be used in a timely fashion in the process of the therapy and patients must be reassured that they do not need to be accomplished artists to use these exercises.

Another type of artwork that is informative is the collage, made up of pictures and words cut out of magazines and pasted on a large piece of paper. The subjects may be as varied as the creation of a healing place (which may then be visualized internally); a map of self-aspects and bridging internal communication (in DID); a visual representation of coping skills; or the separation of the past from the present. When working with potentially powerful affects, it is helpful to add a containing or healing border to the collage.

The construction of a survival kit is another useful art project. The goal is to fill a box (eg, a shoebox decorated as the patient desires) with self-nurturing objects that are intuitively appealing. These objects may include an interesting leaf or rock, a compact disc of soothing music, a postcard or picture of a beautiful scene or painting, a small book, a list of affirmations, or perhaps a list of suggested activities. The kit is a resource to use during times of distress. The selection of objects creates the awareness of "natural antidepressants" in the world and reinforces the right to reach out and claim them for one's own. The kit not only is helpful in undoing the deprivation of the past but also can be part of a safety plan to decrease self-harm impulses.

Summary

Clinical experience over many years has taught that patients who have dissociative disorders routinely experience significant emotional pain and struggle with overall functioning and safety. Finding therapeutic techniques with which to stabilize functioning, create internal safety, alleviate suffering, and further the progress of the treatment within the psychodynamic framework of the psychotherapy is challenging for clinicians who treat this population. This article has discussed useful, skill-building strategies that can be employed judiciously in the treatment, particularly in the early stages of the work.

Several of these interventions derive from the cognitive-behavioral and clinical hypnosis therapies and from the experience of seasoned clinicians who work in the field of trauma and dissociation. Ten areas have been discussed, beginning with suggested topics for psychoeducation that provide a basic understanding of the human response to trauma and the dissociative spectrum, and the road map for stage-oriented treatment. This intervention is followed by the skills of pacing and containment, and grounding. "Talking through" and "internal meeting," two specific and important skills for working with patients who have DID, are included. Patients in the entire spectrum of dissociative disorders have difficulty with traumatic reenactment in the forms of suicidality, self-injurious behaviors, and revictimization. A model for sequenced safety planning is discussed. The installation of an internal "healing place" is valuable because it connotes the power of the process of healing and gives hope. Finally, journaling and artwork are included as therapeutic strategies.

These therapeutic ego-strengthening interventions can help the therapy work proceed more rapidly and with less anguish for the clinician and patient. They are useful strategic skills and techniques that clinicians can learn and apply wisely within the course of psychotherapy with patients who have dissociative disorders.

References

[1] Diagnostic and Statistical Manual of Mental Disorders. 4th edition. Text revision. Washington (DC): American Psychiatric Association; 2000.
[2] Harris M. Trauma Recovery and empowerment, a clinician's guide for working with women in groups. New York: The Free Press; 1998.
[3] Haddock DB. Dissociative identity disorder sourcebook. New York: McGraw-Hill Companies; 2001.
[4] Herman J. Trauma and recovery. New York: Basic Books; 1992.
[5] Napier N. Getting through the day. New York: WW Norton; 1993.

[6] Vermilyea EG. Growing beyond survival: a self-help toolkit for managing traumatic stress. Baltimore (MD): Sidran Foundation and Press; 2000.

[7] Foa E, Davidson J, Frances A, et al. Expert consensus treatment guidelines for posttraumatic stress disorder: a guide for patients and families. J Clin Psychiatry 1999;(Suppl 16):69–76.

[8] Perry B, Pollard R. Homeostasis, stress, trauma, and adaptation. A neurodevelopmental view of childhood trauma. Child Adolesc Psychiatr Clin N Am 1998;7(1):33–51.

[9] Siegel D. An interpersonal Neurobiology of psychotherapy: the developing mind and the resolution of trauma. In: Solomon M, Siegel D, editors. Healing trauma: attachment, mind, body and brain. New York: W.W. Norton; 2003. p. 1–56.

[10] Harris M, Fallot R. Designing trauma-informed addiction services. New Dir Ment Health Serv 2001;(89):57–73.

[11] Courtois CA. Recollections of sexual abuse: treatment principles and guidelines. New York: W.W. Norton; 1999.

[12] Brown D, Scheflin A, Hammond D. Memory, Trauma, treatment, and the law: an essential reference on memory for clinicians, researchers, attorney and judges. New York: W.W. Norton; 1998.

[13] Chu J. Rebuilding shattered lives: the responsible treatment of complex post traumatic and dissociative disorders. New York: Wiley and Sons; 1998.

[14] Linehan M. Skills training manual for treating borderline personality disorder. New York: Guilford Press; 1993.

[15] Kluft R. Playing for time: temporizing techniques in the treatment of multiple personality disorders. Am J Clin Hypn 1989;32:90–8.

[16] Kluft RP. Varieties of hypnotic interventions in the treatment of multiple personality. Am J Clin Hypn 1982;24:230–40.

[17] Putnam FW. Diagnosis and treatment of multiple personality disorder. New York: Guilford Press; 1989.

[18] Braun BG. Uses of hypnosis with multiple personalities. Psychiatr Ann 1984;14:34–40.

[19] Fraser GA. Fraser's "Dissociative Table Technique" revisited, revised: a strategy for working with ego states in dissociative disorders and ego-state therapy. J Trauma Dissociation 2003;4(4):5–27.

[20] Jones E. The life and work of Sigmund Freud, vol. 2. Years of maturity 1901–1919. New York: Basic Books, Inc.; 1955.

[21] Davies J, Frawley M. Treating the adult survivor of childhood sexual abuse: a psychoanalytic perspective. New York: Basic Books; 1994.

[22] Freud A. The writing of Anna Freud: the ego and the mechanisms of defense. New York: International Universities Press; 1966.

[23] Schore A. Early relational trauma, disorganized attachment, and the development of a predisposition to violence. In: Solomon M, Siegel D, editors. Healing trauma: attachment, mind, body and brain. New York: W.W. Norton; 2003.

[24] Koenig L, Doll L, Leary A, et al. Trauma, revictimization, and intervention. In: From child sexual abuse to adult sexual risk. Washington (DC): American Psychological Association; 2004. p. 49–68.

[25] Karpman S. Fairy tales and script drama analysis. Transactional Analysis Bulletin 1968;7: 39–43.

[26] Turkus J. Psychotherapy and case management for multiple personality disorder. Synthesis for continuity care. Psychiatr Clin North Am 1991;14(3):658–9.

[27] Mohawk Valley Hospital. Triangle of Choices for Safety. Presented to Sheppard and Enoch Pratt Hospital Nursing Department. Baltimore, MD, May 1999. First modification by Sheppard and Enoch Pratt Hospital, for the Trauma Disorder Program, May 1999. Second modification by Jennifer Aloe Kahler, PsyD, for The Center-Posttraumatic Disorder Program at the Psychiatric Institute of Washington, D.C., September 2002.

[28] Wilbur CB. Psychodynamic approaches to multiple personality. Presented at meeting of the American Psychiatric Association. Toronto, May 15–21, 1982.

[29] van der Kolk B. The Body keeps the score: approaches to the psychobiology of posttraumatic stress disorder. In: van der Kolk B, McFarlane A, Weisaeth L, editors. Traumatic stress: the effects of overwhelming experience on mind, body, and society. New York: Guilford Press; 1996.
[30] Adams K. The way of the journal: a journal therapy workbook for healing. Baltimore (MD): Sidran Foundation and Press; 1998.
[31] Cohen B, Barnes M, Rankin A. Managing traumatic stress through art: drawing from the center. Baltimore (MD): The Sidran Press; 1995.

ELSEVIER
SAUNDERS

Psychiatr Clin N Am 29 (2006) 263–279

PSYCHIATRIC
CLINICS
OF NORTH AMERICA

A Sensorimotor Approach to the Treatment of Trauma and Dissociation

Pat Ogden, PhD[a],*, Clare Pain, MD, FRCPC[b,c],
Janina Fisher, PhD[d]

[a]Sensorimotor Psychotherapy Institute, 1579 Orchard Avenue, Boulder, CO 80304, USA
[b]Department of Psychiatry, University of Western Ontario, London, Ontario, Canada
[c]Department of Psychiatry, University of Toronto, Toronto, Ontario, Canada
[d]The Trauma Center, Boston, MA, USA

Psychotherapists who work with survivors of psychologic trauma recognize the almost inevitable clinical complexity of trauma-related disorders. Traumatized individuals do not just suffer memories of tragic and horrifying experiences—they demonstrate a number of complicated and debilitating signs, symptoms, and difficulties consisting primarily of bodily responses to dysregulated affects. These bodily responses often have no clear subjective connection to their fragments of narrative memory [1].

Most traumatized individuals fulfill the criteria for a number of coexisting diagnoses that usually include mood disorders, anxiety disorders, substance abuse and dependence disorders, eating disorders, somatoform disorders, and medically unexplained symptoms [2–4]. These complications are reflected in the *Diagnostic and Statistical Manual of Mental Disorders* (fourth edition, revised) by the inclusion of more than 12 associated features of post-traumatic stress disorder (PTSD) [5]. The formal diagnosis of PTSD contains three diagnostic post-traumatic symptom clusters: symptoms indicative of intrusive reliving of the trauma, avoidance and numbing symptoms, and symptoms of increased autonomic arousal. The episodic alternation between the avoidance and reliving symptoms "is the result of dissociation: traumatic events are distanced and dissociated from usual conscious awareness in the numbing phase, only to return in the intrusive phase" [6]. Triggered by stimuli reminiscent of the trauma, these dissociated fragments of past experience return unbidden in the form of psychologic symptoms (amnesia, cognitive schemas of badness or worthlessness, intrusive images,

---

* Corresponding author.
    E-mail address: patogden@comcast.net (P. Ogden).

dysregulated emotions) and somatoform symptoms (physical pain, physical numbing, intrusive sensations, and dysregulated autonomic arousal) [7]. Despite the central involvement of somatoform symptoms in the expression of unresolved trauma, however, the autonomic and somatic components of trauma-related disorders have been relatively neglected in the treatment and understanding of these disorders [8].

Talk therapies and exposure therapy

Although there is evidence to suggest that treatments targeting the various symptoms and problems of trauma-related disorders can promote significant improvement in some patients, full remediation of these disorders is elusive [9,10]. Traditional "talk-therapy" approaches, a category that includes any method that depends on the words of the client as the primary entry point of therapy, tend to address the explicit, verbally accessible components of trauma. They emphasize the role of narrative, emotional expression, and meaning making [11,12]. Because avoidance and withdrawal compose a core diagnostic cluster in trauma-related disorders, it is increasingly recognized that in vitro or imaginal exposure to the potent elements in the patient's experience is usually a necessary ingredient in successful trauma treatment [13]. Although exposure to episodes of past trauma is a potentially effective ingredient, this exposure in any model of therapy can exacerbate rather than resolve symptoms. As the narrative or explicit memory is retold, the implicit, somatosensory components of the memory are simultaneously activated, frequently leading to a re-experiencing of somatoform symptoms that can include autonomic dysregulation, dissociative defenses associated with hyper- and hypoarousal states, intrusive sensory experiences, and involuntary movements. This debilitating, repetitive cycle of mind-body triggering can thwart desensitization regimes and keep past trauma "alive," prolonging rather than resolving trauma-related disorders [14–20]. A considerable number of patients drop out of exposure therapy, perhaps because they are not sufficiently stable to manage it in the face of the threat of retraumatization [21–26].

For clients who are able to sustain exposure-type treatments, two popular and well-researched treatments that address the behavioral avoidance and the reliving and hyperarousal responses in different ways are Prolonged Exposure (PE) [27] and Eye Movement Desensitization and Reprocessing [28]. Both therapies have been studied in treatment trials with patients who are relatively stable or have adult-onset, single-incident trauma. Even in well-run studies of validated treatments, however, only about 50% of patients demonstrate significant improvement. For example, in a study comparing PE versus cognitive restructuring [26], most subjects had experienced a traumatic event lasting less than 1 hour. Results demonstrated that the effects of both treatments were comparable, but at 6 months' follow-up, half of the treated individuals still met the criteria for PTSD and only 25% reported a return to premorbid functioning. In a similarly well-conducted study comparing relaxation training with imaginal exposure, cognitive restructuring, or a combination of both, all but the relaxation training had a beneficial effect in decreasing PTSD symptoms [29]. Although only one third of the subjects still met the criteria for PTSD at termination, less than 50% showed a marked improvement. Strict inclusion and exclusion criteria can serve to increase rates of effectiveness, as demonstrated by an effectiveness study in which PE, stress inoculation, and the combination of PE plus stress inoculation were compared [27]. Despite the superior results for PE in this study, still less than 50% of the subjects (all female assault victims) were found to have good end-state functioning at 1-year follow-up.

Top-down and bottom-up therapies

It is perhaps the sensorimotor symptoms and the autonomic dysregulation of chronic traumatic re-experiencing and avoidance that prove most difficult to ameliorate, even in the relatively straightforward PTSD clients who have single-incident traumatic experience as adults. To address these bodily based symptoms of trauma and the psychologic components, a different approach to treatment may be helpful. The authors propose that it is possible to weave sensorimotor understandings and techniques into existing psychodynamic or cognitive-behavioral models of therapy, including exposure treatments [30]. The working premise in most approaches to psychotherapy, less so with exposure techniques, is that change occurs in a "top-down" direction. That is, a significant change in a patient's thought processes (through insight, exposure, or cognitive restructuring) in conjunction with remembering or therapeutic re-experiencing of the event resolves the problematic emotions, behaviors, and physical symptoms of the patient. Although top-down therapy is effective and necessary in helping patients with many important therapeutic tasks, the addition of "bottom-up" approaches that directly address the effects of traumatic experience on the body may be equally necessary.

Sensorimotor psychotherapy [31,32] is an approach developed to specifically address resolution of the somatic symptoms of unresolved trauma. In sensorimotor psychotherapy, bodily experience becomes the primary entry point for intervention; emotional expression and meaning making arise out of the subsequent somatic reorganization of habitual trauma-related responses. Sensorimotor approaches work from the bottom-up rather than the top-down by attending to the patient's body directly; it becomes possible to address the more primitive, automatic, and involuntary functions of the brain that underlie traumatic and post-traumatic responses. Sensorimotor psychotherapy is founded on the premise that "the brain functions as an integrated whole but [comprises] systems that are hierarchically organized.

The 'higher level' [cognitive] integrative functions evolve from and are dependent [on] the integrity of 'lower-level' [limbic (emotional) and reptilian] structures and on sensorimotor experience" [33].

The capacity of human beings for self-awareness, interpretation, abstract thought, and feeling exists within this developmental and hierarchic relationship to the instinctual and nonconscious responses of the body. These hierarchically organized, interconnected responses range from instinctual arousal and mammalian defenses, feelings, and affective expression to thoughts, reflective self-awareness, and meaning making. Wilbur's [34] notion of hierarchic information processing describes the evolutionary and functional hierarchy among these three levels of organizing experience: cognitive, emotional, and sensorimotor. MacLean [35] conceptualized this hierarchy as the "triune brain," or a "brain with a brain within a brain." In MacLean's theory, the human brain is the product of evolutionary hierarchic development: first to develop in the human infant is the reptilian brain (comprising the brain stem and cerebellum), which governs arousal, homeostasis of the organism, reproductive drives, sensation, and instinctual movement impulses—the heart of sensorimotor experience. The "second" brain is the "paleomammalian brain," or "limbic brain," found in all mammals, which anatomically surrounds the reptilian brain and serves to regulate somatosensory experience, emotion, memory, some social behavior, and learning [36]. Last to develop phylogenetically is the neocortex, which enables cognitive information processing, self-awareness, executive functioning, and conceptual thinking [35]. This hierarchic organization results in two distinctly different directions of information processing (from the top-down or the bottom-up), and the interplay between them holds significant implications for the treatment of trauma [37]. Schore [38] noted that for adults, in nontraumatic circumstances, higher cortical areas act as control centers such that the orbital prefrontal cortex hierarchically dominates subcortical activity, with "veto power" over limbic responses. Thus, top-down processing enables us to outline plans, determine what to accomplish for the day, and then structure time to meet particular goals. Emotions and sensations such as feelings of frustration, fatigue, or physical discomfort may be overridden to accomplish these priorities. It is as though, most of the time, we hover just above our somatic and sensory experience, not allowing it to be the primary determinant of our actions without conscious decision making. For the traumatized individual, however, the intensity of trauma-related emotions and sensorimotor reactions often disorganizes the individual's cognitive capacities, interfering with the ability for cognitive processing and top-down-regulation. This phenomenon has been described as "bottom-up hijacking" and is a frequent source of problems for trauma survivors [37,39].

When bottom-up hijacking occurs, as in recalling trauma, dysregulated autonomic arousal contributes to generating strong waves of body sensations and affects, which in turn are interpreted as current rather than past data that confirm the cognitive conviction of threat, exposure, or helplessness. For example, if a body sensation such as rapid heart rate is interpreted as fear or panic, each of those aspects of the experience—sensorimotor and emotional—inflate and compound the other. If, in addition, they are interpreted as meaning, "I am not safe," then physical sensation and emotion further intensify, and arousal can quickly escalate beyond the person's tolerance or integrative capacity. Adaptive top-down regulation is temporarily lost, leaving the individual at the mercy of bottom-up hijacking.

The idea that "what we think" directs "how we feel" is a fundamentally important development of Cartesian theory that has informed the influential therapies of the Western world. If, however, traumatic memories largely consist of reactivated nonverbal implicit-type memories and habitual procedural responses with limited explicit memory components, then such memories may not be transformed adequately by insight alone [18,40,41]. The authors propose that sensorimotor interventions that directly address the body can work to process implicit-type memories, to challenge procedural learning, and help to regulate dysregulated autonomic arousal. Not only is what we feel a robust predictor of what we will think but it may also predict how we will interpret what we experience.

In sensorimotor psychotherapy, clients' cognitions are engaged to evoke mindful observation of the interplay of their perceptions, emotions, movements, sensations, impulses, and thoughts. In the act of noticing their bodily experience, innate somatic regulatory capacities, or "resources," become spontaneously available or can be evoked by the therapist: taking a breath, adjusting the spine, making a movement, or orienting perceptually and physically to the environment. For example, with the help of his therapist, "Jim" realized that the perpetual slump in his spine had served to maintain his feelings of inferiority, helplessness, and passivity. As this component of his early abusive experience was addressed somatically, his posture gradually became more erect, transformed from a physical liability to a physical resource that supported his newly found sense of well-being and competency. His thoughts correspondingly started to become less negative, his emotions more buoyant. In the hands of an informed body-oriented psychotherapist, the client's body gradually becomes his ally rather than his enemy in the process of healing from trauma. Such somatic changes, in and of themselves, often help to resolve the habitual trauma-related responses or provide enough stability to allow more intense exposure to traumatic material.

Bottom-up dysregulation and the window of tolerance

The characteristic components of the trauma response—a poor tolerance for stress and arousal with consequent affect dysregulation—render traumatized individuals hyperaroused, experiencing "too much" activation, or hypoaroused, experiencing "too little" [42]. Information cannot be processed effectively in either state, top-down-regulation is lost as the patient feels en-dangered, and meaning making becomes biased by the danger signals. The hyperaroused patient is tormented by intrusive re-experiencing of the trauma. The perceptual distortions and losses in the hypoaroused patient can involve not only a sense of separation from the self (as in derealization and depersonalization) but also motor weakness, paralysis, ataxia, numb-ing of inner body sensation, and cognitive abnormalities such as amnesia, fugue states, and confusional states [43]. Although hyperarousal symptoms and intrusive re-experiencing are commonly considered the hallmark symptoms of trauma, not all trauma patients respond to trauma reminders with hyperarousal. In one study, 30% of subjects responded with hypoar-ousal and emotional symptoms when hearing their trauma scripts read to them [44].

To put the past in the past, it is necessary to process traumatic experience in a state of "optimal arousal." The ideal zone between the two extreme physiologic states of autonomic hyper- and hypoarousal was described by Siegel [18] as the "window of tolerance"—the range of activation within which the individual can experience psychophysiologic arousal as tolerable or manageable. In this optimal range, the patient can integrate information on cognitive, emotional, and sensorimotor levels. All of the interventions characteristic of sensorimotor psychotherapy seek to develop or to enlarge an existing stable and generous window of tolerance.

The extremes of autonomic arousal that might have been adaptive at the moment of danger ultimately become a potential source of therapeutic im-passe when the patient cannot maintain arousal within the window of toler-ance [45]. As a threat is first perceived, an instinctive mind/body chain reaction is set in motion, involving cascades of stress hormone responses that mobilize the sympathetic nervous system and prepare the individual for flight, fight, and freeze defenses. When adaptive responses are successful, the body uses and metabolizes the neurochemicals, and arousal may gradu-ally return to an optimal zone when the threatening stimulus has receded or disappeared. In the wake of a traumatic experience, however, this return to baseline does not always occur. In cases of extreme or prolonged trauma or in the context of subsequent inadequacies in soothing and relational sup-port, the individual may have difficulty recalibrating autonomic arousal [42,46–48].

Chronic hyperarousal creates a vicious cycle: a hyperaroused nervous sys-tem increases vulnerability to state-dependent memory retrieval triggered by trauma-related stimuli, which results in "increased access to traumatic mem-ories and involuntary intrusions of the trauma, which lead in turn to even more arousal" [20]. These intrusive perceptual memories appear as symp-toms such as flashbacks and nightmares, causing a rapid heart rate, elevated blood pressure, and altered skin conductance associated with hyperarousal [49–51]. Because repeated traumatic responses can result in the kindling of survival-related neural pathways, traumatized people tend to become increasingly more vulnerable to progressively minor triggers [52]. They remain autonomically "on guard" against danger (hyperaroused and hypervigilant or hypoaroused and numbly passive), and they fail to notice or integrate new data from the present that tells them that the danger is over. People who have trauma-related disorders lose somatic connection to present reality: at a body level, these responses are experienced as the past event happening again and again [42]. In sensorimotor psychotherapy, connection to the present is maintained through the use of mindfulness-based techniques. By keeping the treatment focused on the patient's here-and-now somatic experience in the session (by mindfully noticing the trauma as it manifests in changes in heart rate, breathing, and muscle tone), the individual is encouraged to experience being "here now" while acknowledging the "there and then" of traumatic experience.

Defensive subsystems

In the context of threat, hyper- and hypoarousal states are accompanied by one of two general types of defensive responses or a combination of both: mobilizing defenses (such as fight or flight) or immobilizing defenses (such as freezing or collapse/submission). No one defensive response is "better" than another; all are potentially adaptive and effective at diminishing threat, depending on the situation and the capabilities of the individual. The authors propose that inflexibility among these defensive subsystems and their overactivity in the absence of threat involves chronic dysregulated arousal and contributes to the traumatized person's continued distress after the traumatic event is over.

Mobilization

The mobilizing defenses of fight and flight are characterized by arousal of the sympathetic nervous system and the corresponding neurochemically mediated physical reactions. Flight is probably the most common response to threat when successful escape is probable [53]. When the flight response is activated, the large muscles are primed and ready to mobilize for flight and awareness of any pain or injury is diminished. Flight can be understood not only as running away from danger but also as running toward the person or place that can provide safety [54]. Versions of the flight response can be observed in patients in a variety of additional, less obvious behaviors such as twisting, turning, or backing away from a perceived source of danger. If the chance of escape is remote and the threat closes in, the potential victim's attempts at flight may become increasingly frantic. When flight becomes impossible, fighting may provide the alternative of self-defense [55]. The fight response is often provoked when the victim feels trapped or whenever aggression might effectively secure safety.

Mobilizing defenses also include innumerable patterns of skilled responses that are learned or spontaneous and enacted automatically in the course of safely performing physical activities. For example, the ability to drive or operate machinery requires the incorporation of complex movements that, through repetition, become action tendencies that can be executed without thought, such as putting on the brakes and turning the steering wheel to prevent an accident. Such defensive actions anticipate and correct for possible difficulties without invoking flight/fight systems and include such motor acts as engaging the righting reflexes during a near fall, raising an arm for protection from a falling object, avoiding a rock in a downhill ski run, and so on.

Immobilization

In the animal kingdom, the mobilizing defenses give way to immobilizing responses when the former are ineffective or cannot ensure survival [55,56]. For example, according to Nijenhuis and Van der Hart [55], a child who is being sexually or physically abused by a caregiver is not in a psychologic position that enables flight. In some situations, running or fighting (mobilizing defenses) would worsen the situation for the child being physically or sexually abused or who witnesses violence, increasing the danger and provoking more violence.

The authors identify three main immobilizing defenses: freezing, limp passivity or feigning death, and submissive behaviors. There seem to be several somatosensory states that have been described as freezing. These states are briefly reviewed here, although it is the last description that is most clearly aligned with the immobilizing defense. Clients who have experienced freezing frequently report that they were very aware of the environment, especially of threat cues, potential escape routes, or protective impulses; they felt energized and tense; and were ready and able to run if needed. Misslin [56, p. 58] described freezing as "alert immobility," where there is complete cessation of movement except for respiration and movement of the eyes. This freezing appears to involve a highly engaged sympathetic system in which "muscle tone, heart rate, sensory acuity, and alertness are all high [57], with the individual waiting for more data from the threat before taking action. Freezing may be the best defense when the threat is a possibility rather than a certainty, in which case flight would be most effective. Another version of freezing occurs when the predator is still at a distance and motionless behavior may prevent detection. This kind of freezing occurs as a "preventative" measure in nature, as when baby deer are left camouflaged in tall grass while the mother is away foraging for food. For children growing up in traumatogenic environments, freezing behavior often accompanies hiding from threat, for example, in the closet, behind a chair, or under the stairs. Freezing promotes safety in these instances because when the child is still and quiet, it increases the likelihood that he or she will remain un-noticed.

Clients also describe a third type of freezing as feeling "paralyzed," terrifyingly incapable of moving and unable to breathe. This version is associated with a sense of being "trapped." There is a concurrently high level of arousal that is combined with an inability to take action [18,58]. Siegel [18] postulated that with this kind of freezing, the sympathetic and the parasympathetic systems are aroused simultaneously, which produces muscular constriction paired with a feeling of paralysis.

Freezing is accompanied by sympathetic nervous system arousal, whereas the immobilizing defenses of feigning death, behavioral shutdown, or fainting are powered by the parasympathetic dorsal branch of the vagus nerve [59]. These defensive variants (feigning death, behavioral shutdown, or fainting) of the immobilizing defensive responses are apparent states of passivity that involve the subject becoming "limp": the muscles become flaccid rather than tense and breathing becomes shallow [58,60,61]. Patients often describe this condition as feeling "trancelike or dreamlike." It is accompanied by a reduced capacity to simultaneously attend to the external environment and the internal phenomena. Anesthesia, analgesia, and the slowing of muscular/skeletal responses [53,58,62] often co-occur in this group of responses.

Submissive behaviors (such as crouching, avoiding eye contact, and generally appearing physically smaller and therefore nonthreatening) are also common among traumatized individuals. Submissive behaviors serve a protective and preventative function because they "aim at preventing or interrupting aggressive reactions" [56, p. 59]. Body language in these circumstances is characterized by nonaggressive movements, automatic obedience, and helpless compliance in which the eyes are lowered and the back is bowed before the perpetrator. A version of this condition, described as "robotization," has been noted in Nazi concentration camp survivors; it includes mechanical behavior and automatic obedience, without question or thought, to the demands of others [63]. Elements of the behavior, such as downward flexion (head ducking), appear to be part of the fixed action patterns of fear. As a result of chronic abuse, it is not uncommon for patients to characteristically respond to threat cues with mechanistic compliance or resigned submission, which may be wrongly understood as collusion or agreement. This mechanistic compliance or resigned submission can be seen, for example, in the patient who perfunctorily allows a male relative into her apartment despiteknowing he will rape her as he has done in the past. Predatory or abusive individuals often seek to evoke these behaviors in others, taking advantage of the instinctive defensive response to elicit automatic compliance with the abuse [12].

Incomplete mobilizing defenses

When the cascade of mobilizing and immobilizing defensive actions is evoked, some of the actions (in particular, the mobilizing defenses) that might enable escape or the warding off of danger are rendered ineffective or interrupted and left incomplete. An automobile accident victim might have felt the impulse to turn the steering wheel but was unable to execute the action before hitting the oncoming car. The sexual abuse survivor might have wanted to fight her perpetrator but was overpowered and unable to follow through. These incomplete actions of defense may subsequently manifest as chronic symptoms. As Herman [12] stated, "each component of the ordinary response to danger, having lost its utility, tends to persist in an altered and exaggerated state long after the actual danger is over" (p. 34). When an endangered person experiences the instinct to fight back or to flee but is unable to execute these actions, this unfinished sequence of possible defensive actions may persist in distorted forms. Individuals may experience their fight and flight muscles held in a chronically tightened pattern, have heightened and unstable aggressive impulses, or have a chronic lack of tone or sensation in a particular muscle group. It is as if part of the brain does not know that the trauma is over and is still responding bodily "in the moment of the trauma." In addition, many patients come to therapy exhibiting chronic immobilizing defensive tendencies in their bodies that, in turn, profoundly influence their emotions and cognitions.

In sensorimotor psychotherapy, these patients are helped to rediscover their truncated mobilizing defensive impulses through tracking their bodily movements and sensations that emerge during the therapy session. For example, a patient who had to submit to her caregiver's sexual abuse as a child discovered her forgotten, dormant impulse to push away and flee to protect herself. As she mindfully re-experienced how her body ultimately did not resist the abuse and automatically submitted, she noticed a tightening in her jaw accompanied by muscle tension that went from the jaw down the neck into her shoulder and arm. In response to the therapist's encouragement to continue studying her tension, the tightening continued to increase and her hands curled up into a fist. Being able to observe and attend to how her body wanted to respond, she became aware of the previously aborted physical urge to not only punch at her caregiver but also to run away, reflected in a tightening and feeling of energy in her legs. These physical impulses on which she did not and could not act at the time of the abuse appeared spontaneously as she became meticulously aware of her physical sensations and impulses during recall of her abuse in therapy. She later discovered how her truncated, lost impulses to resist had become encoded not only in the praxis of submission but also as beliefs or automatic assumptions of "I don't deserve to defend myself."

The healing transformation of defensive styles

Sensorimotor psychotherapy thus addresses the failed processing of the old trauma as it is directly "found" in the present moment in the embodied experience of the patient. The sensorimotor-informed therapist carefully observes, with the patient, how the impulses for active or mobilizing defenses are overwhelmed and how they unconsciously resort to the immobilizing defenses (freezing, submitting, or becoming hypoaroused and "floppy"). Lewis and colleagues [57] described this mammalian immobilizing defense as feigning death. By evoking somatic responses to the trauma, in the session, the therapist helps the patient transform immobilizing defenses into mobilizing defenses. The patient can feel the full, completed experience of his or her capacity to defend through physical action, within her window of tolerance, instead of repeatedly re-experiencing the truncated, aborted, active defense or the frozen, dissociated, or submissive immobilizing responses. Thus, before treatment, unresolved trauma insidiously predicts the individual's future before the future has happened. The future has been prescribed as hopeless by the past. Under the sway of this anticipation, there is little room for living in the present. Until an abused patient can experience the satisfaction of performing her active defensive actions fully, her future seems to hold only further abuse and disappointment as she continuously fails to defend herself. As the patient consciously distinguishes her mobilizing physical defensive action from her immobilizing physical response to the original trauma, her new actions can become conscious and available to her, and as a result, the future can hold more promise. Rather than insight alone, it is the actual experience of mobilizing action with conscious intention and awareness while simultaneously addressing the cognitive distortions and emotional reactions that helps effect such change.

Sensorimotor treatment: bottom-up interventions

Thus, instead of focusing on the verbal description of traumatic events, sensorimotor treatment focuses on the re-activation of autonomic hyper- or hypoarousal and defensive action tendencies as these occur within the therapy hour. In a bottom-up approach, the narrative becomes a vehicle for activating these physiologic responses and movements so that they can be studied and ultimately transformed. The therapist and client have an opportunity to work with the implicit elements of traumatic memories by directing the client's awareness away from the verbal components of memory to the nonverbal residue of the trauma. Somatic bottom-up interventions that address the repetitive, unbidden, physical sensations of hyperarousal and hypoarousal together with movement inhibitions can then be integrated with more traditional top-down interventions that help to transform the narrative of the trauma and facilitate the development of a reorganized somatic sense of self. The sense of self is represented not only in beliefs and emotional responses but also in physical organization, postural habits, and movements of the body. An integrated approach to soma and psyche helps these patients regulate their physical experiences so that their corresponding sense of self feels grounded, resourced, and oriented toward present experience.

Sensorimotor psychotherapy builds on and adds to traditional, widely accepted psychotherapeutic understandings and principles. For instance, sensorimotor psychotherapy, along with talk therapies (regardless of the theoretic model), recognizes the necessity of a good therapeutic alliance between therapist and patient. The alliance in a sensorimotor treatment, however, is built bottom-up as the therapist supplements the patient's bodily sensings with another pair of eyes and thoughtful appreciation of the patient's somatic experience through careful observation of "bodily language," taking on the role of an "auxiliary cortex" for the client [64]. The therapist becomes a kind of somatosensorially attuned "affect regulator of the patient's dysregulated states to provide a growth-facilitating environment for the patient's immature affect-regulating structures" [65]. That is, as the therapist tracks the patient's sensorimotor experience, he or she notices the physiologic signs of dysregulation and applies the appropriate interventions to settle or increase arousal: adjusting voice tone, energy level, pacing, choice of vocabulary, mindful observation, movement, and the amount of emotional or cognitive content. As the patient experiences the calm and relief that accompanies optimal arousal or a return to their window of tolerance, the therapeutic alliance is strengthened. With an increase in the sense of safety, the client's exploration of his or her experiences becomes less inhibited. Alternatively stated, as the client's chronic fear subsides, the client is freer to explore both inner and outer worlds like a child with a secure attachment base.

Activating neural systems that enhance exploration

In the traumatized client, chronically activated somatic defenses and their corresponding fears tend to override and inhibit the exploratory system that is also a wired-in mammalian motivational system. Panksepp [66] maintained that the SEEKING system "drives and energizes many mental complexities that humans experience as persistent feelings of interest, curiosity, sensation seeking, and, in the presence of a sufficiently complex cortex, the search for higher meaning (p. 145)." Evoking the patient's seeking system in therapy stimulates curiosity about how they can combat or inhibit habitual fear-based survival responses. At the moment of threat, instinctual survival defenses take precedence over cognitive functions. Long after the traumatic events are over, activation of the prefrontal cortices and cognitive functions can be intermittently inhibited in response to trauma-related stimuli [20,39], hindering the capacity for successful self-observation, exploration, and new learning. The therapist's job is to "wake up" the exploratory capacities by promoting a somatic sense of safety and cultivating the capacity for observation, curiosity, and mindfulness in the client. Observation of the present moment's experience engages the executive and observing functions of the prefrontal cortex, and the capacity to maintain this observing focus prevents clients from becoming overwhelmed by the reactivation of a traumatic event. For example, as a client discusses a traumatic motor vehicle accident in therapy, she is asked by her therapist to become interested in how she is "organizing" the experience—what is happening inside her—as she begins to talk and think about her accident. The therapist gently and empathically interrupts the story to direct the client's awareness away from their verbal dialog to her inner body sensations, movement impulses, and sensory experience. In a state of mindful observation, she notices that as she talks about the accident, she has the thought that she is going to die. Next, she observes her body tensing in response to the thought and she notes a feeling of panic. Rather than reliving this experience, as she might have if the therapist had not carefully directed her attention to the present moment's organization of it, she steps back, observes it with curiosity, and reports how it is manifesting internally now. The panic subsides, her heart rate returns to normal and she "knows" at a body level that she did not die, she survived. With this somatic differentiation of "having" an experience and exploring how she has organized it, the traumatic event is relegated to the past, it no longer causes her to have the experience again, and she experiences the felt sense that it is over: "I thought I was going to die, but I didn't."

Often, just by uncoupling trauma-related emotion from body sensation and attending exclusively to the physical sensations of the arousal (without attributing meaning or connecting emotion to it), the physiologic responses diminish and settle. This conveys at a bodily level that the danger is past and all is now safe [58]. Uncoupling emotion from sensation is critically important because it eliminates physiologic cueing for a trauma response in the presence of a sensory recollection that is a priori a somatic experience. These transformations at the sensorimotor level result in improvements in emotional and cognitive processing (ie, emotions can be better tolerated), and cognitive processing reflects the incorporation of information from the body.

"Martin," a Vietnam War veteran, came to therapy to "get rid of" nightmares and feelings of being chronically emotionally overwhelmed. In the course of sensorimotor psychotherapy, Martin learned to track his physiologic arousal as he experienced it in his body. He learned to pay active attention to his rapid heart rate and to the shaking and trembling that occurred after the original combat and that he had subsequently re-experienced intermittently over the years. Over the course of several therapy sessions, he learned to describe his inner body sensations, noting the tingling in his arms preceding the shaking, the slight accelerated heart rate, and the increase of tension in his legs. As his capacity to observe and describe bodily sensations developed, he learned to accept these sensations without trying to inhibit them. The therapist instructed him to track these sensations as they moved or changed or "sequenced." Martin noticed that as he tracked the sequence of sensations progressing through his body, the shaking gradually became quiet, his heart rate returned to baseline, and the tension in his legs diminished. Martin's body relaxed, his arousal quieted, he was less afraid and hopeless, and he experienced a somatic feeling he described as "calm" and "safe."

Left brain cognitive functions are integrated with right brain sensorimotor experience

Thus, in sensorimotor psychotherapy, top-down, cortically mediated functions are harnessed to observe and facilitate sensorimotor processing. Clients observe and report (both of which are cognitive functions) the interplay of physical sensations, movements, and impulses and notice their internal reactions as they try out new physical actions. They also learn to observe the effects of their thoughts and emotions on their body; noticing in which part of the body they feel the impact of a particular thought or how the body organizes a particular emotion. Meaning making emerges from the observing and subsequent transformation of habitual response tendencies. For example, as Martin's body experienced the completion of the trembling and shaking, he finally achieved the somatic experience of "peacetime" decades after the end of the Vietnam War. He finally recognized that the feelings of calm and safety meant the events that had continued to torment him were in the past. For the incest survivor who was able to finally execute mobilizing defensive responses, the meaning that emerged was, "I can defend myself." Integrated meaning making was possible for these patients when they experienced a transformation of sensorimotor, emotional, and cognitive responses to their traumatic experiences.

Thoughts and emotions are viable targets of intervention that can support resolution of the traumatic experience. Top-down approaches that attempt to regulate arousal, emotions, and cognitions are a necessary part of trauma therapy, but if such interventions overmanage, ignore, or suppress body processes, then traumatic responses may not be resolved. Similarly, bottom-up interventions that reinforce bottom-up hijacking or fail to include cognitive processing can sabotage integration of the effects of trauma and may lead to endless repetitive flashbacks, hyposarousal states, retraumatization, or chronic trauma kindling.

Summary

The authors believe that the complex effects of trauma are more likely to respond to treatment when the use of insight, understanding, and somatically informed top-down management of symptoms is thoughtfully balanced with bottom-up processing of trauma-related sensations, arousal, movement, and emotions. Effective treatments for trauma involve evoking the fragmented, cognitive, emotional, and sensorimotor responses within the patient's window of tolerance and facilitating new, adaptive responses that can lead to the integration of past and present, of belief and body, and of emotion and meaning.

References

[1] North CS, Nixon SJ, Shariat S, et al. Psychiatric disorders among survivors of the Oklahoma City bombing. JAMA 1999;282:755–62.
[2] Davidson JR, Jughes D, Blazer DG, et al. Post-traumatic stress disorder in the community: an epidemiological study. Psychol Med 1991;21:713–21.
[3] Faustman WO, White PA. Diagnostic and psychopharmacological treatment character-istics of 536 inpatients with posttraumatic stress disorder. J Nerv Ment Dis 1989;177: 154–9.
[4] Kulka RA, Schlenger WE, Fairbank JA, et al. Trauma and the Vietnam War generation: report of findings from the National Vietnam Veterans Readjustment Study. New York: Brunner/Marzel; 1990.
[5] American Psychiatric Association. Diagnostic and statistical manual of mental disorders. 4th edition, revised. Washington, DC: APA; 2000.
[6] Chu JA. Rebuilding shattered lives: the responsible treatment of complex post-traumatic and dissociative disorders. New York: John Wiley & Sons; 1998.
[7] Brewin CR, Dalgleish T, Joseph S. A dual representation theory of post traumatic stress disorder. Psychol Rev 1996;103(4):670–86.
[8] van der Kolk BA. The body keeps the score: memory and the emerging psychobiology of post traumatic stress. Harv Rev Psychiatry 1994;1:253–65.
[9] Bradley R, Greene J, Russ E, et al. A multidimensional meta-analysis of psychotherapy for PTSD. Am J Psychiatry 2005;162(2):214–27.
[10] Ursano RJ, Bell C, Eth S, et al. Practice guideline for the treatment of patients with acute stress disorder and posttraumatic stress disorder. Am J Psychiatry 2004;161:3–31.
[11] Brewin CR, Holmes EA. Psychological theories of posttraumatic stress disorder. Clin Psy-chol Rev 2003;23(3):339–76.
[12] Herman J. Trauma and recovery. New York: Basic Books; 1992.
[13] Foa EB, Rothbaum BO. Treating the trauma of rape: cognitive-behavioral therapy for PTSD. New York: Guilford Press; 1998.
[14] Aposhyan S. Bodymind paychotherapy: principles, techniques and practical applications. New York: WW Norton; 2004.
[15] Kepner J. Body process: a gestalt approach to working with the body in psychotherapy. New York: Gestalt Institute of Cleveland Press; 1987.
[16] LeDoux J. The emotional brain: the mysterious underpinnings of emotional life. New York: Simon & Schuster; 1996.
[17] Rothschild B. The body remembers: the psychophysiology of trauma and trauma treatment. New York: W.W. Norton & Co.; 2000.
[18] Siegel D. The developing mind. New York: Guilford Press; 1999.
[19] Van der Hart O, Steele K. Relieving or reliving childhood trauma? A commentary on Miltenburg and Singer. Theory Psychol 1999;9:533–40.
[20] van der Kolk B, McFarlane AC, Weisaeth L, editors. Traumatic stress: the effects of over-whelming experience on mind, body and society. New York: Guilford Press; 1996.
[21] Burnstein A. Treatment noncompliance in patients with posttraumatic stress disorder. Psychosomatics 1986;27:37–40.
[22] Devilly GJ, Foa EB. The investigation of exposure and cognitive therapy [comment on Tarrier et al, Br J Psychiatry 1999;175:571–5]. J Consult Clin Psychol 2001;69:114–6.
[23] Pitman RK, Altman B, Greenwals E, et al. Psychiatric complications during flooding therapy for posttraumatic stress disorder. J Consult Clin Psychol 1991;52:17–20.

[24] Scott MJ, Stradling SG. Client compliance with exposure treatments for posttraumatic stress disorder. J Trauma Stress 1997;10:523–6.

[25] Tarrier N. What can be learned from clinical trials? [reply to Devilly and Foa]. J Consult Clin Psychol 2001;69:117–8.

[26] Tarrier N, Sommerfield C, Pilgrim H, et al. Cognitive therapy or imaginal exposure in the treatment of posttraumatic stress disorder. Twelve-month follow-up. Br J Psychiatry 1999;175:571–5.

[27] Foa EB, Dancu CV, Hembree EA, et al. A comparison of exposure therapy, stress inoculation training, and their combination for reducing posttraumatic stress disorder in female assault victims. J Consult Clin Psychol 1999;67(2):194–200.

[28] Shapiro F. Efficacy of the Eye Movement Desensitization procedure in the treatment of traumatic memories. J Trauma Stress 1989;2:199–223.

[29] Marks I, Lovell K, Noshirvani H, et al. Treatment of posttraumatic stress disorder by exposure and/or cognitive restructuring: a controlled study. Arch Gen Psychiatry 1998;55(4):317–25.

[30] Chefetz RA. The paradox of detachment disorders: binding-disruption of dissociative process. Psychiatry 2004;67(3):246–55.

[31] Ogden P, Minton K. Sensorimotor psychotherapy: one method for processing traumatic memory. Traumatology 2000;VI(3).

[32] Ogden P, Minton K, Pain C. Trauma and the body: the theory and practice of sensorimotor psychotherapy. New York: W.W. Norton & Co., in press.

[33] Fisher A, Murray E, Bundy A. Sensory integration: theory and practice. Philadelphia: Davis; 1991.

[34] Wilber K. A brief history of everything. Boston: Shambhala; 1996.

[35] MacLean PD. Brain evolution relating to family, play, and the separation call. Arch Gen Psychiatry 1985;42:405–17.

[36] Cozolinno L. The neuroscience of psychotherapy: building and rebuilding the human brain. New York: W.W. Norton & Co.; 2002.

[37] LeDoux J. Synaptic self: how our brains become who we are. New York: Penguin Putnam, Inc., 2002.

[38] Schore AN. Dysregulation of the right brain: a fundamental mechanism of traumatic attachment and the psychopathogenesis of posttraumatic stress disorder. Aust N Z J Psychiatry 2002;36(1):9–30.

[39] Rauch SL, van der Kolk BA, Fisler RE, et al. A symptom provocation study of posttraumatic stress disorder using positron emission tomography and script driven imagery. Arch Gen Psychiatry 1996;53:380–7.

[40] Grigsby J, Stevens D. Neorodynamics of personality. New York: Guilford Press; 2000.

[41] Sykes WM. The limits of talk: Bessel van der Kolk wants to transform the treatment of trauma. Psychother Networker 2004;28(1):30–41.

[42] van der Kolk BA, Pelcovitz D, Roth S, et al. Dissociation, somatization, and affect dysregulation: the complexity of adaptation of trauma. Am J Psychiatry 1996;153(Suppl): 83–93.

[43] Van der Hart O, Nijenhuis E, Steele K, et al. Trauma-related dissociation: conceptual clarity lost and found. Aust N Z J Psychiatry 2004;38:906–14.

[44] Lanius RA, Williamson PC, Boksman K, et al. Brain activation during script-driven imagery induced dissociative responses in PTSD: a functional magnetic resonance imaging investigation. Biol Psychiatry 2002;52:305–11.

[45] Chefetz RA. Affect dysregulation as a way of life. J Am Acad Psychoanal 2000;28(2): 289–303.

[46] Cloitre MK, Stovall-McClough MR, Chemtob C. Therapeutic alliance, negative mood regulation and treatment outcome in child abuse-related posttraumatic stress disorder. J Consult Clin Psychol 2004;72(3):411–6.

[47] Herman JL. Complex PTSD: a syndrome in survivors of prolonged and repeated trauma in psychotraumatology. New York: Plenum Press; 1995.

[48] Nemeroff CB. Neurobiological consequences of childhood trauma. J Clin Psychiatry 2004; 65(Suppl I):18–28.

[49] Lanius RA, Bluhm RL, Lanius U, et al. A review of neuroimaging studies of hyperarousal and dissociation in PTSD: heterogeneity of response to symptom provocation. J Psychiatric Res, in press.

[50] Orr S, McNally RJ, Rosen GM, et al. Psychophysiological reactivity: implications for conceptualizing PTSD. In: Rosen GM, editor. Posttraumatic stress disorder: issues and controversies. Chichester, England: John Wiley & Sons; 2004.

[51] Rosen GM, editor. Posttraumatic stress disorder: issues and controversies. Chichester, England: John Wiley & Sons; 2004.

[52] Post RM, Weiss SRB, Smith MA. Sensitization and kindling: implication for the evolving neural substrates of post-traumatic stress disorder. In: Freidman MJ, Charney DS, Deutch AY, editors. Neurobiological and clinical consequences of stress: from normal adaptation to PTSD. Philadelphia: Lippincott-Raven Publishers; 1995.

[53] Nijenhuis ERS. Somatoform dissociation: phenomena, measurement, and theoretical issues. The Netherlands: Van Gorcum; 1999.

[54] Bowlby J. A secure base: parent-child attachment and healthy human development. New York: Basic Books; 1988.

[55] Nijenhuis ERS, Van der Hart O. Forgetting and reexperiencing trauma: from anesthesia to pain. In: Goodwin J, Attias R, editors. Splintered reflections: images of the body in trauma. New York: Basic Books; 1999.

[56] Misslin R. The defense system of fear: behavior and neurocircuitry. Neurophysiol Clin 2003; 33(2):55–66.

[57] Lewis L, Kelly K, Allen J. Restoring hope and trust: an illustrated guide to mastering trauma. Baltimore (MD): Sidran Institute Press; 2004.

[58] Levine P, Frederick A. Waking the tiger: healing trauma. Berkeley (CA): North Atlantic Books; 1997.

[59] Porges SW. Orienting in a defensive world: mammalian modifications of our evolutionary heritage. A polyvagal theory. Psychophysiology 1995;32:301–18.

[60] Holman EA, Silver RC. Getting 'stuck' in the past: temporal orientation and coping with trauma. J Pers Soc Psychol 1998;74:1146–63.

[61] Scaer RC. The neurophysiology of dissociation and chronic disease. Appl Psychophysiol Biofeedback 2001;26(1):73–91.

[62] Van der Hart O, van Dijke A, van Son M, et al. Somatoform dissociation in traumatized World War I combat soldiers: a neglected clinical heritage. J Trauma Dissoc 2000;1(4): 33–66.

[63] Krystal H. Integration and self-healing: affect, trauma, alexithymia. Hillsdale (NJ): Analytic Press; 1988.

[64] Diamond S, Balvin R, Diamond F. Inhibition and choice. New York: Harper and Row; 1963.

[65] Schore A. The effects of early relational trauma on right brain development, affect regulation, and infant mental health. Infant Ment Health J 2001;22:201–69.

[66] Panksepp J. Affective neuroscience: the foundations of human and animal emotions. New York: Oxford University Press; 1998.

ELSEVIER
SAUNDERS

PSYCHIATRIC
CLINICS
OF NORTH AMERICA

Psychiatr Clin N Am 29 (2006) 281–304

Dealing with Alters: A Pragmatic Clinical Perspective

Richard P. Kluft, MD[a,b,*]

[a]Temple University School of Medicine, Philadelphia, PA, USA
[b]Private Practice, 111 Presidential Boulevard, Suite 238, Bala Cynwyd, PA 19004, USA

Alternate identities or personality states are core phenomena of dissociative identity disorder (DID) and found in several forms of dissociative disorder not otherwise specified (DDNOS) [1]. Whether they are called identities, personalities, personality states, ego states, subpersonalities, parts, disaggregate self-states, alters, or any number of other descriptive terms (hereafter termed alters), they form a central and often colorful and controversial feature of these disorders.

Clinicians confronted with DID and related forms of DDNOS (hereafter referred to collectively as DID) must determine how they will approach and address the alters. Working with alters has long been an important aspect of DID treatment, but many mental health professionals have been (and remain) reluctant to elicit or work directly with the alters. Such colleagues prefer to understand the alters as obstacles, distractions, or artifacts to be bypassed or suppressed; they may endeavor to address the issues raised by the alters and their activities obliquely, employing allusive circumlocutions but without dealing directly with the alters.

Although these stances are not without their supporters, they are buttressed more by strongly held and vigorously voiced opinion than by scientific data or clinical experience. A longitudinal study [2] demonstrated that 97% of those patients who had DID (termed multiple personality disorder at the time of the study) and received treatments that did not work directly with the alters still satisfied diagnostic criteria for DID on follow-up. To date, no substantial scientific literature or major series of successfully treated cases has been published that describes the definitive psycholytic treatment of DID (ie, a treatment to the point of eliminating the condition) without addressing the alters. In contrast, available reports of successful treatment (eg, Coons [3],

---

* 111 Presidential Boulevard Suite, #238, Bala Cynwyd, PA 19004.
  E-mail address: rpkluft@aol.com

0193-953X/06/$ - see front matter © 2005 Elsevier Inc. All rights reserved.
doi:10.1016/j.psc.2005.10.010   *psych.theclinics.com*

Kluft [4,5]) have involved therapies in which the alters are addressed. There-fore, despite the support voiced for treatments that avoid working with the alters in DID, those who follow such plans of action are implicitly following an experimental path that is likely to prove therapeutically futile and may ex-pose the patient to danger and excess morbidity [6,7].

Those experienced in the treatment of DID do not regard the alters as mere curious phenomena. They understand the alters to "express the struc-ture, conflicts, deficits, and coping strategies of the DID patient's mind" [7]. As Coons [8] and Kluft [9] have observed, the personality of a patient with DID is to have multiple personalities. Kluft [7] observed that

> Bypassing or disregarding the alters creates a therapy in which major areas
> of the patient's mental life and autobiographic memory will be denied an
> empathic hearing. Furthermore, it is rarely sufficient simply to address
> the alters as they emerge. The alters are aspects of a process of defense
> and coping. It would be naïve in the extreme to imagine that the patient
> will predictably present in those alters most relevant to the conduct of
> the therapy. Considerations of facilitating day-to-day function, shame,
> guilt, and apprehension dictate otherwise. Therapists who await the emer-
> gence of alters to work with them may prolong the treatment considerably.

When voices are raised to dispute the practice of eliciting or working with the alters, the objections make two basic and closely related forms of argu-ment. The first starts with the assumption that the alter phenomenon is iat-rogenic [10,11]. From this perspective, it is reasonable to propose that alters have (usually) emerged in response to inappropriate therapeutic pressures, subtle or overt, and if their manifestations do not receive attention, then they will cease to exist. Deprived of reinforcements believed to instigate and to sustain the alters, it is assumed that they will wither into oblivion. The second argument starts with the assumption that there are more impor-tant therapeutic goals than treating the core phenomena of DID and that diverting attention from the alters while prioritizing the attaining of stability and function directs the treatment toward these more important or reason-able therapeutic objectives. It shares the implicit assumption that attention to the alters reinforces them and makes them a more prominent and difficult clinical problem to address.

The first objection is a matter of strong opinion, but definitive proof of the iatrogenesis of DID/DDNOS has yet to be presented [6]. There is wide-spread agreement that DID can be worsened and complicated by iatrogenic errors, and that additional personalities may be formed in response to a therapist's expectations and pressures [12–17]. Many also agree that a pa-tient who has a form of DDNOS that falls just short of the diagnostic cri-teria for DID may be "promoted" to fulfill DID criteria by therapist expectation/pressure or by the pain inherent in the treatment of traumatic issues. The laboratory studies purporting to demonstrate the reality of iatro-genesis, however, fall far short of doing so [6,18] and are conceptually flawed by the assumption that inducing an individual to manifest behavior consistent with DID is the same as the creation of DID. The following helps to illustrate the problem: if a person is induced to behave like a chicken under hypnosis, it does not follow that he should be given a diet appropriate for a chicken, kept in a chicken coop, or cooked for dinner.

The second objection is more complex and nuanced. Indeed, there are many times in the treatment of DID when concerns other than the phenomena of DID per se must be the center of clinical attention [7,19]. The treatment of the DID is only one aspect of an overall therapeutic strategy and may be a minor or incidental concern for long periods in some therapies. A strategy of omitting attention to the phenomena of DID, however, leaves the patients who suffer DID only partially treated and may condemn them to lives in which a definitive treatment and a complete cure is deliberately withheld from them. To initiate a course of treatment that from the first denies a patient a definitive resolution of his or her difficulties remains a questionable course of action [6,7,19].

In this article, I offer a perspective on working with alters in the treatment of DID. I draw on my experience in treating hundreds of patients who have DID and my clinical study of the treatments of thousands of others seen in consultation for colleagues or observed during their inpatient treatment at the Dissociative Disorders Program at The Institute of Pennsylvania Hospital, where I served as director for 8 years. My personal series of DID cases includes just under 170 DID patients who have achieved stable integration [5] in the course of our work together. Many others have reached integration but could not be followed up or re-evaluated in a manner that allows me to state that their integrations fulfilled criteria for stability [4].

What are alters?

Many attempts have been made to define and describe alters in DID patients. It is well appreciated that the minds of normal subjects and of psychiatric patients have a certain degree of differentiated modularity [20]. Concepts such as ego states [20,21], representations of interactions that have become generalized [22], affect scripts [23], and core conflictual relationship themes [24] address, from different perspectives, the phenomenon of persistent patterns of structure and behavior that can be found to underlie aspects of human psychology. One of the most widely accepted approaches to describing such phenomena is Watkins and Watkins' [20,21] work on ego states. They defined an ego state as an "organized system of behavior and experience whose elements are bound together by some common principle but that is separated from other such states by boundaries that are more or less permeable" [21].

Normal ego state phenomena have very permeable boundaries; the more pathological ego states that are found in DID have boundaries that are often relatively impermeable. All alters necessarily fall under the broad rubric of ego states, but most ego states are not alters. Ego states that are also alters generally have four characteristics that are not intrinsic to the ego state phenomenon per se [19]: (1) they have their own identities, involving a sense of self (a center of initiative and experience [25]); (2) they have a characteristic self-representation, which may be discordant with how the patient is generally seen or perceived; (3) they have their own senses of autobiographic memory, distinguishing what they understand to be their own actions and experiences from those done and experienced by other alters; and (4) they have a sense of ownership of their own experiences, actions, and thoughts, and may lack a sense of ownership of and a sense of responsibility for the action, experiences, and thoughts of other alters. Clinicians often find this latter point unsettling.

In 1988, Kluft [26] attempted to define the phenomenon of alternate identities or personality states:

> A disaggregate self-state (i.e., personality) is the mental address of a relatively stable and enduring particular pattern of selective mobilization of mental contents and functions, which may be behaviorally enacted with noteworthy role-taking and role-playing dimensions and sensitive to intrapsychic, interpersonal, and environmental stimuli. It is organized in and associated with a relatively stable (but order effect dependent) pattern of neuropsychophysiologic activation, and has crucial psychodynamic contents. It serves both as recipient, processor, and storage center for perceptions, experiences, and the processing of such in connection with past events and thoughts, or present and anticipated ones as well. It has its own identity and ideation, and a capacity for initiating thought processes and actions.

Alters are complex phenomena not easily encompassed by simple descriptions or definitions that may acknowledge some of their features but that fail to address the full range of their characteristics.

The development and nature of alter systems

Over a period of time, a person in the process of developing DID is likely to generate a number of alters in his or her attempt to cope with life situations and to find ways to live with intolerable circumstances. The alters may be understood as being developed in the service of sustaining a more fundamental "multiple reality disorder" that includes alternate and often incompatible ways of understanding and trying to live in a difficult world, including gross distortions of autobiographic experience and the debasement of concepts of safety and causality [4,5,26–28] in the interests of security and the protection of important relationships.

Illustration of an alter system

Lois (see references [6,27,28]) was the daughter of good, religious, but rigid and undemonstrative parents. The light of her life was her Uncle Ben, who was warm, effusive, generous, and playful. His visits and her weekly excursions with him became the emotional center of her life. Over a period of time, Uncle Ben became more seductive and introduced several "games" into their times together. These games became "secret games" that progressed to sexual acts that Lois experienced as sometimes frightening, painful, pleasant, or stimulating but always overwhelming and confusing.

Table 1 illustrates the roster of alters discovered when Lois was mapped in treatment some 30 years later. Each alter had emerged to play a role in keeping Lois going and in protecting her from the loss of Ben, the person she most loved and the person by whom she was most abused. It is apparent that coping styles that served Lois well in her family during her difficult childhood and adolescence are prescriptions for disaster in dealing with the world at large and generally dangerous when used by an adult individual. For example, having sexually receptive and aggressive personalities such as Sherri and Vickie exerts a form of damage control under circumstances of chronic abuse by accepting sexual advances rather than being hurt or made to submit. Such stances, however, may lead to self-destructive and unstable relationships under other circumstances.

Alters' understanding of themselves and one another

Although situations are encountered in which alters are completely unaware of one another, it is more common to find varieties of asymmetric amnesia in which some alters know about others but are not known by all of those about whom they are aware. In a given patient, one may encounter

Table 1
Coping strategies and alter formation

Coping strategy	Alter or alters created
This did not happen	A Lois who knows, and a Lois who does not
I must have deserved it	Bad Lois, whose behavior would explain trauma as punishment
I must have wanted it	A sexual alter, Sherrie
I can control it better if I take charge	An aggressively sexual alter, Vickie
I would feel safe if I were a boy	Louis, Lois' male "twin"
I wish I were a big man who could prevent this	Big Jack, based on some person of power
I wish I were the one who could hurt someone and not be hurt	Uncle Ben, or a more disguised identification with the aggressor
I wish I could feel nothing	Jessie, who endures all yet feels nothing
I wish someone could replace me	"The Girls," who encapsulate specific experiences of trauma unknown to Lois
I wish someone would comfort me	Angel, with whom Lois imagines herself to be while the body is being exploited and "The Girls" are experiencing the trauma

From Kluft RP. Reflections on the traumatic memories of dissociative identity disorder patients. In: Lynn S, McConkey K, editors. Truth in memory. New York: Guilford; 1998. p. 315; with permission.

instances of mutual unawareness, directional or asymmetric amnesia, and alters aware of most or even all of the others.

When alters share a degree of mutual awareness of one another, they may understand themselves to have all manner of relationships with one another. For example, certain parts often care for or try to protect scared child parts. In addition, life experiences may be recapitulated in the alter system; for example, an alter based on an abuser may see itself entitled to hurt alters based on the patient's experiences of being unable to prevent or interrupt victimization by the abuser or abusers.

The alter system frequently replicates the DID patient's experience of the relationships and circumstances that prevailed in his or her family of origin. An "inner world" is commonly developed in which the alters interact. It is common that some alters active in the inner world may never assume executive control of the patient as the patient interacts with external others and may never manifest themselves in therapy unless they are sought out. Furthermore, events in this inner world constitute a "third reality" to the patient and may be experienced as just as real as events that take place in external reality [27]. Stored together in memory with autobiographic memory of "real world events" and often severed from indicators of their source or origin (source amnesia), events from the inner world may be reported as if they had occurred in external reality, often seriously complicating life and treatment.

The issue of complexity

Many clinicians have difficulty coming to grips with reports of large numbers of personalities. Patients with hundreds or even thousands of alters have been reported [26]. Often the large numbers in and of themselves evoke shock and disbelief, with countertransferential disparagement of the patient who claims such complexity and the clinician who reports such phenomena. My perspective is that reacting to the number itself rather than what the number signifies is counterproductive. Claims of a large number of alters should be heard empathically and explored thoughtfully. Kluft [26] listed 20 pathways into extreme complexity. These pathways can be condensed into four general mechanisms: (1) coping with particularly severe, sustained, and vicious abuse over a long period, (2) employing coping strategies that in themselves generate large numbers of alters, (3) using coping strategies driven by character issues, and (4) the sequelae of unique patient response patterns.

It stands to reason that more abuse may generate more alters to cope with and sequester the additional overwhelming experiences; however, the role of coping strategies in and of themselves in generating large numbers of alters may not be as apparent. Let us assume for the moment that Lois, who sequestered much abuse into a group of alters called "The Girls," had been taught by her religious parents to pray every night. Lois prayed every night after an abuse episode that God would make her into a "better little girl" so good and sweet and loveable that no one would ever want to hurt her. This prayerful wish involved the creation of a new, "better" alter after each occasion of mistreatment, with the goal of preventing further abuse. Each newly created alter would encounter the same fate as its predecessors because what drove Uncle Ben to abuse Lois was not under Lois' control. One patient in Kluft's [26] 1988 series of complex DID patients was abused several times per week by two male relatives for over 10 years and developed over 1000 alters in that manner.

Other DID patients may create a caretaker, protector, or consoling friend for each new trauma-based alter. Imagine an increasing number of abused child alters, as in the previous example, of which each would also have its own version of Big Jack. Numbers in the hundreds or thousands would be reached easily. Finally, some patients who have DID harbor rebirth fantasies. At some junctures, they may replicate their systems of alters, replacing those who endured "the bad old days" with new and undamaged versions of themselves, hoping to start all over and put their pasts behind them. Kluft [26] termed such events "epochal division." The superceded group of alters often becomes inactive or is relegated to the inner world. In one patient known to the author, the same 20-plus alter system was replicated when the patient went from elementary school to junior high school, junior high school to high school, high school to college, and finally on the occasion of her marriage, leading to well over 100 alters. This process was repeated during the course of a painful divorce.

DID patients who are extremely avoidant, obsessive, or without strong nondissociative defenses are prone to develop larger numbers of alters. For the group without strong nondissociative defenses, dissociation is not a last-ditch defense—it is their first response to stress. In addition, some idiosyncratic patterns are encountered in which patients come up with unique strategies that lead to large numbers of alters. Some create elaborate inner worlds or multiple inner worlds and populate them with alters designed to have specific functions and roles in those inner worlds. Others imaginatively transform their histories to conform to myths, movies, television shows, or pieces of literature and generate large numbers of alters to play roles in them. Rarely, DID patients become involved with some system of symbolism or numerology and generate enormous systems of alters consistent with these systems. For example, one DID patient believed that seven was a powerful number for her and generated clusters of seven alters whenever severely overwhelmed beyond the capacities of the alters already in place.

In such cases, the large number of alters is a potentially unsettling distraction, but when placed in perspective, it need not be disquieting. With some unique exceptions, large systems based on considerations other than the characteristics of the abuse that had been experienced generally collapse uneventfully as the treatment moves forward. A large number of alters derived from the extensiveness of the abuse suffered generally indicates a prolonged and difficult course of treatment because it may prove necessary to process all or most of that abuse, but it does not necessarily indicate a worse long-term outcome. Some complex DID patients demonstrate astonishing resilience.

A rationale for working directly with the alters

Working with the alters remains an unfamiliar area of practice to many mental health professionals. When a clinician accepts the possibility of working with the alters, a whole new avenue of interaction with the patient is possible. Exploring the alters and their meanings, like exploring a patient's other productions such as fantasies and dreams, may be stabilizing and encouraging for a patient who otherwise has never before felt heard and understood so completely. Toward this goal, a number of pragmatic considerations that are derived from personal clinical experience and from doing thousands of consultations over the course of 30 years are presented.

In working with DID, should a clinician work with the alters? If so, should the clinician try to elicit or bring to the surface the various alters, or simply to work with them as they present themselves spontaneously in the treatment setting? Those who question the genuineness of DID or believe that working with the alters reifies or concretizes the condition would respond to both concerns in the negative, maintaining that attention to such sociopsychologic artifacts, often iatrogenic, makes a bad situation worse. In contrast, those who are convinced that the condition occurs naturalistically would generally recommend working with the alters and eliciting alters to facilitate the treatment. Between these perspectives are those who believe that the condition occurs naturalistically and will talk to alters if they present spontaneously but hold the opinions that the condition can often be treated without directly accessing and working with the alters and that efforts to do so may reinforce the condition.

When I began my work with DID, I sought the advice of an eminent authority. This person believed that DID was an artifact and confidently predicted that nonreinforcement of the alters would lead to their disappearance. I followed his recommendations for months. One of two things happened: my patients who had DID stopped talking about their DID phenomena but were still miserable or their alters became more frantic and driven in their efforts to communicate their concerns to me, and the patients' situations deteriorated. Confronted with uniformly negative responses to my use of this strategy, I rethought the issue. I appreciated that the strategy I had used inflicted ongoing narcissistic injuries to my patients and was detrimental to the formation of a therapeutic alliance. I began to communicate with the alters and to make deliberate efforts to establish and maintain dialogs with them. With this approach, my patients uniformly stabilized and began to improve. A series of articles drawn from this work [4,5,29,30] reflects the positive impact of treatments that work with and elicit the participation of alters. Summarizing the results of this work, 89% of the patients who had DID in this series achieved stable integration. This work also identified three groups of DID patients: one group that had relatively little comorbidity and moved rapidly toward improvement and integration; a second group that had considerable comorbidity and progressed more slowly and might or might not achieve full integration, and a third group that had serious comorbidity and external impediments to recovery and that progressed slowly and chaotically, rarely achieved integration, and generally would have been better served by a supportive treatment [31,32]. Similar groupings have been recognized by other investigators [33].

My experience has taught me again and again that approaching DID as if the alters were completely separate persons or as if the patient were a person whose subjective experience of having separate selves can be discounted is counterproductive. These approaches deny, dismiss, and disavow the nature of DID phenomenology and the subjective world of the DID patient. Such stances lead to failures of empathy and profound difficulties if not overt disruptions of the therapeutic alliance. The patient is a single individual whose personality is to have multiple personalities [8,19]. Although the personality systems of some patients who have DID may be sufficiently accessible for treatment to proceed with no need to access and address individual alters, others may be organized in a way that will not allow treatment to move forward without such efforts. In my experience, the former group is much smaller than the latter, making it more appropriate to assume that such efforts may prove necessary.

There are many reasons that might move a therapist to address and access alters individually or in groups instead of working on their issues through the apparent host personality. The host personality is the personality in apparent executive control most of the time over a particular period [34]. Many clinicians and theoreticians assume that the host constitutes the patient's true identity and should be regarded as the core of who the patient really is, but there is no scientific or clinical reason to proceed on this basis. Twenty such reasons for working with and accessing the alters are noted Box 1. The list could easily be longer. This list and the discussion that accompanies it draw heavily on Kluft [35].

Potential contraindications for working with alters

Having noted the advantages to be had from working with and accessing alters, it is important to acknowledge that there are reasons for avoiding such approaches that are not based on mere opinion and abstract theory but have a substantial legitimacy and merit under certain circumstances.

1. Notwithstanding the controversy raised in some forensic cases surrounding allegations that DID can be caused iatrogenically, the requirements of forensic assessments may preclude making any interventions that might later be vulnerable to the assertion that they may have created rather than investigated dissociative phenomena.

Box 1. Twenty reasons for working with and accessing the alters

1. Acknowledging the dissociative surface. The more the concept of the host personality is studied, the clearer it becomes that what has been understood to be the host personality is often the manifestation at the "dissociative surface" [28,35] of a far more complex phenomenon than is generally appreciated and represents an aggregation rather than a single entity. Many clinicians attribute to the host a strength, persistence, resilience, and face validity as "the real person" on the basis of the theoretic orientation of the therapist or the unconscious defensive efforts made by the therapist to make the strange and different feel more familiar and manageable. There is no basis in science or clinical experience to justify this stance. Such attributions also are often more a tribute to the presentation of a "good act" and a survival-oriented camouflaging of the DID due to the actions of many alters than to the stable presence of an actual core identity.

2. Decoding the dissociative surface. Working with and identifying alters allows us to decode the dissociative surface, which therapists are more likely to encounter than a host personality in pure culture. Unless efforts are made to access the alters and learn their manifestations, the therapist will not develop the capacity to interpret complex phenomena of the dissociative surface, appreciate the interactions within the alter system that are giving rise to them, and enlarge his or her capacity to understand and intervene effectively with the DID patient. The "decoding" process is addressed later.

3. Making alters stakeholders in the treatment. Engaging alters is likely to make them stakeholders in the therapy and more invested in, rather than oppositional to the treatment and its outcome. Because alters have senses of themselves, they are sensitive to narcissistic wounds, rejection, and dismissive treatment—all of which is inherent in any strategy that does not strive to reach out to them and instead promotes their being bypassed or neglected. Making efforts to reach them and solicit their participation and their perspectives holds the potential to diminish such difficulties and to enhance the therapeutic alliance.

4. Putting the "host" in perspective. Often the host is simply another alter and may not be seen by the other alters as constituting or representing the essential core of the patient.

In many if not most alter systems, the host is scorned and perceived as a "wimp," a "human shield," or "cannon fodder" by other alters. In some situations, one aspect of the host's role is to shield a part or parts understood to be the true core or identity of the person. Any proclamation by the therapist to the effect that the host is the patient's center and reason for being may encourage disruption rather than cooperation by other alters. It may convince them that the therapist does not understand what is going on, and is trying to impose an unwelcome and illegitimate authority on them.

5. Approaching reluctance respectfully. Most of what is withheld by DID patients is withheld by conscious decisions rather than by unconscious resistances to treatment. That is, the withholding is due to reluctance rather than to resistance. Alters may have knowledge that they withhold for a wide variety of reasons. Reluctance is best addressed with persuasion, and persuasion is more easily accomplished when one acknowledges and treats with respect the subjective reality and the perspectives of those (the parts) that one is trying to persuade. An ego state therapy "family of self" model [20,21,33] is very effective here.

6. Declining to collude with avoidance. If all alters are not directly accessible, then the failure to address them and their perceived experiences and concerns, which may play important roles and contain crucial mental content, constitutes a decision to leave major aspects of mental content, structure, and function unaddressed. Such a collusion with the patient to avoid addressing important issues and materials is what Langs [36] eloquently described as "lie therapy" and is usually ineffective. The problem is very analogous to what Freud [37] observed about secrets in psychotherapy. When there is an agreement to avoid the exploration of any particular area of the mind, all manner of mischief will congregate in that area, escaping exploration and undermining treatment.

7. Understanding alters/alters' behavior as communications. Alters are more than sociopsychologic phenomena. In expressing, personifying, and enacting wishes, defensive operations, object relationships, and the dynamics and genetics of symptomatic behaviors, enactments, and re-enactments, alters bring crucial material into the treatment. They express themselves in the transference, elicit countertransference, and are a major source of projective identification "from behind the scenes." That is, they embody

and communicate material essential for a meaningful treatment. Their neglect constitutes lie therapy [36] and may cause the alters to initiate dysfunctional "interventions" to bring attention to their concerns or to punish the other alters or the therapist for their neglect and its perceived consequences.

8. Eroding amnesia by engaging alters. When the therapist asks the alters to talk about themselves, their attitudes, and their experiences and listens carefully and respectfully, it is easier to obtain history or undo amnesia due to withholding without making intrusive interventions that have the potential to generate inaccurate recollections. This approach avoids the perceived need for more intrusive or potentially "leading" techniques and efforts to "pull out" or extract the material against resistance/reluctance and reduces the risks of censorship, contamination, and confabulation.

9. Exploring and relieving symptoms due to alters' intrusions. Often the most rapid path to symptomatic relief is to address or access the alter or alters "behind" a problematic symptom, behavior, affective state, or perplexity and to negotiate with the alters for relief [38–40]. An alter-driven intrusion into the dissociative surface is the most common source of such disruptions. An hallucination may be the voice of an alter trying to make itself heard or issue a command; a "made" feeling or action may be an alter's efforts to impose its will on another; an unexplained pain may be the somatic discomfort component of a memory, the narrative structure of which remains obscure; and so forth.

10. Disabling "being normal" as self-sabotage. As the host strives to pass for "normal," it often engages in such vigorous disavowals of present or potential problems that indicators of potential danger that might prompt preventive measures are banished from awareness or minimized and not communicated to the therapist. This pseudonormality and defensive disavowal facilitates revictimization [41]; the process of the therapy may falter and stall when the possibility of true understanding is avoided by the patient's presenting and trying to believe in a pseudo-normal facade. Regular efforts to access the alters and to draw on their perceptions, knowledge, and perspectives is useful in anticipating and avoiding crises [40].

11. Enhancing the impact of empathy. Empathic expression in direct conversation with an alter is much more effective

in eroding dissociative barriers and provides a more convincing corrective emotional experience than that alter's experiencing the therapist's empathy vicariously as it is expressed with, to, and through other alters. It helps to bear in mind that alters regularly cannot or will not own the experiences of other alters of whom they may not be aware and for whose experiences they may have amnesia. One of my workshop axioms is that "DID is that form of psychopathology that dissolves in empathy."

12. Bringing "abuser alters" into treatment. Alters based on abusers often cause chaos and instigate self-injury behind the scenes but are more likely to become amenable when regularly accessed and brought into the therapy. Their defensive narcissistic constellations often preclude their feeling included in approaches that do not address them directly. Their experience of the clinician's caring and empathy are crucial to their changing in a constructive manner. This concern may be problematic with alters of all sorts. Their not being directly addressed is often perceived as a rejection and a narcissistic insult.

13. Negotiating with alters as an aspect of treatment. Many approaches to the treatment of DID that are understood to be very useful by a consensus of those who treat dissociative disorders, such as ego-state therapy [20,21], Fine's version of tactical integrationalism [42,43], and hypnotic and nonhypnotic safety, containment, and shut-down techniques (eg, see [44–47]) require negotiating with the alter system. To discard such important and well-regarded interventions may imperil rather than improve the treatment of the DID patient.

14. Mobilizing currently inaccessible skills. Often a DID patient who is currently overwhelmed gives a history of significantly higher function in the past and indicates that the resources (such as job-related knowledge and skills) essential for better function are associated with a particular alter or alters that are currently not available. Accessing and mobilizing alters with such strengths may prove essential to the rehabilitation of a DID patient. The patient creates his or her own sense of safety through the application of his or her own skills.

15. Creating interactions that anticipate integration. Alters can be helped to overhear and view one another in action. Initial preoccupation with their differences from one another ultimately yields to an appreciation of their connections and commonalities. This awareness moves them toward better

communication, collaboration, mutual empathy and identification, and ultimately toward integration. The usual pathway by which this occurs is through the alters' shared experience of their encounters with the therapist [48].

16. Reaching out to and enlisting alters in the third reality. Often the reality of the inner world, the third reality [27], is so compelling that much of the patient's emotional energy and interest may be withdrawn from the here and now, leading to prolonged and painful difficulties in helping the patient address pressing concerns in external reality. The inner world may be inaccessible to or through the host for long periods. In fact, those in the inner world may see the host as an enemy of the inner world or a mere drone necessary to deal with the mundane or painful reality from which many alters have withdrawn. It may be possible for the therapist, by addressing the parts that have turned away from the external world, to communicate with those immersed in the third reality and bring them into the here and now or enlist their help in addressing problems in the here and now.

17. Resolving shame face-to-face. Work on shame dynamics [23] is crucial to the resolution of traumatic insults to one's identity and one's self. Work on shame with particular alters about experiences and actions they consider mortifying is more effective face-to-face. Such encounters challenge the shamed part's perception that it is "shorn from the herd" and unwelcome by others. Efforts to reduce the shame of a particular alter by working through another alter, the host, are less effective than working directly with the alters who are experiencing the shame as their own. Without the direct subjective experience of the therapist's empathic attunement with their plight, shame-bound alters may not believe that they are truly accepted despite their difficulties, that their issues have actually been addressed, and that they have truly mastered their concerns.

18. Enlisting more mature alters to care for child alters. The treatment of DID is often complicated by the deeply felt needs of child alters, often expressed in their wishes or efforts to create a tangibly more gratifying childhood in a regressive relationship with the therapist. Putnam [49] wisely observed that the most appropriate person to respond to such perceived needs is not the therapist but the patient, who should be helped to mobilize more grown-up alters to provide the requested nurture and play experiences.

Addressing the patient as a family of self and helping particular alters work with the child alters facilitates this process and reduces the extent to which child alters obstruct the psychotherapy.

19. Avoiding re-enactments of rejection and neglect. For many patients who have DID, their experiences of neglect, not being listened to, empathic failure, and rejection have been as important or more important than overwhelming trauma in the development and perpetuation of their disorders. Attachment issues may prove to be major concerns. When a decision is made to avoid dealing directly with individual alters, the DID patient's childhood mistreatments by the omission of appropriate attention and consolation are recapitulated, re-enacted, and legitimized under the aegis of therapy.

20. Paving the way for integration. Integration involves the bringing together of alters. Integration occurs or can be facilitated when the reasons for maintaining the separateness have been resolved and when each alter has received what had been sequestered in the other alters and, in turn, has shared its unique experiences, reactions, and perspectives [48]. Without accessing, consulting, and working with individual alters, it is very difficult to be sure that these issues and concerns have been addressed. Follow-ups on such patients are discouraging. In 1985, I reported [2] that less than 3% of patients who had DID treated in this manner achieved and maintained integration. Many cases referred for consultation for distress subsequent to purported integrations or for the failure of apparent integrations are found to be related to alters that were never encountered in the treatment or that assumed to have spontaneously integrated but had merely absented themselves from the treatment process [50,51]. During the 1-month period in 2005 in which I wrote this article, I evaluated three female patients in their 50s whose prior therapists believed that they were integrated after the spontaneous presentation of alters in therapy and everyday life appeared to have ceased. The natural history of DID is that its manifestations wax and wane [2]. It is common for therapists who are unaware of this phenomenon and who do not make efforts to access alters to mistake fluctuations and reconfigurations of the DID process for improvements and cures. Therapists who make efforts to access alters and to follow their responses to treatment are less likely to make such errors.

2. In some DID personality systems, it may be found that all available alters are currently overwhelmed or trauma based and that the system is without parts able to function or to contain disruption and protect stability. In such cases, bringing other alters forward brings a risk of worsening the disequilibrium and should be avoided until the patient becomes more stable.
3. The patient's circumstances may necessitate that therapy should address issues in external reality and defer any exploration of the DID itself.
4. Patients who demonstrate compromised ego strength or whose ego strength resources are stretched to their limits by their life circumstances, situational stressors, comorbid mental disorders, medical illness, and other burdens must be discouraged from opening up their systems and their histories because they do not, at least at that point in time, have the psychologic resources to address the alters or trauma work [7,52]. They already "have too much on their plates."
5. In a therapy that must be supportive, it often is best to avoid deliberately bringing out alters that bring with them too much pain and concern for a patient who is already struggling to get by. When alters of this sort emerge spontaneously, they should be addressed supportively when necessary, but in general, their issues and memories should not be raised by the therapist. In some uncommon situations, such alters and their issues may intrude in a manner that is disruptive and may not respond to supportive and shut-down interventions. Under these circumstances, sometimes they have to be worked with until they are more settled and unburdened and the situation can be restabilized [53].
6. Many therapists begin work with DID patients without having become conversant with the dissociative disorders field, its literature, and its opportunities for training. Therapists should not proceed with exploratory work of any sort, access alters, or press for historical material until they have the expertise to undertake these endeavors in a manner that is safe for the patient.

Learning to identify manifestations of the alters at work

When an argument is being made that it is useful to work with alters, it is useful to wonder, "What does this mean in practice?" Patients who have DID are often under clinical observation for many years before they are diagnosed with DID. It is not unusual for clinicians to encounter a patient who has received the DID diagnosis from other diagnosticians and emerge with the impression that the disorder is not present. Clearly, the alters that one is urged to work with do not appear to be making themselves manifest in a recognizable way most of the time. To work with the alters, one must learn how to recognize and find them.

A study of the natural history of DID [2] found that most patients who have DID spend most of their time manifesting little or no evidence of DID.

With the exception of a small minority of DID patients who are consistently and dramatically florid in their presentations, DID is, as Thomas Gutheil observed, "a psychopathology of hiddenness" [2]. For most patients who have DID, there are certain "windows of diagnosability" (due to stress, loss, retraumatization, injury, illness, a contemporary situation that triggers a strong connection to the traumatic past, or when the alter system has been opened up by psychotherapy) during which the symptoms of DID can be more readily observed or elicited [2].

Most of the time, even in treatments by mental health professionals who are working with DID patients whose diagnosis has already been made and confirmed, the clinicians who work with DID patients are confronted with the "dissociative surface" [28,35] referred to earlier. "Overt switches constitute a small minority of the alters' actual behavior" [35]. The dissociative surface is the external manifestation of the alters' behaviors and interactions with the external environment and with the third reality—the inner world of the alters [27]. The inner world may be accorded equal or superior importance than the outer world of external reality.

Without an appreciation that much of the alters' behavior is expressed indirectly by their impacts upon the host from behind the scenes and an approach to beginning to decode and work with their impact upon the dissociative surface, clinicians are restricted to dealing with the "host" (the alter in apparent executive control most of the time over a period of time) and those alters that assume executive control after overt switches. The dissociative surface, however, is composed of manifestations more complex and varied than these (Box 2).

Alters may pass for the host or be copies of the host. Several may switch off in a tag-team manner but fail to change in appearance. Clinicians often encounter mixed combinations of alters. These combinations may include a dominant alter's (1) showing aspects of one or more other alters that are copresent, (2) following the instructions of another alter, (3) response to the impact of intrusions of other alters, and (4) being overwhelmed and experiencing its behavior as made or imposed from elsewhere. These influences may come directly from one alter to another, from an alter itself influenced or commanded by a more powerful alter (up the food chain), and from the inner world of alters that often includes alters that rarely or never take over executive control in the external world and may be unknown to most of the personality system.

The most productive way to go about decoding the dissociative surface is to take careful note of the appearance, voice, and mannerisms of each alter one encounters and to observe the patient when one has reason to believe that a particular alter is active but its manifestations are somewhat different or inconsistent. The clinician may make an observation of a change in these qualities to the host or to whichever alter is understood to be primarily present and ask for clarification. This interaction may be followed by a request to talk directly to the present alter or the alter whose

---

Box 2. The dissociative surface

The Host or the "Usual Patient"
The Semblance of the Host or "Usual Patient"
    Passing For the Host
    Isomorphism
    Tag-Teaming
Copresence Combinations
    Mixed Presentations
        1. Cooperations
        2. Clashes
        3. Vectors
        4. Temporary Blendings
    Fluctuating Presentations
    One-Plus Presentations
    Shifting One-Plus Presentations
Instructed Behavior
Intrusions
    Simple
    "Up the Food Chain"
    From the "Third Reality"
Imposed or "Made" Behavior
    Simple
    "Up the Food Chain"
Switching, Rapid Switching, and Shifting

---

influence is changing the appearance or behavior of the one ostensibly in control.

For example, if a clinician understands himself to be speaking to Lois but notices that she is becoming somewhat confrontational, appreciates that her voice has become somewhat deeper, and notes that her body language has become less explicitly feminine, then the dialog might proceed in the following manner:

> Doctor: Lois, as we have been talking about these issues, I have noticed that you are seeming to be more assertive and opinionated than you usually are and taking issue with some matters that usually are not a problem for you. Your voice and manner seem to have changed a bit. Are you aware of anything out of the ordinary?
>
> Lois: I don't know, but I am feeling and thinking a little different from usual. A little out of it, detached.
>
> Doctor: Are you aware of anything that might be influencing your point of view?

Lois: Well, I hear a voice telling me to be careful, not to just go along with what you were saying.

Doctor: Please tell me all that you can about this voice.

Lois: It is male. And it seems worried, and angry.

Doctor: Is this voice familiar to you?

Lois: It sounds like Jack (usually referred to as "Big Jack"). But I'm not sure.

Doctor: OK. Well, Jack, or whoever else it might be if it is not Jack, I do want to understand what is concerning you and to take your concerns into account.

Lois: It is Jack. [Switches to Big Jack] You keep on getting her to talk about the stuff that happened, and she goes along 'cause that's what she does. But I don't think you get it. She can't handle this right now. She isn't telling you that she is still upset about the last things she talked about, and you didn't notice that. She's trying to give you what you ask for even if it messes her up. She can't say no to you.

Doctor: Well, that's important Jack, and I thank you for the information. Let me talk to Lois again, while you stay nearby and pitch in, and let's try to figure things out.

After a series of such encounters with various alters, the clinician would be in a position to make a reasonable guess when Lois (or some other alter) was being intruded on by particular others, even if the others were not taking over. With such awareness, the clinician could make remarks and observations that take into account the concerns and issues of the alters that seem to be playing a covert role in the conversation. For example, some months later, the clinician might notice some signs that Big Jack was near the surface while the clinician was discussing a possible medication change with Lois.

Doctor: It seems that Big Jack is taking some interest in this conversation. Big Jack, if you have some concerns about this medication I am recommending, I'd like to hear from you.

Lois: [In Big Jack's demeanor] You know she is going to look it up on the Internet, and if she's afraid it'll make her gain weight, she is not going to take it. And I'll be stuck with all of them little ones screaming inside about how bad they feel, and they will be angry as hell at Lois. They'll sneak out and take the medicine. If Lois finds out she'll stop eating and she'll be too afraid of getting you angry to really tell you what is going on. Do you think you really know what the hell you are doing with these pills and how they mess up these girls inside?

After following up on several changes in appearance in the host or other alters who are not being replaced but are being influenced by still other alters, the clinician can develop an increasingly rapid and accurate appreciation of which alters are becoming involved with certain issues and concerns.

This ability to infer the involvement of alters which have not assumed complete executive control but which are exerting important influences from behind the scenes allows the clinician to follow the alters' actions even in the absence of overt switching and makes it possible to follow and to treat DID in a more knowledgeable and nuanced manner.

Accessing alters for the purposes of treatment

Accessing alters is a venerable topic, discussed in depth in classic texts on the treatment of DID (eg, see reference [49]). After access has occurred—by an alter's spontaneous emergence in response to a direct request by the therapist or as a result of a hypnotic intervention—it is often possible to access an alter again by direct request or by initiating discussion of an issue or event that concerns them. At times, one or more alters may oppose the therapist's efforts to speak to a particular alter; this failure to gain access should be followed by inquiry about why access is being denied. The many possible rationales for refusal of access include all manner of apprehensions about the potential consequences of the anticipated interaction between the therapist and the alter he or she is trying to reach and concerns about this interaction's impact on the inner world. The therapist should (1) appreciate that these blockages are indications of important work that must be done before the alter system is ready to move forward into whatever material may be coming up next and (2) almost always work with the apprehensive alters rather than exert pressure for compliance with his or her request. The exceptions to this approach involve circumstances under which the therapist has reason to be concerned about the safety of the patient or about someone whom the patient may be at risk for harming.

The importance of working with alters to optimize pharmacotherapy for dissociative identity disorder

Many of the symptoms suffered by patients who have DID appear to be reasonable targets for psychopharmacology, but before prescribing, it is useful to try to learn what is behind the target symptom [54]. This determination is often impossible until one has established some relationship with the patient and has become at least somewhat familiar with the alter system. In his classic review of the psychopharmacologic treatment of DID, Loewenstein [54] discussed the importance of appreciating that many symptoms suffered by DID patients are best approached with other therapeutic modalities. Hypnosis is often useful to explore and control problematic symptoms in patients who have DID.

It is often useful to ask for feedback from all alters about the impact of a medication that has been prescribed or about the effects of a medication given the patient by a prior prescriber. The personality of the DID patient with whom one is conversing may or may not have all of the memories relevant to assessing the safety or the effectiveness of a medication. On dozens of occasions, I have learned that I was about to prescribe or had actually already prescribed a medication to which the patient had had a serious reaction that was unknown to or had been forgotten by the alter or alters to which I was speaking.

It is also useful to ask for alters' perceptions of why particular symptoms are occurring when they occur and to inquire whether any alter has an idea of whether the symptom has been experienced before. The latter inquiry raises a fascinating differential: is the symptom recurrent because it is part of a recurrent autonomous process such as an affective disorder? Or, is the symptom recurrent because it is (1) part of a memory/body memory that has been triggered by some material in the treatment? (2) part of a flashback or revivification? or (3) experienced as being created in the here and now due to a reenactment of a past trauma or one analogous to it in the inner world of the alter system?

The psychopharmacologist who determines that the symptom is the epiphenomenon of the DID patient's response to trauma or to problematic interactions among the alters next has to determine whether the symptom is within striking distance of the psychotherapeutic process itself. It does the patient and the therapy no good to withhold medication because a psychotherapeutic cure may be possible if, at present, the symptom is problematic and the treatment process itself does not yet have the capacity to contain the symptom. It may be safer to prescribe knowing that one may, at best, elicit a response from an active placebo than to withhold medication and insist that the DID patient resolve the symptoms in question when one knows that such a solution may be months or years in coming.

Case 1

Beverly was subject to profound panic attacks that were frequent and only partially responsive to massive doses of selective serotonin reuptake inhibitors and benzodiazepines. Her psychiatrist learned from the alters that the panic attacks reflected Beverly's experience of the panic of two child personalities. The psychiatrist asked all alters to listen in and participate in a discussion of treatment options. The alters came up with the strategy of creating a safe place to which these child alters could be sent, along with some protective and consoling alters. Furthermore, a wall would be created that would protect the remaining alters from experiencing the disruptive panic. The psychiatrist helped the patient create these images with the use of hypnosis, and made a tape that could be used to reinforce and strengthen this approach. When the patient demonstrated the ability to use autohypnosis to repeat his interventions successfully, Beverly was sent home with the instruction to use the tape and to practice the autohypnotic containment strategy she had been taught. Medication was not prescribed for the symptoms of panic.

Case 2

Early in the treatment of Wendy, a talented professional woman who had DID, her psychiatrist became convinced, in contrast to the opinions of Wendy and her primary care doctor, that her painful and disabling somatoform symptoms were recapitulating the pain associated with particular abuses. Wendy had reported painful traumatic experiences, aspects of which might have been recreated in these symptoms; however, preoccupied with matters of safety; maintaining her function as a wife, mother, and professional person; and dealing with contemporary stressors, she was by no means prepared to explore the terrible experiences her psychiatrist believed to underlie and determine her many severe pain problems. The psychiatrist, in consultation with Wendy's primary care physician, made the decision to treat the severe pains with moderate doses of oxycodone. Wendy became able to carry on her personal and professional lives. After 3 years of additional psychotherapy while maintained on oxycodone, Wendy was a much stronger individual and had demonstrated her capacity to work through painful memories without decompensating. At this point, the memories the psychiatrist thought were associated with her pains were accessed and processed. As the power of these memories diminished, Wendy's opiate analgesic medications could be gradually tapered and then discontinued uneventfully. She has remained free of these symptoms for several years.

Summary

The treatment of DID is facilitated by therapists' being prepared to work directly with alters. Interventions that access and involve the alters in the treatment are vital components of the successful treatment of DID and should be a part of the therapeutic armamentarium of those who treat this patient population.

References

[1] American Psychiatric Association. Diagnostic and statistical manual of mental disorders. 4th edition, revised. Washington, DC: APA; 2000.
[2] Kluft RP. The natural history of multiple personality disorder. In: Kluft RP, editor. Childhood antecedents of multiple personality. Washington, DC: American Psychiatric Press; 1985. p. 197–238.
[3] Coons P. Treatment progress in 20 patients with multiple personality disorder. J Nerv Ment Dis 1986;174:715–21.
[4] Kluft RP. Treatment of multiple personality disorder. Psychiatr Clin North Am 1984;7:9–29.
[5] Kluft RP. Treatment of dissociative disorder patients: an overview of discoveries, successes, and failures. Dissociation 1993;6:87–101.
[6] Kluft RP. Current issues in dissociative identity disorder. J Pract Psychiatry Behav Health 1999;5:3–19.
[7] Kluft RP. An overview of the psychotherapy of dissociative identity disorder. Am J Psychother 1999;53:289–319.

[8] Coons P. The differential diagnosis of multiple personality. Psychiatr Clin North Am 1984;7:
51–67.

[9] Kluft RP. An update on multiple personality disorder. Hosp Community Psychiatry 1987;
38:363–73.

[10] Piper A. Hoax and reality: the bizarre world of multiple personality disorder. Northvale
(NJ): Aronson; 1997.

[11] Merskey H. The manufacture of personalities: the production of multiple personality disorders. Br J Psychiatry 1992;160:327–40.

[12] Braun BG. Iatrophilia and iatrophobia in the diagnosis of MPD. Dissociation 1989;2:66–9.

[13] Coons P. Iatrogenic factors in the misdiagnosis of MPD. Dissociation 1989;2:70–6.

[14] Fine CG. Treatment errors and iatrogenesis across therapeutic modalities in MPD and allied
dissociative disorders. Dissociation 1989;2:77–82.

[15] Kluft RP. Iatrogenic creation of new alter personalities. Dissociation 1989;2:83–91.

[16] Torem M. Iatrogenic factors in the perpetuation of splitting and multiplicity. Dissociation
1989;2:92–8.

[17] Greaves G. Observations on the claim of iatrogenesis in the promulgation of MPD: a discussion. Dissociation 1989;2:99–104.

[18] Kluft R. Current controversies surrounding dissociative identity disorder. In: Cohen L,
Berzoff J, Elin M, editors. Dissociative identity disorder: theoretical and treatment controversies. Northvale (NJ): Aronson; 1995.

[19] Kluft RP. Multiple personality disorder. In: Tasman A, Goldfinger S, editors. Annual review
of psychiatry, vol. 10. Washington, DC: American Psychiatric Press; 1991. p. 161–88.

[20] Watkins J, Watkins H. Ego states: theory and therapy. New York: Norton; 1997.

[21] Watkins HH, Watkins JG. Ego-state therapy in the treatment of dissociative disorders. In:
Kluft RP, Fine CG, editors. Clinical perspectives on multiple personality disorder. Washington, DC: American Psychiatric Press; 1993. p. 277–99.

[22] Stern D. The interpersonal world of the infant. New York: Basic Books; 1985.

[23] Nathanson DL. Shame and pride. New York: Norton; 1992.

[24] Luborsky L, Crits-Cristoph P. Understanding transference: the core conflictual relationship
method. 2nd edition. Washington, DC: American Psychological Association; 1998.

[25] Kohut H. The restoration of the self. New York: International Universities Press; 1977.

[26] Kluft RP. The phenomenology and treatment of extremely complex multiple personality disorder. Dissociation 1988;1(4):47–58.

[27] Kluft RP. Reflections on the traumatic memories of dissociative identity disorder patients.
In: Lynn S, McConkey K, editors. Truth in memory. New York: Guilford; 1998. p. 304–22.

[28] Kluft RP. Diagnosing dissociative identity disorder. Psychiatr Ann 2005;35:633–43.

[29] Kluft RP. Varieties of hypnotic intervention in the treatment of multiple personality. Am J
Clin Hypn 1982;24:230–40.

[30] Kluft RP. Personality unification in multiple personality disorder. In: Braun BG, editor.
Treatment of multiple personality disorder. Washington, DC: American Psychiatric Press;
1986. p. 29–60.

[31] Kluft RP. Treatment trajectories in multiple personality disorder. Dissociation 1994;7:
63–76.

[32] Kluft RP. Clinical observations on the use of the CSDS Dimensions of Therapeutic Movement Instrument (DTMI). Dissociation 1994;7:272–83.

[33] Horevitz R, Loewenstein R. The rational treatment of multiple personality disorder. In:
Lynn S, Rhue J, editors. Dissociation: clinical and theoretical perspectives. Washington,
DC: American Psychiatric Press; 1994. p. 289–337.

[34] Kluft RP. An introduction to multiple personality disorder. Psychiatr Ann 1984;14:19–24.

[35] Kluft RP. The inevitability of ego state therapy in the treatment of dissociative identity disorder and allied states. In: Peter B, Bongartz W, Revenstorf D, et al, editors. Munich 2000:
the 15th International Congress of Hypnosis. Munich, Germany: MEG-Stiftung; 2002.
p. 69–77.

[36] Langs R. Resistances and interventions. New York: Jason Aronson; 1981.

[37] Freud S. Introductory lectures on psycho-analysis. In: Strachey J, editor. The standard edition of the complete psychological works of Sigmund Freud, vols. XV & XVI. London: Hogarth; 1961, 1963.

[38] Braun BG. The BASK (behavior, affect, sensation, knowledge) model of dissociation. Dissociation 1988;1(1):4–23.

[39] Braun BG. The BASK model of dissociation: clinical applications. Dissociation 1988;1(2): 16–23.

[40] Kluft RP. Hypnotherapeutic crisis intervention with multiple personality. Am J Clin Hypn 1983;26:73–83.

[41] Kluft RP. Dissociation and subsequent vulnerability. Dissociation 1990;3:167–73.

[42] Fine CG. Treatment stabilization and crisis prevention: pacing the treatment of the MPD patient. Psychiatr Clin North Am 1991;14:661–75.

[43] Fine CG. A tactical integrationalist perspective on multiple personality disorder. In: Kluft RP, Fine CG, editors. Clinical perspectives on multiple personality disorder. Washington, DC: American Psychiatric Press; 1993. p. 135–53.

[44] Kluft RP. On treating the older patient with multiple personality disorder: race against time or make haste slowly? Am J Clin Hypn 1988;30:257–66.

[45] Kluft RP. Playing for time: temporizing techniques in the treatment of multiple personality disorder. Am J Clin Hypn 1989;32:90–8.

[46] Kluft RP. Applications of hypnotic interventions. Hypnos 1994;21:205–23.

[47] Phillips M, Frederick C. Healing the divided self. New York: Norton; 1995.

[48] Kluft RP. Clinical approaches to the integration of personalities. In: Kluft RP, Fine CG, editors. Clinical perspectives on multiple personality disorder. Washington, DC: American Psychiatric Press; 1993. p. 101–33.

[49] Putnam F. Diagnosis and treatment of multiple personality disorder. New York: Guilford; 1989.

[50] Kluft RP. On giving consultations to therapists treating multiple personality disorder: fifteen years of experience—part I (diagnosis and treatment). Dissociation 1988;1(3):23–9.

[51] Kluft RP. On giving consultations to therapists treating multiple personality disorder: fifteen years of experience—part II (the "surround" of treatment, forensics, hypnosis, patient-initiated requests. Dissociation 1988;1(3):23–9.

[52] Van der Hart O, Boon S. Treatment strategies for complex dissociative disorders: two Dutch case examples. Dissociation 1997;10:157–65.

[53] Kluft RP. On the treatment of the traumatic memories of DID patients: Always? Never? Sometimes? Now? Later? Dissociation 1997;10:80–90.

[54] Loewenstein RJ. Rational psychopharmacology in the treatment of multiple personality disorder. Psychiatr Clin North Am 1991;14:721–40.

ELSEVIER
SAUNDERS

PSYCHIATRIC
CLINICS
OF NORTH AMERICA

Psychiatr Clin N Am 29 (2006) 305–332

DID 101: A Hands-on Clinical Guide to the Stabilization Phase of Dissociative Identity Disorder Treatment

Richard J. Loewenstein, MD[a,b]

[a]Trauma Disorders Program, Sheppard Pratt Health Systems, 6501 North Charles Street, Baltimore, MD 21204–6819, USA
[b]Department of Psychiatry, University of Maryland School of Medicine, Baltimore, MD, USA

This article provides clinical examples in the stabilization phase of the treatment of dissociative identity disorder (DID), formerly known as "multiple personality disorder." I bring the reader into the clinical session with representative dialogs from clinical material with DID patients. Since Putnam's [1] classic 1989 work systematized the treatment of DID in one salient reference, a great deal has been written about DID treatment. For example, both Putnam [1] and Ross [2] give detailed clinical examples illustrating how they discuss a variety of issues with patients, ranging from informed consent for DID treatment to specific interventions related to working with alters, mapping, abreaction of trauma material, cognitive therapy, attachment issues, and fusion and integration, among others. Overall, however, these works, like most of the clinical literature, are more prescriptive than descriptive about many clinical problems. This article gives the reader a "window" into the clinical session as a trainee might experience it in a treatment program.

Every year, in The Trauma Disorders Program at Sheppard Pratt Health Systems, new psychology postdoctoral fellows rotate through the inpatient and outpatient programs, along with an occasional psychiatric resident on elective. This is a tertiary-quaternary care referral center with a patient population primarily consisting of severely symptomatic, multiproblem trauma patients, most with DID or severe forms of dissociative disorder not otherwise specified, referred for stabilization of acute safety problems or overwhelming dissociative and posttraumatic symptoms. They present with major problems in stage one trauma treatment, the phase in which the

E-mail address: rloewenstein@sheppardpratt.org

doi:10.1016/j.psc.2005.10.005

patient develops basic stability and safety to pursue the goals of long-term treatment [3,4]. Even those patients referred for putative stage two issues, such as intensive memory work, abreaction to stabilize, and so forth, are almost always found actually to need major stage one work.

As part of their initial training, postdoctoral fellows and residents are required to sit in with experienced clinicians to observe sessions with DID patients. This hands-on learning is often crucial for the trainee to see how interventions are used in actual clinical practice. The trainee can observe in vivo the stance of the therapist toward the patient, how the experienced clinician structures the interaction with the patient and helps resolve (or does not succeed in resolving) the seemingly intractable conflicts, contradictions, dilemmas, and predicaments commonly produced by DID patients. The trainee and mentor then discuss what has occurred.

This article presents something of that process: practical didactics to help the neophyte clinician develop a framework for clinical work with DID, based on specific clinical vignettes that illustrate common problems in negotiating stabilization. Case vignettes are drawn from my own clinical experience, illustrating modal themes and clinical problems. These vignettes are amalgams of several patients. Dialogue is not verbatim from clinical sessions, but is meant to represent typical interactions, tidied up to read fluently. Interventions described should not be taken as biblical pronouncements or viewed as applicable to all DID patients. Readers should use these notions as templates to adapt what seems helpful into their own style. Other clinicians may have far more efficacious and parsimonious ways than mine of handling these (and other) clinical problems. They represent, however, interventions and approaches that have helped me in assisting many DID patients achieve a modicum of safety and stability.

Case history 1

Ms. A is a woman in her 30's diagnosed with DID and posttraumatic stress disorder, referred to the Sheppard Pratt Trauma Disorders Inpatient Unit because of violent behavior toward herself and others. The outpatient therapist reported that the patient had had episodes of dyscontrol including shouting, fighting with her spouse, trying to jump from a moving automobile, stabbing herself in the legs with sharp objects, and switching to alter identities who were disoriented to current circumstances. These alters denied knowledge of the patient's husband, children, therapist, and job, and threatened violence to the therapist. By history, this symptom exacerbation began after the patient's accidentally meeting a male relative whom the patient reported had molested her throughout childhood. She had had several unsuccessful brief hospitalizations in her local community. In each, she had been in restraints for several days because of violent attacks on herself, threats against staff, and attempts at elopement.

On admission, the patient presented as a wiry, anxious woman who became increasingly agitated as the admission interview progressed. As she described the recent contact with her relative, she began to rock back and forth, appeared to go into a trance, and began to laugh inappropriately and repeatedly smashed a fist violently into her thigh. As the admitting psychiatrist, I attempted to use symptom containment techniques to de-escalate the situation and attempt to reground the patient. At this, however, the patient became more physically agitated, laughing more wildly, smashing her fist even more violently against her leg. She leaned forward threateningly, and hissed, "You're lucky I'm here. The other one wants to kill you. He's coming now." I quickly left the room and initiated an all-staff call.

The patient required a large number of staff to subdue her as she screamed, kicked, bit, and scratched at the nursing staff. Eventually, she was placed in five-point restraints and given intramuscular sedatives. The staff was upset and worried about the patient's potential for additional violence and disruption of the hospital milieu, especially with the history of dyscontrol in prior hospitalizations.

Shaken and scared, I decided, albeit reluctantly, to talk to the patient again to process the events and to see if a repetition of the situation could be avoided. The patient was more subdued, denied recall of the events precipitating being placed in restraints, and seemed very sad and scared by what had happened. She discussed finding herself in restraints in the other hospital and her fear, bewilderment, and profound shame at being told of her behavior. She did say that she found it difficult to look at me because I bore a physical resemblance to "my perpetrator."

I asked if the situation of being in restraints reminded her of anything in the past. The patient answered, "Yes. When my perpetrator took me away when I was 11. He tied me to the bed, and put me in child pornography." I asked if the patient could tell me any more about this, adding, "You don't have to tell me all the detail or feelings of this event, just a brief overview." The patient looked anxiously at me as if unsure how to do this.

RJL: "Do you have any idea how to talk about scary or traumatic stuff without going into flashback?" The patient shook her head, "No," looking increasingly scared and sick.

I then asked the following: "Have you ever read a newspaper?" The patient assented. I continued (the patient nodding assent with each idea), "You know how there is the big, big headline on the first page, 'Peace Declared! Soldiers to Return Home,' something like that. Then, under that, there's a headline in somewhat smaller type, and then another one in a little smaller type, then finally the story. Then the story might continue onto page 12 and onto page 14 and so on and so on. All you need to talk about today is the first two levels of headline, maybe the third. You don't need to go into the details of the story and definitely not anything continued on the inside pages. Makes sense?"

The patient looked relieved. In a more detached way, she described how, when she was 11, she had fought the perpetrator to prevent being tied to the bed, even escaping her bondage and trying to run away. She cursed him and threatened to kill him when he caught her. Eventually, she stopped fighting because of his violent rage and threats to do "worse" if she did not do as she was told. She wasn't sure but thought that she had been drugged during this episode. She added that she "knew" that he let her go home later, and that she had "bits and pieces" of what happened after being tied to the bed.

I responded, "I'd like everyone to listen, especially the ones who were threatening me and trying to attack me. We, the staff and I, seem to have walked into your flashback with you here in the hospital. In trying to help you we have recreated what some of you must feel is just like what happened before, including many elements of what has gone on here today. We really want to help you all to separate that time and place from here."

I gave my name and the name of the hospital and the date, asking for assent by nodding or saying "yes" out loud to indicate that I was heard. The patient nodded. I repeated the information and the request for assent. The patient nodded more intently.

RJL: "It's important to recognize that the one's who were threatening me were actually trying to protect all of you, but in a way that would only make things more difficult, and maybe even more traumatic in the present. They need to know that they are in a place where people want to help and don't want to hurt anyone or be hurt by you. This is not a hurting place."

Patient (in an angry voice): "Why are you punishing us then? Why are you grabbing us and tying us up and all that. It's not help. You just want to do punishment!!"

RJL: "I'd like all of you to listen, please. Psychiatry is a very primitive medical specialty. We have very limited ways of preventing people from hurting themselves or others if they are not in control. Maybe in a hundred years we'll have a little gizmo, like in Star Trek. We'll just go 'zap' and you'll stop being unsafe and we can talk about what's bothering you. But nowadays, all we can really do when you're an immediate danger is stuff that's almost certainly going to remind you of punishments and mean things that have happened to you before, like the stuff you were talking about a moment ago about what your relative did to you.

"For example, we get a bunch of people, including big men, to grab someone, hold them down, give them medicine in their butt, wrap them in a big blanket, carry them to a room, and either lock the door or tie them up to a bed. For someone who's had a lot of trauma, it's likely that in all that will be a reminder of something that's happened before. Even if not, it's likely that the person will feel traumatized more by all this. That's why we really try to avoid all this stuff. We want to work with you to find ways not to have you be in restraints and all that, but we can't do it without your helping! We're going to ask you to check things out, talk about what your concerns are, not act in such a way that to protect you, and all the other people here, all of whom also have backgrounds of trauma, we have to do things that are going to remind you of upsetting stuff from the past. We would like all of you to be able to decide freely whether we are planning to behave in a mean or hurtful way with you, or just trying to do our best to help you recover from all that has happened to you before."

Patient (in a deep voice): "You look like him. How do we know you aren't trying to trick us? He always tricked us. He told us it would be 'OK.' It was safe. That he was sorry. He wouldn't do it anymore. We could trust him. Then, he just got us worse." She gazed away with a sick, sad look.

RJL: "That's a really hard thing. It makes it hard to trust one's own judgment when that kind of thing happens, doesn't it? Makes it hard to trust anyone else inside who might get you into a terrible situation by trusting. It makes it hard to trust anyone who suggests that you trust him. It's all a big trigger." The patient nodded assent vigorously.

RJL: "It's really a matter of risking, isn't it? Risking that we can all work together on solving some of these problems. You took a risk in talking to me so openly just now, even though you were very mistrustful. How did it go?"

Patient: "I guess OK. You don't sound mean or nothing, but I still can't look at you, you look like him. I keep seeing him here."

RJL: "Sounds like your mind, by having his image stay so strong for you, is still trying to warn you about being tricked. Maybe there are parts inside who are still very concerned that no one gets co-opted too easily. I think they are really concerned for your safety and should be appreciated for being so caring and concerned."

Patient in a different voice: "But I hate them, some of them sound just like him, cursing, threatening all the time. They hurt me, cut me, and put things up me. I can't stand them. They won't let me talk about him. They just threaten me."

RJL: "How did they feel about what you told me about him and the child pornography?"

Patient: "They didn't get too mad about that because you didn't make me get all into the details. It was a relief to say something about it."

RJL: "What would have bothered them about the details?"

Patient: "That gets too much into the really big secrets that he told us he'd kill us for sure if we told, and kill my parents too."

RJL: "Again, it really sounds like they're trying to protect you from something they see as worse: threats to you and your family. I really think they care and want to help. It's just that their methods make it hard for many of you to see that. I think we can help all of you find ways to be protected from harm, but do it in ways that you are not harming yourselves or others. What do they think about what I'm saying?"

Patient: "They say that you make sense, but they're really not sure about all of this. It's all so different from how it's been. They're confused."

RJL: "Confused is good about all this, thinking about stuff is good. You can begin to keep an open mind about things you've been so sure of for a long time. I know it's a lot of new stuff. How about if they agree to think seriously about what we've talked about and back off from the threats, if we agree to not have anymore discussion about this right now, and just work on separating what happened before from what's going on here in the hospital?" The patient nodded intently and her expression changed again.

Patient (in the voice that she first manifested): "This is what I hate. How can I get better when they stop me from knowing about all the important stuff all the time? How am I going to remember? They can't control what I say or do!! I need my memories! I need to just get it all out of me, once and for all, so I don't have to live with this shit!!"

RJL: "Well, how has it gone so far working on the memories by doing it the way you describe"?

Patient: "Not so good. I wind up lost in my car so I can't get to my sessions. I hurt myself. I've been in restraints a lot in hospitals before...."

RJL: "So, it's safe to say that it hasn't gone so well, right?"

Patient: "I guess."

RJL: "Let me suggest a different approach, because if you try the same thing over and over and it just doesn't work, it might be time to try something different, don't you think?"

Patient: She nods assent with a sad smile. "Yeah," she said, "that's what I tell my students. I'm a special education teacher for learning disabled children."

RJL: "OK. I'd like everyone to listen. Everyone listening? When everyone is listening, nod your head 'yes.' " Patient nods. I repeated this request and received the assent several times. "Everyone listening? It's important that we have some good listening. Everyone, inside, outside, known or unknown, anywhere in creation, please listen now.

"First, it's important for all of you to understand that the purpose of working on memories is not to just 'get it all out.' If that were so, we'd have everyone on this unit lined up just getting it all out. I know it really feels like that's what has to happen, like it's just this big thing inside that just should burst, but it doesn't work like that. You have to get safe and know how to work together with your system of selves before you can work on the memories with all the details and all the feelings. Even then it's not just letting it all hang out. It's a long slow process that is designed to overwhelm you as little as possible. We can discuss it in depth at a later time. Right now, your situation reminds me of a bunch of folks on a big sailboat that's taking on water. No one knows where the life vests are, or how to put them on. Half the crew is below decks refusing to come out, and the other half is fighting with each other. Then someone says, 'Ooh there's a hurricane, let's sail into that!' Doesn't sound likely that the ship and the crew are going to do very well there, does it? Sometimes, even if you're not prepared, a hurricane hits, but that's different from deliberately sailing into one.

"The first thing is that everyone needs to work on working together, getting safe from harm to yourselves and others. I really believe, from everything you've all said, that you've all been hurt enough. You don't need any more harm coming to any of you or your body. You don't have to like everyone, love everyone, or even trust everyone inside. It's just a matter of seeing how you can begin to risk to work together."

The patient began to look very tired and weary. I continued, "You look pretty tired, we've done a lot of work and you're still in restraints."

Patient: The patient nodded ruefully. "When can I get out of these?" she asked.

RJL: "When you've really processed with the staff: how everyone is going to maintain safety here, that everyone has worked on understanding that this is a helping place, not a hurting place. If you're not sure, you wait before you go off and check out what's really going on, ask why people are doing what they are doing, OK?"

Patient: Nods assent. "Everybody agree to that?" She nods assent more vigorously.

RJL: "I'd like to teach all of you something to help keep things here more separate from before. Do you know what a split screen is?"

Patient: "Not really."

RJL: "Like on television. Daffy Duck is doing something on one side of the screen and Bugs Bunny is doing something on the other. There's a line down the middle separating them. You could put me on one side and your relative on the other and compare and contrast the two of us." The patient looked puzzled.

"Another way is to think of one of those big life-size cutouts of Ronald Reagan, George Bush, and Bill Clinton. You superimpose one on me. Then, we move it over across the room, over into that chair over there, and you check out the similarities and differences between us." Again the patient looked confused.

RJL: "Another way is the 'Highlights for Children' way."

Patient: The patient looked oddly younger. In a pleased childish voice, she said, "I know about Highlights for Children!!"

RJL: "OK, you know they have that section where you compare two pictures. You know, one house has two chimneys and the other has one; one has a square window and the other has a rectangular window...."

"I get it," said the patient in her first voice, looking relieved. "You have different eyes. Your eyes are a different color, and you have a lot more grey hair...."

RJL: "Thanks a lot!"

The patient laughed. "And your eyes are nice, not mean like his." She shivered. "He has these cold, dead eyes." She settled back, looking calmer.

RJL: "OK, so we have a plan. You guys are going to work on separating the hospital and me from the perpetrator and the place where he took you. You're going to work on getting to know the staff here as people in 2005, not back when you were a kid. If everyone can agree not to do anything to hurt themselves or anyone else and really mean it, and agree to get help from staff before you do anything to harm anyone, you'll be able to get out of restraints. Does everyone really hear me, especially those who were violent when we first met? I hope you guys really think about this too, because I don't think you need any more time in your life being tied up, even if it's to protect you now." The patient nodded vigorous assent.

I added: "I'm going to ask the one's who were threatening violence before to be more aware, closer by, observing what goes on here, so you can decide if we can be counted on to do as we say, within the limits of our being fallible humans working with 19 other patients in the hospital. If you have concerns or questions, I'm going to ask you to raise them by talking with me or the staff, not by action." As I said this, the patient's expression began to subtly change, looking more like the face of the patient before she lost control. She maintained control, however, and nodded assent thoughtfully.

Before leaving, I asked "those who were just 'up close' now, I'd like you to 'step back' now, on the count of three, to allow the one who was here at the beginning to be fully forward. One, two, three." The patient's expression changed back to the sad perplexed one I had encountered originally. She stated that she felt "tired out, but calmer. I don't really know why."

I asked Ms. A what she remembered of the discussion that we had had. She said that she remembered very little of it. She asked me to tell her what had been said by the "others". Instead, I suggested that she ask her "mind", or the "others" inside, to tell her what they felt she was able to know of the conversation with me. I pointed out that I could tell her, but if I did so, she wouldn't learn anything new about communicating with her "parts". If she relied on "outside people" to keep her informed, then, when she was alone, she would have no ability to find out things within her. In addition, the "others" might have a better sense than I of what she could tolerate knowing. I asked the others if they were comfortable with what I proposed. The patient nodded in a trance-like way. Then, I asked Ms. A to "listen inwardly" and to tell me what she learned.

She said, "They said, they had had a talk with you that they were going to think about a lot. They had heard about a lot of new ideas. They think we might learn some things here. That's all." I told her we would stop for now, but that I would see her the next day.

I concluded the interview and left the room. I talked with the staff about a plan to help the patient get out of restraints. The staff was to work on helping the patient maintain orientation in the present and to continue to separate past and present about feeling imprisoned by her relative, and other matters as they came up.

The patient rapidly came out of restraints and did not require them again during a month-long hospitalization. In therapy, the alter personality system was directly engaged to work on becoming more aware of a variety of reminders that precipitated flashbacks, switching, loss of current reality orientation, and urges to behave violently. She was helped to make connections to many aspects of her experience that served as subtle traumatic triggers and reminders of her reported abuse. For example, she became more and more panicky as the day went on, usually feeling overwhelmed, asking for multiple extra medications, starting around 4 PM. When simply asked what occurred to her about this time of day, related to her earlier life experience, she recalled that, as a child, 4 PM was approximately the time that she would go after school to her abusive relative's house for "child care" while her parents worked. She was frequently left there alone with this man. She reported that this was when much of the early abuse with him occurred.

As the hospitalization progressed, she worked on strategies for real-world self-protection in her current life from her relative, who was said to be involved currently in a variety of criminal activities. She was also able to express anger at her family for having failed to protect her as a child and for rationalizing visible evidence that she was being hurt. Work was done with the patient and her husband to help him have a better appreciation of the patient's reaction to seeing the relative and to help him take more seriously her fear and distress about this.

Discussion

Reframing and the therapeutic alliance

Throughout my meeting with Ms. A, I continually reframe symptoms as psychologically explicable responses to her situation, especially those that she experiences as distressing and devastating. The alters, especially those who seem the most alien to the "everyday" self-states, must be understood as embodiments of the patient's survival, not evil or alien beings. To do otherwise serves to buttress rather than to moderate the delusional separateness so common in DID patients [5,6]. Similes and metaphor are helpful in making this comprehensible to the patient, using the DID patient's highly developed capacity for abstraction and self-observation (see the article by Brand et al elsewhere in this issue) [7,8].

For example, the patient can be asked: "If you were in the Underground in Nazi Germany, and someone asked for your identification, would you say, 'Oh, yeah. I'm in the Underground?' No. You'd act like the most convincing Nazi you could. That may help explain why [so and so, the persecutory alter] doesn't just acknowledge what he's actually all about when I suggest that he's really trying to help and protect with all his strength. He doesn't believe or doesn't trust that he's free of the Nazis now, or that I'm not just the cleverest Nazi he's met yet."

As I explain to patients, DID is a very logical disorder. The trick, however, is to understand the underlying logic. Patients find this process both relieving and disconcerting. They say things like, "This makes a lot of things in my life make sense for once. But I don't like any of this at all."

In addition, I begin working on the therapeutic alliance in the first interactions with the patient. Work on reframing, communication, and cooperation among the alters can be understood as development of a kind of internal therapeutic alliance among the self-states to work toward recovery by becoming more tolerant, collaborative, and decent toward one another. Kluft [5,6,9] in particular has cited the development of the therapeutic alliance as one of the most crucial elements in successful DID therapy.

As described by most experienced DID therapists, I am very active with the patient, talking a lot, anticipating problems, suggesting solutions, and changing directions when new issues come up. I have very specific ideas about the basic issues that will be encountered in therapy: safety concerns, the need for improved internal communication and collaboration, separation of past and present, reframing, therapeutic alliance, responsibility for behavior, among many others. This does not preclude my listening with great care, however, and responding thoughtfully to what the patient presents.

Unconscious flashbacks

Putnam [1], among others, has discussed the seemingly uncanny way in which DID patients unconsciously recreate personally specific traumatic scenarios in their contemporary life, including the involvement of others in complementary roles in these situations. Blank [10] has described this as an "unconscious flashback" in which

> manifest psychic content is only indirectly related to [traumatic experiences].... The individual's state of consciousness, outwardly observed may or may not be altered. Memories, affects and impulses...come forth...without conscious visual or other registration. The subject...[carries] out complex integrated actions based on past experiences that are not consciously remembered, with no awareness that he is repeating anything.... As in post-hypnotic suggestion, the subject invents rationalizations for his or her behavior.

In discussing this phenomenon, in 1993 [11] I stated

> It is less commonly realized, however, that unconscious flashback experiences permeate the life of the multiple personality disorder patient and are frequently omnipresent in the therapy. In addition, projective identifications in the dissociative transference field may give rise to an uncanny phenomenon in which the patient and therapist appear to have "walked into the flashback together" as one of my patients described it.

Another window into the pervasiveness of complex, often multilayered, posttraumatic responding in DID is found in research on the psychologic structure of DID patients using psychologic assessment (see the article by Brand et al elsewhere in this issue) [7,8]. For example, the researchers had to develop a "traumatic content' score on the Rorschach, because repeated traumatic intrusions into projective testing were ubiquitous in DID, including going into full flashback with the Rorschach card as a stimulus.

Inquiry about whether the situation reminds the patient of something from the past is a surprisingly simple way to find out about posttraumatic responding. At least a basic narrative of the material may be readily available to the patient's consciousness. Alternatively, a more specific question can be asked, such as "Is there anything significant (distressing, upsetting, traumatic—potentially more suggestive terms) that comes to mind about that 4 PM time, or late afternoon, that seems to be associated with getting so upset every day?" It may help to give a classical free association suggestion: "Tell me whatever goes through your mind, even if it seems silly or irrelevant. Just reflect inwardly, let your mind open up to your inner experience, and share with me whatever you may think, see, hear...." To be sure, cautions about the complexities of memory and its reliability should inform inquiries of this nature [4,6,9].

Talking over

I repeatedly use the technique of "talking over" [1] to communicate with alters without inducing a frank switch. This approach skims the dissociative surface [12], mobilizing the copresence of alters, frequently experienced as passive influence symptoms by the patient. As described by Kluft [6], Putnam [1], and Ross [2], I assume that alters need to be prompted to listen, often repeatedly, and that many alters experience themselves as disoriented to current circumstances, requiring concrete reorientation. Ideomotor signaling [13], asking the patient to assent nonverbally, can be quite helpful when using talking-over interventions. To be sure, the clinician must use other forms of data (verbal, behavioral, and so forth) to decide how to understand these ideomotor responses, just as one does with any communication by the patient.

With Ms. A, I targeted the violent and persecutory alters immediately and began to reframe their behavior and to attempt more of an alliance with them. In a patient who is not in an acute safety crisis, where these alters may be more hidden, I usually go more slowly, allowing the material develop with less active prompting by me. Nonetheless, one of my first tasks is to identify, access, and talk to the seemingly persecutory, self-harming, violent, dangerous, shaming, so-called "bad" alters. It is essential for the patient's stabilization to communicate with these self-states and to begin to understand their crucial helping function [1,2,6]. In addition, this kind of intervention is a kind of provocative test to begin to see how responsive the patient is likely to be to reframing interventions and attempts to engage the alter system to form an alliance with me and among its members. This allows me to begin to form initial hypotheses concerning the difficulties that may be encountered in the therapy, especially the depth of entrenched internal conflicts and the tenaciousness with which the patient holds onto his or her multiple realities [9,12]. Asking if there are any objections to a particular new strategy is especially important because these can be immediately addressed in direct or indirect conversation with an alter or group of alters. Often, objections are not volunteered and remain hidden. Accordingly, they are much easier to work with if they are anticipated and inquired about, rather than waiting for sabotage of a healthier new strategy (and another crisis) to announce the presence of the objection.

Posttraumatic intrusions

The therapist needs to be active in detecting early signs that the patient is becoming overwhelmed by intrusive posttraumatic stress disorder symptoms. Here, the therapist must actively intervene to back off intrusive material and help the patient begin to develop strategies to distance or attenuate its impact. Ms. A's history and current dyscontrol indicated that she had limited skills to manage DID, let alone discussion of the trauma history. At the same time, however, in many situations in which the patient is overwhelmed by intense, inexplicable reactions, it can help the patient make sense of the experience to allow a brief, cognitive, distanced report of aspects of the event to connect the past trauma with current response [14]. Here one is attempting to help the patient separate past from present by understanding something specific about the traumatic memories that are affecting responses to current circumstances. This is in contrast to stage two therapy, where the goal is to bring the past into the present in an affectively intense and cognitively detailed way.

For example, another patient was packing to move to a new apartment. She became panicky, shaky, and kept having an intrusive thought that this activity was "dangerous." Suddenly it occurred to her that, as a child, packing was usually associated with vacation travel to visit relatives in another city where, over many years, she reported being molested by a family friend. She also recalled that by the age of 6, her family put her alone on the Greyhound bus, with her little suitcase that she learned to pack, to travel by herself for hundreds of miles to visit these relatives. Despite the distress at the recollections, she reported being, "Happy. Well, not really happy," at this recollection because it allowed her to understand why she had always panicked at the idea of moving. She had felt, "stupid, crazy, wacko," and deeply ashamed about this. Retrieval of the cognitive component of the memories reduced her sense of shame and ineffectiveness because of her inability, until now, to "make it go away" by repeatedly berating herself for having "these stupid feelings." The recollection made explicable her intense, seemingly perplexing emotional response. In turn, this allowed her to be more able to pack "in the present" without feeling endangered by doing so.

This process can sometimes be explained to the patient as an emotional flashback in which the affective component of the dissociated trauma memory [15] returns without the sensory or cognitive components. This term can also describe a pervasive emotional response to a current situation that fits the current situation, but is much more intense and compelling than can be understood by the current situation alone. This is illustrated in the next case study.

Imagery

With Ms. A, I began to use a distancing image very quickly when she showed signs that she was having an increase in posttraumatic stress disorder reactivity. The newspaper image seems to be one that most patients grasp readily. This kind of imagery, and the patient's ready acceptance of it, mobilizes the often-described high hypnotizability and dissociativity of the DID patient without formal induction of hypnosis [16,17]. These interventions can be immediately reassuring to the patient that there are tools to help reduce highly distressing symptoms that seemed without anodyne in the past.

It is important to tailor the imagery to the patient and to the clinical situation. Alternatives to the newspaper may include a more typical screen image as described by Putnam [1] with a mental remote control to modify the screen. As an initial quick intervention, I tend to use the newspaper image, and introduce the screen image later to help the patient work more systematically on containment of posttraumatic stress disorder intrusions. Some patients, however, especially those with a reported history of being in child or adult pornography, may have trouble using a movie or television screen image. A computer screen may be a useful substitute (with file folders to close, and so forth). Kluft (in Hammond [13]) has described the library image with a book that prints the painful material onto a blank page, only showing the patient as much as he or she can tolerate knowing at a given time.

These interventions may be crucial in giving the patient a sense of control over trauma material. A successful distancing intervention may be the first experience the patient has had that traumatic memories can be managed safely in a clinical context.

With Ms. A, I also introduced the idea of being in the flashback together and needing to separate past from present. Subsequently, I worked on the issue of free choice: the patient being able to decide freely that we want to help her, but she needs to separate from the past to do so. I often point out to patients that being in a flashback, conscious or unconscious, robs them of their freedom to choose responses to a given person or situation. I sometimes add, "You are free to judge that I am a jerk or a mean person, but please separate me from that person who lives rent-free in your head first. At least decide that I am a bozo on my own merits." For many DID patients, like Ms. A, the notion of trusting is associated with being repeatedly betrayed. I tell them that I have no intention of harming them or exploiting them, but that they must judge for themselves over time that I live up to that pledge.

As Ross [2] and others have described, I frequently ask the most suspicious alters to watch carefully and to speak up if they have any questions or concerns about what is transpiring. Further, I immediately start working on reframing the intent of the angry, violent, persecutory alters as attempts to help and protect, although being careful not to validate their means (usually self-harm, internal emotional abuse, and so forth), and to support those alters who feel harmed as having a legitimate complaint.

Further, I introduced to Ms. A the idea that the alters may mistrust one another, not just outside people. In particular, this is a common occurrence when the patient reports that he or she has been prevailed on to trust abusive individuals, only to have this trust shattered. This may be especially difficult for the patient who reports that the abuser apologized, asked the patient to trust him repeatedly, then violated the trust. This may also occur under other circumstances (eg, believing a mother who promises repeatedly to leave an abusive spouse, but never does so). The intense shame, demoralization, and despair at giving trust and being betrayed repeatedly can lead to difficulty in trusting one's own judgment about many important life issues. In DID, this is often manifested as an internal war among the alters, sometimes resulting in complete paralysis and global withdrawal.

The idea of the patient taking a risk to work on issues is a helpful one that may better connect with the patient's experience of hopelessness about anything being helpful and fear that connections with others can only lead to disaster. The intense shame at being repeatedly tricked ("like Charlie Brown with Lucy holding the football," as one patient reported) may result in a person who completely doubts his or her own judgment about whether to trust again (she added, "and, she was Charlie Brown's psychiatrist!") Some sadistic abusers are reported deliberately to inspire trust in the victim to take pleasure in the repeated betrayal: "He only wanted to see the look in my eyes when he betrayed me one more time."

Similarly, in some DID patients, a motivation for repeated "snatching defeat from the jaws of victory" results from a belief that any confidence in the continuation of something good inevitably will be unpredictably shattered when the good thing is discovered and taken away or destroyed by the abuser. Accordingly, to control what is thought to be the inevitable outcome, the patient (in an alternate personality) sabotages himself or herself whenever the possibility arises of success, better relationships, improvement in treatment, and so forth. This may be a tenacious dynamic to overcome, because overcoming it results in the patient tolerating the anxiety associated with the idea of getting better, increasing the fear of having the "good" taken away again. In this situation, any adversity or obstacle, traumatizing or quotidian, can be seen by the patient as proof that this cognitive distortion is the truth.

Safety

Finally, I set clear limits about demonstrating safety before coming out of restraints. I made clear that there are expectations about the patient's maintenance of safety and, most importantly, honesty about difficulty managing safety. I also insisted that the patient is not given a free pass on issues of personal responsibility (eg, getting out of restraints). Ms A had to demonstrate that she had made concrete efforts to change before a behavioral contingency would be modified.

I gave homework about this to work on separating past from present, dealing with fear by talking not acting, and working on specific goals for increased safety. I also discussed with the unit nursing staff the clinical situation, the safety issues, and what the patient needed to do to come out of restraints. In inpatient settings, particularly when a patient has been unsafe, it is vital that the treating clinician involve the nursing staff in understanding the treatment plan. If we are to ask the DID patient to communicate and collaborate effectively among the members of the inner team, we cannot ask less of the outside clinical team.

Case history 2

Ms. B is a woman in her early 40's who sought treatment with me for DID, posttraumatic stress disorder, depressive symptoms, recurrent self-mutilation, and repeated self-destructive behaviors in which she would, with great creativity, undermine any business enterprise that she started, once it became successful. Because she was a talented businesswoman with a gift for inspiring others, she created and then demolished a number of successful enterprises. This resulted in a kind of recurrent Phoenix-like pattern to her life. She began treatment with trepidation, having seen me in consultation some years before. At that time I had confirmed the diagnosis of DID. The patient spent the consultation switching continuously, however, returning to the bewildered, amnestic host alter self-state at the end of the consultation session. She fled from the office insisting that I was "crazy" for confirming her treating psychiatrist's tentative DID diagnosis.

Before the DID diagnosis being suspected, Ms. B had spent years in unproductive psychiatric treatment for refractory affective symptoms, requiring hospitalization after lethal suicide attempts on several occasions. Even after the DID diagnosis, she had seen several therapists over the years with little progress. When she contacted me again for treatment, she had begun a new business venture that was prospering. She had also hired her daughter and son-in-law, however, both of whom had major substance abuse problems. They had looted one of her last businesses, ultimately writing a variety of bad checks on her accounts. Despite costly legal problems that resulted from this fiasco, she believed she could not refuse her daughter employment. She blamed herself for the daughter's troubles, relating them to her deficiencies as a parent because of her psychiatric problems and tumultuous life history.

Ms. B grew up in a slum neighborhood in a large Midwestern city. Her memory for her early life was limited. She knew more about it than she remembered. Her mother had died before she was 2 years old. Her father was unknown. Her uncle and aunt had adopted her. The uncle was reported to be a violent, cruel alcoholic. The aunt, a compulsively religious woman, was reported to have heard voices, believed that God spoke to her through the television, and that the neighbors could be heard talking about her through the walls. Ms. B had flashes of a memory, when she was 6 years old, of a violent fight with her uncle destroying the furniture, grabbing her, and taking her into the bedroom while her aunt screamed at both of them. She knew that during her childhood she was seen in the emergency department of the "charity" hospital in her home city for broken bones, vaginal bleeding, and infections. She knew also that she had been removed from her adoptive family's custody when she was 6, but had no recall of how or why she was returned to them when she was 8. She gave birth to her daughter at 15 and was married to a violent alcoholic by 16. She gave birth to a son when she was 17. Despite all this, she had excelled at school, finding it an island of peace. Several teachers recognized her intelligence, befriended her, and supported her intellectual endeavors, even after she was forced to leave school when she became pregnant at 14.

The uncle and aunt both died when she was 18. She divorced her husband and began to make her way in the world. While working several jobs, she obtained a high school equivalency degree, attended college, and eventually attained a master's degree in philosophy. She married again and moved with her husband to the Baltimore area. Divorced from him, she obtained better and better jobs. Eventually, she was able to move her family to a prosperous, suburban neighborhood and began her career as a businesswoman.

Ms. B's symptoms on initial evaluation included recurrent, dense, dissociative amnesia resulting in a variety of problems. These included buying clothing and other items that she could not afford; driving long distances and finding herself in other cities and states without recall for her journey; and finding herself cut and bleeding from cuts to her arms, legs, and genitals. Also without recall, she found that she had made a variety of brilliant business decisions, held successful meetings with customers, and introduced several new computer innovations to her company.

She heard voices in her head, arguing, berating her, and threatening her. Some voices spoke calmly and soothingly to her. Other voices sounded like those of her uncle and aunt, respectively. The uncle voice cursed her and called her a "whore," a "slut," and a "stupid cunt." The aunt voice spoke in religious homilies. Ms. B was filled with shame at her belief that she had utterly failed to live up to these latter directives.

In the second session with me, Ms. B sat nervously discussing her recent history. She had found herself in Washington, DC, the night before, about 50 miles from her home. She had lost a number of hours for which she had no recall. As she discussed this, she began to complain of a headache, looked stricken, fell silent, then looked away. When she looked up again, she spoke in a soft voice with a slight British lilt. She introduced herself as "Mrs. J," her former married name.

Mrs. J: "Oh, she is so confused and getting more depressed, the poor child. She doesn't know what has gone on. I have to tell you, Doctor, that the driving is the least of the problems; she has been cut again, on her arm. Not that she needs stitches, this time, I can assure you. She's too ashamed of it to tell you herself. I think she's getting dangerous again, like those other times when she was in the ICU. That's really why I called to make the first appointment."

She told me that she knew a number or alter self-states, but could do little to control them. She described several child self-states, a caretaker for them, a worker who "built up these businesses for her, but has no social finesse," a driver who was said to be responsible for the long-distance travel, and several others. When asked about internal aunts and uncles, because of the voices that seemed to embody their traits, at least as Ms. B had described them, Mrs. J smiled and said, "Nobody talks to them, they're so mean. They never come out."

In a sad voice, she told me that she could not give me any information about who was responsible for the self-injury or the prior suicide attempts. "B is the most suicidal one right now, that I can tell you," she said. She refused to show me her arm because "they" felt this was a private matter. When I stated that I would need to talk with "them" immediately to work on safety, Mrs. J replied, "They won't talk to you. I assure you of that. I don't know why they insist on things being unpleasant. It's all so unnecessary."

RJL: "I'd like all of you to listen. Your safety is very important. I want to be your doctor and help you. I want the opportunity to listen to all of you and hear what you have to say. But, as long as there's an immediate threat to your safety, that's all we can focus on right now. I need to speak directly to the ones who have hurt your arm." This was followed by silence.

Ms. J: "I'm sorry for their rudeness, but, they're just not going to speak with you."

RJL: "I'd like everybody to listen, Let me explain your problem to you. In order for you to not be hospitalized immediately, I need to know, in words that a simple-minded psychiatrist can understand, who is harming the body and who, in addition to B, intends to suicide, what is going on that led up to these events, and a plan for your safety from any sort of injury or death, at least until our next face-to-face meeting." Again there was silence.

RJL: "I really want to talk this out with all of you to find a solution. You all came here today to see me, suggesting that, overall, there is a wish to get help. If you are silent, I can only assume that, deep down, you really feel you can't manage safety as an outpatient and that I'm going to need to hospitalize you today."

Ms. B again seemed to look dazed for a moment, then shifted in her chair, her expression intent and angry. In a tough, deep voice, with a Midwestern accent, she said: "I ain't going back in no damn hospital, I have a damn business to run. Maybe she needs that shit. But I don't. She's so damn wimpy and candy ass. *She* needs a psychiatrist. You help her. I don't need any help. Besides, I have to be on the lookout that her damn junkie daughter doesn't steal the carpets off the floor. I've already locked up the checkbooks, pass protected the business accounts on the computer, and made it really hard for that little thief to start up again. And that J woman? All she knows is 'shop till you drop.' You don't know what I've had to do to keep up with her damn credit card bills!'' This alter was named "TCB." She described herself as "the businesswoman." TCB acknowledged that J, despite her spending, was good at business meetings, talking with clients, and handling employees. "I hate that shit. Just let me be with the computers and a spread-sheet and I'm happy!"

RJL: "I really appreciate what you're saying. It sounds like you're working hard and trying to help everybody by working and protecting the finances. I would like to work with you as your psychiatrist. I prefer outpatient treatment for you too. But, if you're severely injured or dead, you won't be able to work either."

Ms. B: "*Her* psychiatrist. I don't need a damn psychiatrist. But they're a whole bunch of depressed and upset people in there. They really need a shrink too. Or, you can just get rid of them. That would be the best solution. Then I could do my work in peace. But, I'll tell you what, that dead thing. I don't like that. But, the other, makes the trains run on time, honey. They're wailing and carrying on in there, and this stuff just quiets right down when they get to sawing on each other. They go to sleep."

RJL: "You don't seem to think that the injury to the body affects you, although you do believe that if she suicides you'll die."

TCB: "Quit getting me all confused! A little sawing never really hurt nobody if things get quiet. It's just a means to an end. Calms everything down. Of course, there is all the blood and shit. I don't do no cleaning, though. That Aunty creature screaming all that 'cleanliness is next to Godliness' shit. Jesus H. Christ. Then B who don't know nothing about nothing feels so screwed up about it, she cleans it all up so no one will see it. It's a mess."

RJL: "What do you know about how it happens, the "sawing," as you put it."

TCB: "I don't pay much attention to all that. I know that there's about five of them that do it, for different reasons."

RJL: "Who did it last night"?

TCB: "I think it's time for me to leave." Despite my attempts to get her to continue, calling her name, saying how important it was for us to continue to talk, the patient switched back to Ms. B. She was panicky, looking all around her. She said, "What did I do? Did I do something wrong? Am I in trouble"?

RJL: "Some of the others were here. No one has done anything wrong. You're not in any trouble. What's most important, though, they indicated that you're thinking a lot about being dead."

Ms. B, breaking down into tears: "I can't stand this! I've been losing more and more time! I was in Washington, DC, last night and I don't know how I got there. I was in some terrible neighborhood and thought I was going to get killed. My daughter is starting to ask me for money again, and I have to give it to her, even though my head tells me it's just going to be a big mess again if I do. I wake up and find that I've been hurt and I don't know how it's happened. I just feel so tired and lost all the time. I don't want to go on like this, I just want to sleep."

RJL: "That tired and lost feeling, waking up finding yourself hurt, finding yourself in strange places, wanting to sleep, does this bring anything to mind, remind you of anything in the past?"

Ms. B, looking surprised: "It's like my whole life. When I was a kid, that's what would happen. I'd wake up and I'd be hurt or I'd be in that horrible hospital hurt. I just wanted to have some peace, get away from it all."

RJL: "Did you want to die as a kid"?

Ms B: "How did you know that? I've never told anyone that. I used to pray that I'd be taken to heaven." When asked if she attempted suicide as a child, Ms. B again seemed surprised. Ms. B: "I never told anyone. When I was 8, I took the pills in the medicine cabinet. I just slept for a day and when I woke up again, my aunt shouted, 'Idle hands make work for the devil!' and made me clean the whole house. I tried to get hit by the cars in the street, but I'd always find myself on the other curb and not know how I got there safely."

RJL: "Do you know what an emotional flashback is?" Ms. B shook her head in puzzlement. "You know what a regular flashback is, right? It's an intense reliving of something, usually with the sensations related to the event, with emotions from that event, seeing it, hearing it, feeling it, like you are in it again, pretty much. An emotional flashback is an intense emotion that belongs to a time long ago, but without the sensory or narrative part. For example, the kinds of thing you're going through now, the time loss, finding yourself hurt, you describe as very similar to what you went through as a kid. It results in the same feelings of loneliness, helplessness, hopelessness, not wanting to live. It's as if you're going through the sequences simultaneously in both the present and in the past.

"It's kind of a double whammy, like something is piggy-backing or supercharging your emotions in the present situation leading to more intensity than would be evoked by just the current circumstances. What helps is to begin to work on recognizing it, by working on separating the emotions from the past from those of the present, looking at what goes with what. It can be quite a challenge if the situations are reminiscent of each other and evoke very similar emotions, but the strongest cases are often the most helpful in the long run. For example, you can begin to get perspective if you think about getting some distance on all this. You can imagine that you are up in an airplane or on a mountaintop, looking down at the landscape. Things that seemed so large and overwhelming before, now become small. You can see the relationships between things more easily, that previously were obscured when you are on the ground.

"For example, even though you feel overwhelmed now, among the differences are that you are a grown up person now with resources and supports that you didn't have as a kid to get help. You have your own friends, house, business, shrink, and so on. When you're real little, you have to depend on your family for everything. Early on, you couldn't read, write, get food for yourself, cross the street by yourself, let alone pack up and move out. You depended on your family for your whole reality.

"I'd like to work on all this with you. There's a lot of new stuff to think about. I can't work with you on this, however, unless you stay alive. I'm going to ask you if you'll agree not to hurt yourself or kill yourself, or anyone else inside or outside, accidentally or on purpose, at least until we see each other next. In addition, before you hurt yourself or kill yourself, and so on, you will call me, have me paged, and wait for me to call you back before doing any harm to yourself or others, inside or outside. If you can't wait for my call back, you'd go to the emergency room. If you can commit to this, I would like to see you tomorrow. I can fit you in at the end of my day." (This safety agreement structure is based on that described by Braun [1,18].)

Ms. B looked relieved. She said that she agreed. I helped her to repeat the words of the safety promise. I continued: "B, I really need to make sure that when you promise something like this, you really mean it. If you asked me to do something important as part of your treatment, and I agreed that it was clinically appropriate, and made a commitment to do it, and turned around the next day and did the opposite, how would you feel"?

Ms. B: "Angry. Betrayed. Hurt."

RJL: "Right. Well, trust is a two-way street. You guys have huge issues with trust, and I absolutely don't expect that any of you trust me now, or any time soon, actually. When you make a commitment to me, however, I have to have confidence that you're being honest with me, most especially about issues of safety. That is, if you really can't be safe, that you let me know that.

Ms. B: "I understand. I don't break my word. I can last another day. I've survived this long. If I get in trouble, I'll call you. I don't want to have to go back to the hospital again.

RJL: "Everybody listen, please. We still have to resolve the problem of the ones who cut and to see whether anyone else is planning to kill themselves. It is 1:20 now. Our session is over at 1:50. If I haven't gotten a safety commitment from the rest of you by 1:30, I'm making arrangements for you to go to the hospital, either voluntarily or by 911. You have 10 minutes."

Ms. B switched suddenly. In an angry voice, she said: "I'll be *fine*!" This alter refused to identify herself by name.

RJL: "Listen, everybody, just saying that is not going to work. I need to know very specifically how we are going to set things up so that everybody is safe from harm to themselves or others, at least until our next meeting, which is scheduled tomorrow."

Ms. B, tearfully: "I don't know what you want. All I know is that I get peace when I do that. What's wrong with that? Nothing else stops it. I can sleep then."

RJL: "The problem is that hurting yourself is a short-term solution to a long-term problem. It's like an alcoholic who drinks to solve problems. He drinks a quart of scotch, numbs out his problems, and passes out. In the morning, however, all his problems are all still right there. Plus, he feels sick and ashamed that he's gotten drunk again. Because a lot of what people commonly want to numb themselves from is shame, you wind up with more of the problem you were starting out to solve. If this was a medicine that I prescribed for you, you'd sue me."

Ms. B: "But it's the only thing I know how to do to stop all this chaos inside. Why should I give up the one thing that helps. All those pills and junk you guys give me never helped like this."

RJL: "When an alcoholic or any other kind of addict hits bottom and decides to quit their drug of choice, you can predict one thing. They're going to feel worse. First, there's whatever withdrawal they're going to go through. Then, they have no coping skills other than drinking to handle problems. They have to learn new skills, even though they're feeling terrible. That can take a long time. In the long run, building new problem-solving skills that affirm life and safety feels much better than those old addictive short-term ways."

Ms. B: "I don't know what the big deal is. I didn't even get stitches this time. Why are you making such a big deal out of it. I even stopped her from taking all the pills this time by putting us to sleep."

RJL: "Consider this: if you're walking down the street and someone knocks you down and grabs your purse, you've been mugged. If someone knocks you down, steals your purse, and beats you up, you've been mugged. I agree that in the second case you've been harmed physically more, but in either situation, you've been hurt and traumatized, and who's to say which will be worse psychologically in the long term. Thinking that being unsafe to make yourself safe comes from living with trauma all the time. You don't get the sense that getting hurt is optional; you just want to control the timing and intensity as best as you can."

Ms. B: "That's exactly right. How did you know that? Oh, all right, they're telling me that you've got a good point."

RJL: "Also, you're setting up what I gather is a familiar situation: someone is hurting someone else all the time and no one can do anything about it. You're asking me to be a bystander who knows that someone is being hurt and doesn't do anything about it. I think these are old roles and scripts you guys are playing out, and I won't be a part of it. If you really can't work on safety, at least from session to session, or agree to go into the hospital, then I don't think that I'm the right doctor for you right now. Maybe you aren't ready for the kind of therapy that requires an honest commitment to safety."

Ms. B: "OK. I'll try."

RJL: "Trying really isn't enough. If a drunk "tries" to get sober, it just means he's bargaining about when he's going to drink again. Like my colleague, Richard Kluft, says, 'Saying "you'll try" means that you're planning to fail, but you want to be approved of for your efforts.' There's only one way to get sober and that's to stop completely. For example, in A.A. you don't just quit and that's it. One gets a sponsor, goes to meetings. They're not asking one to stop so much as to delay acting while one does the alternative plan. I really believe that you can delay hurting yourself. You've sat here for almost 30 minutes and you haven't hurt yourself, right? What we're talking about here is all the unsafe parts delaying acting, at least until you all see me tomorrow at 6:00 PM.

Ms. B: "What do I do about all these scared kids? They don't know about all these big words you're spouting. I can make an agreement like that for now, but they're out of control."

RJL: "Has anyone taught you guys how to find a safe place, or a safe place for them?"

Ms. B: "No. What's that?"

I proceeded to discuss how each self-state could find a safe place, by imagining a place that could encompass all of them, or a unique place for each one; a place that the alter had been to, never been to, read about, heard about, always wanted to go to, was just thinking about it right now. Even a "no place place," if places were not OK. Then, once this was imagined, entering into the safe place and absorbing themselves in everything about it: temperature, light, colors, time of day, time of year, and bringing with them whatever they need to make that place personally right just for them. Then letting a protective shield or barrier come down around them. A shield with a special quality: it immediately transports out all that is difficult, troublesome, worrisome, and so forth, and allows all that is safe, peaceful, quiet, serene, and so forth to enter into it. I discussed how only those alters who wanted to participate would do so. The rest could watch and listen to make sure that nothing untoward was occurring (Richard P. Kluft, MD, personal communication, 1988).

Ms. B entered a trance-like state while I discussed this. She indicated when asked that many self-states wished to participate. I repeated the imagery suggestions. Ms. B visibly relaxed. When asked how things were inside, she said: "Peaceful, quiet." I asked if any wished to sleep in their safe places, with no need to awaken at least until a few minutes into our next session tomorrow. Ms. B nodded yes.

I said that first they could do whatever they needed to do to get ready for sleep, brush their teeth, find their stuffed animals, get a drink of water. Then they could settle down into their sleeping places, their eyes closing as they drifted down into a deep, safe, healing sleep, without any dreams or images, not to awaken at least until a few minutes into our next session, sitting down for therapy.

RJL: "Are they OK?" She nodded yes. I suggested that she could open her eyes gradually, letting the others go even deeper into sleep as she gradually came back to her usual state of awareness, keeping the relaxed, peaceful feeling with her.

Ms. B, opening her eyes, looking more relaxed for the first time that day: "That's much better. How did you do that?"

RJL: "I didn't do that, you did. I just helped you use a talent for imagery that you didn't know you had. In our next sessions, we're going to have some discussions about your gift for imagery and trance, and how you can learn about this to help you in therapy For now, we still have to make sure everyone agrees to be safe before we can conclude for today. What about it?"

Ms. B: "They say they will never make any kind of agreement with a man, but that they'll make an agreement among themselves to keep their promise. They don't want to go to the hospital." I repeated exactly what was being agreed to, and the patient reported that "they" all agreed.

I rechecked again that no "part, person, presence, force, or entity, known or unknown, anywhere in creation" (Richard P. Kluft, MD, personal communication, 1988) was unable to agree to the agreement to not suicide or self-harm. There was no objection.

I continued, "Is Ms. B here, or does she need help in coming back? She walked in, she should walk out at the end."

Ms. B appeared to go into a brief trance, then looked up, and, with Mrs. J's accent, said, "She had to go to sleep too. She was so exhausted and overwhelmed. I'll take us home. She needs to come back tomorrow to see you, but I'll keep her safe until then." The session was over.

Mrs. J paged me urgently that night. Some of the "little ones" had "awakened" and were "agitating everyone." A brief discussion revealed that the patient's daughter had called asking for money. TCB had answered the phone and "told her off." Ms. B had "woken up" and was feeling guilty. I spoke with the Ms. B self-state about the need to find ways to work on this problem, together with the whole "system," to forge more of consensus about handling the situation. She was able to reaffirm her safety commitment. She was able to return to "sleep inside," along with the other newly awakened alters. Mrs. J asked: "Does Verizon know that you do this on the phone?"

Despite these positive responses in the early sessions, the therapy continued to be stormy. A variety of safety crises continued to occur. Ms. B needed urgent hospitalization on several occasions because of severe self-mutilation, suicidal threats, and rageful, homicidal threats from the "Uncle" self-state. A far more elaborate set of "safety plans" was put in place to help the patient delay action. These included improved communication and collaboration among the alters. This allowed the patient to be more proactive in "internal" problem solving. She found activities that soothed the upset alters, learned to use self-hypnosis, and found some helpful as-needed medications. She used supportive friends, who understood something of her situation, as supports. She made progress in setting limits with her daughter and making the daughter take more responsibility for her addiction problem.

Gradually, over the next 2 years, she was more and more able to maintain safety. This occurred despite a long series of life crises that resulted from prior self-destructive decisions she had made about her business, her daughter, and her finances. Self-states began to work together more efficiently. For example, TCB and Mrs. J worked out a budget for clothing and household items and began actively to cooperate about business issues. "The Driver" was allowed to take drives as long as there was prior agreement about where and when he drove. He was enlisted to help with driving, especially when other self-states were overwhelmed after leaving therapy. "Older" self-states were enlisted to do caretaking for the child alters. Child alters began to "grow up" and a variety of self-states fused as therapy progressed.

We began to understand more fully the traumas, abuse, and neglect that the patient had suffered throughout her development, including massive failures of the child welfare system to remove her from her aunt and uncle. Ms. B eventually found documented evidence that the authorities had returned her to her family, despite knowledge of the maltreatment by her aunt and uncle. Her current self-defeating, self-destructive behavior patterns, and certain phobic behaviors and other symptoms, often involved uncanny repetitions of specific traumatic events and scenarios that she recalled, or reactions to these.

Discussion

Safety management

In this case, I doggedly keep the focus on the patient's safety. I had to work on both suicidal ideation and parasuicidal behaviors. The emphasis is on a clear-cut, no loopholes agreement with a plan for dealing with an inability to maintain safety. The patient is not allowed to just affirm that he or she is safe ("I'll be fine"). Instead, the patient must give a more detailed and psychologically convincing discussion of what led to the lack of safety and how this will be managed subsequently. Otherwise, the patient is presumed to be a danger to self or others. Safety agreements are fundamentally about delaying action and having an alternative repertoire of skills and supports to manage difficulties that previously led to self-harm. One patient of mine calls her safety agreement "the no-immediate-action plan," because the word "safety" is upsetting to her.

It is vital that the therapist become an advocate for safety and nonabusive values [11]. Compromise with the patient who attempts to bargain about how much "unsafety" is okay inevitably leads to the patient seeing the therapist as corruptible around basic values. DID patients often describe many people including family members, doctors, teachers, and therapists who had some awareness that the patient was being hurt and did nothing. It is vital that the therapist does not fall into this trap and replicate this traumatic relationship theme [11]. I understand that, in many communities, DID patients must be hospitalized in general psychiatric units where DID is not recognized as a legitimate disorder, or, even if the diagnosis is accepted, there are limited resources for definitive DID therapy. However, the DID patient needs to understand this as part of the realistic consequences of being unsafe. In general, the DID patient may embody the values of those who hurt them: harming someone's body to solve your problems is without apparent consequence. I point out to the patient that, by harming his or her own body, he or she replicates the stance of the perpetrator: that it is okay for someone to solve their problems by messing up another person's body. As long as the DID patient engages in self-harm, he or she keeps himself or herself in the "trauma world," reinforcing these old messages, delaying meaningful recovery.

I carefully structure sessions where I become aware of safety issues to attempt to resolve them within the scheduled therapy time. There are several reasons for this. First, if at all possible, it maintains the therapeutic frame, even in a situation of danger to self or others. Next, in most cases, it helps to preserve the structure of my day, and the next patient's session, if the index patient does require hospitalization (taking time to call to make arrangements, call 911, and so forth). It prevents interminable discussion about the patient's internal struggles that rarely produces a timely result. It emphasizes the patient's responsibility for safety, even if the patient has a limited understanding of this ("Let me explain your problem to you...."). It treats these issues as solvable, relatively routine, practical clinical problems, rather than matters of cosmic significance.

As in Case 1, I worked very rapidly on issues of the patient's responsibility for honesty and safety, building the therapeutic alliance, reframing alters as helpers and protectors, educating the patient about what is required in therapy, interpreting the traumatic transference around safety issues, and helping provide concrete alternatives to self-destruction for self-soothing [5, 6,9,11]. Also, my availability was crucial in developing an outpatient safety contract and safety plan with a patient who was an acute danger to self and at risk for emergency hospitalization [19]. If an urgent appointment is not possible immediately, the therapist should be available by telephone or schedule brief, safety-focused telephone contacts with the patient until the next session. Scheduled calls can help reduce the possibility that the patient will feel that only a renewed crisis allows a telephone call. If, however, the safety plan begins to evolve into a situation where only frequent telephone contact seems to prevent hospitalization, this is not a stable long-term, outpatient solution to safety issues. In this situation, a more restrictive level of care, such as day hospital or inpatient hospital, should be considered. Similarly, extended telephone calls with additional lengthy negotiations about safety generally suggest that outpatient management is not workable.

Posttraumatic responding

As in Case 1, I focused on the patient's multifaceted posttraumatic responding, here pragmatically conceptualized as an "emotional flashback." This is a very helpful concept for DID patients. Commonly, in DID intense emotional reactions to present circumstances are infused and influenced by affects and emotions from the past. If the patient can be made aware of these, and cognitively separate the different sources of emotion, it can be a very valuable intervention.

For example, the concept of emotional flashback can be particularly helpful with the patient who, under the weight of working on trauma, experiences the process as one without end: "every time I think it's finished, there's more," "I don't think I can survive doing this," and so on. The therapist should become attuned to these sorts of statements as possible representations of the patient's emotional experiences in the past, while undergoing the original traumatic events, now embodied in adult cognitive form.

Many DID patients report that they were suicidal as children, although usually acknowledge this only when asked specifically. Often, suicide is described as wanting to have control, to be free of intolerable danger and cruelty, to be at peace, out of unending misery, to be "in Heaven where grown-ups do not hurt little children," and so on. When a patient describes this sort of early history, I sometimes refer to it as "the life-affirming function of suicide." In its essence, this kind of suicidality often represents a wish to be free from trauma, cruelty, and abuse; to find some last modicum of control when all of it seems to have been taken away. As with so many DID symptoms, it can be helpful in working with suicidal self-states to reframe this as a logical response to trauma and as a wish to get relief and control in some way. The same aspiration can be pursued by living better in the present, becoming safe from exploitation, abuse, and trauma, at the hands of others or of oneself. Getting well is the best revenge.

Summary

I have presented two in-depth, clinical vignettes that illustrate basic issues from early sessions with DID patients in phase one therapy. In these examples, I show how themes that present in initial sessions, and work on their resolution, can set the framework for successful stabilization of the DID patient. Major themes have included unconscious posttraumatic responding, the therapeutic alliance, the patient's responsibility for safety, skill building and management of symptoms using imagery, and structuring the treatment frame to work on acute crises.

Acknowledgements

I cannot claim originality with any idea presented here. I have been influenced by and learned from many clinicians in both the dissociative disorders field and elsewhere. I cite specifically when I know the origin of a specific intervention. Many others by now, however, have been subjected to dense source amnesia: to the extent that I have adopted the ideas of others and believe them to be my own, I have stolen them fair and square. Accordingly, I would like to express gratitude in advance to many of the clinicians who have contributed to my clinical development and the work described here. They include but are not limited to Richard Kluft, Frank Putnam, Susan Wait, Judith Armstrong, Catherine Fine, Stephen Marmer, David Caul, Cornelia Wilbur, Kathy Steele, Ono van der Hart, Bennet Braun, Colin Ross, D. Corydon Hammond, Joan Turkus, Christine Courtois, Constance Dahlenberg, James Chu, Anna Salter, Judith Herman, Besel van der Kolk, George Frazier, Elizabeth Bowman, Phillip Coons, Arthur Blank, Jr., Bethany Brand, Richard Chefetz, the late Paul Kaunitz, and the late Robert Byck.

References

[1] Putnam FW. Diagnosis and treatment of multiple personality disorder. New York: Guilford; 1989.
[2] Ross CA. Dissociative identity disorder: diagnosis, clinical features, and treatment of multiple personality. New York: John Wiley & Sons; 1997.
[3] International Society for the Study of Dissociation (Chu JA, Loewenstein R, Dell PF, et al). Guidelines for treating dissociative identity disorder in adults. Journal of Trauma and Dissociation, 2006;6(4):in press.
[4] Brown D, Scheflin AW, Hammond DC. Memory, trauma, treatment, and the law. New York: Norton; 1998.
[5] Kluft RP. Basic principles in conducing the psychotherapy of multiple personality disorder. In: Kluft RP, Fine CG, editors. Clinical perspectives on multiple personality disorder. Washington: American Psychiatric Press; 1993. p. 19–50.
[6] Kluft RP. Dissociative identity disorder. In: Gabbard GO, editor. Treatment of psychiatric disorders, vol 2. 3rd edition. Washington: American Psychiatric Press; 2001. p. 1653–93.
[7] Armstrong JG, Loewenstein RJ. Characteristics of patients with multiple personality and dissociative disorders on psychological testing. J Nerv Ment Dis 1990;178:448–54.
[8] Armstrong JG. The psychological organization of multiple personality disordered patients as revealed in psychological testing. Psychiatr Clin North Am 1991;14:533–46.
[9] Kluft RP. Overview of the treatment of patients alleging that they have suffered ritualized or sadistic abuse. In: Fraser GA, editor. The dilemma of ritual abuse: cautions and guides for therapists. Washington: American Psychiatric Press; 1997. p. 31–63.
[10] Blank AS. The unconscious flashback to the war in Vietnam veterans: clinical mystery, legal defense, and community problem. In: Sonnenberg SM, Blank AS, Talbott JA, editors. The trauma of war: stress and recovery in Vietnam veterans. Washington: American Psychiatric Press; 1985. p. 293–308.
[11] Loewenstein RJ. Posttraumatic and dissociative aspects of transference and countertransference in the treatment of multiple personality disorder. In: Kluft RP, Fine CG, editors. Clinical perspectives on multiple personality disorder. Washington: American Psychiatric Press; 1993. p. 51–85.

[12] Kluft RP. Diagnosing dissociative identity disorder. Psychiatr Ann 2005;35:633–43.
[13] Hammond DC. Handbook of hypnotic suggestions and metaphors. New York: Norton; 1990.
[14] Horevitz R, Loewenstein RJ. The rational treatment of multiple personality disorder. In: Lynn SJ, Rhue JW, editors. Dissociation: clinical and theoretical perspectives. New York: Guilford; 1994. p. 289–316.
[15] Braun BG. The BASK (behavior, affect, sensation, knowledge) model of dissociation. Dissociation 1988;1:4–23.
[16] Frischholz EJ, Lipman LS, Braun BG, et al. Psychopathology, hypnotizability, and dissociation. Am J Psychiatry 1992;149:1521–5.
[17] Williams TL, Loewenstein RJ, Gleaves DH. Exploring assumptions about DID: an investigation of suggestibility, hypnotizability, fantasy proneness, and personality variables. Presented at the Annual Meeting of the International Society for the Study of Dissociation. New Orleans, November 17–20, 2004.
[18] Braun BG. Aids to the treatment of multiple personality disorder on a general psychiatric inpatient unit. In: Kluft RP, Fine CG, editors. Clinical perspectives on multiple personality disorder. Washington: American Psychiatric Press; 1993. p. 155–75.
[19] Linehan MM. Cognitive-behavioral treatment of borderline personality disorder. New York: Guilford Press; 1993.

ELSEVIER
SAUNDERS

Psychiatr Clin N Am 29 (2006) 333–342

PSYCHIATRIC CLINICS
OF NORTH AMERICA

Index

Note: Page numbers of article titles are in **boldface** type.

A

Alcohol abuse, dissociative disorders and, 135–136

Alcohol use, in posttraumatic personality disorder-organized and posttraumatic personality disorder-disorganized, 104

Alexithymia, and secondary dissociation, in chronic childhood physical and sexual abuse, 120–121
dissociation versus, 236

Altered states of consciousness (ASC), culture-bound, medical models of, 214–215
in nonpossession trance, 215–219
in possession trance, 219–222

Alters, abuser, bringing into treatment, 293
accessing for treatment, 300
addition or multiplication of in dissociation, 31–32
as stakeholders in treatment, 290
avoidance of, in dissociative identity disorder, 281
awareness of presence of, 2, 4–5
behaviors as communications, 291–292
collusion with patient in avoidance of, 291
complexity of, 286–288
conversion seizures in, 201–202
dealing with, **281–304**
definition and characterization of, 283–284
development and nature of, illustration of, 284–285
ego states and, 283–284
enlisting in third reality, 294
hiddeness of, as host or copies of host, 297
iatrogenesis of, 282–283
in avoidance of re-enactments of rejections and neglect, 295
inner world of, 286
in shame work, 294
integration of, 295

interactions of in anticipation of integration, 293–294
manifestations of at work, learning to identify, 296–299
mature, enlistment for care of child alters, 294–295
mechanisms of, 286
mobilizing for inaccessible skills, 293
negotiation with in treatment, 293
numerous, in avoidant, obsessive dissociative identity disorder patients, 287–288
objections to working with, 282–283
understanding of themselves and one another, 285–286
working directly with, rationale for, 288–289
20 reasons for, 290–295
working with, contraindications to, 289, 296
importance for optimizing pharmacotherapy for dissociative identity disorder, 300–301
case examples, 301–302
working with to optimize pharmacotherapy for dissociative identity disorder, 300–302
and to access and work through painful memories, 301–302
panic attack case, 301

Amnesia, alters in erosion of, 292
as criteria for dissociative identity disorder, 235–236
dissociative, 195–196
in dissociative identity disorder, 2–3, 8–10
in pathologic dissociation, 8–10
retrograde, organic and dissociative forms of, 236

Anterior cingulate cortex (ACC), diminished response in posttraumatic stress disorder, 114–115
in primary dissociation, 114–116

doi:10.1016/S0193-953X(06)00009-8

Changing Your Address?

Make sure your subscription changes too! When you notify us of your new address, you can help make our job easier by including an exact copy of your Clinics label number with your old address (see illustration below.) This number identifies you to our computer system and will speed the processing of your address change. Please be sure this label number accompanies your old address and your corrected address—you can send an old Clinics label with your number on it or just copy it exactly and send it to the address listed below.

We appreciate your help in our attempt to give you continuous coverage. Thank you.

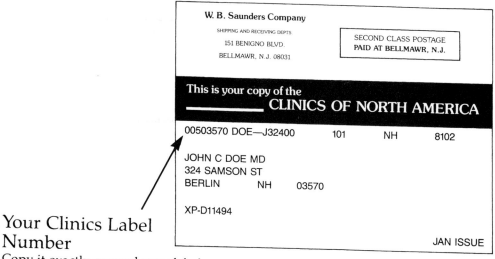

W. B. Saunders Company

SHIPPING AND RECEIVING DEPTS.
151 BENIGNO BLVD.
BELLMAWR, N.J. 08031

SECOND CLASS POSTAGE
PAID AT BELLMAWR, N.J.

This is your copy of the
_____ CLINICS OF NORTH AMERICA

00503570 DOE—J32400   101   NH   8102

JOHN C DOE MD
324 SAMSON ST
BERLIN   NH   03570

XP-D11494

JAN ISSUE

Your Clinics Label Number

Copy it exactly or send your label
along with your address to:
W.B. Saunders Company, Customer Service
Orlando, FL 32887-4800
Call Toll Free 1-800-654-2452

Please allow four to six weeks for delivery of new subscriptions and for processing address changes.